FONDATION HARDT
POUR L'ÉTUDE DE L'ANTIQUITÉ CLASSIQUE

ENTRETIENS
TOME XLIX

GALIEN

ET

LA PHILOSOPHIE

ENTRETIENS SUR L'ANTIQUITÉ CLASSIQUE

TOME XLIX

GALIEN
ET
LA PHILOSOPHIE

HUIT EXPOSÉS SUIVIS DE DISCUSSIONS

PAR
JONATHAN BARNES, R.J. HANKINSON
MICHAEL FREDE, TEUN TIELEMAN,
DANIELA MANETTI, JACQUES JOUANNA,
VÉRONIQUE BOUDON, GOTTHARD STROHMAIER

Entretiens préparés et présidés par Jonathan Barnes et Jacques Jouanna

Avec la participation de Vincent Barras

Index rédigé par Lavinia Galli Milić

VANDŒUVRES – GENÈVE
2-6 SEPTEMBRE 2002

ISSN 0071-0822
ISBN 2-600-00749-0

PRÉFACE

Le sujet des Entretiens de 2002 a été proposé par le professeur Jacques Jouanna. À sa demande, le professeur Jonathan Barnes lui a été adjoint par le Comité scientifique de la Fondation Hardt pour les préparer et les diriger.

Les savants invités, quand ils acceptent de participer à une série d'Entretiens, s'engagent non seulement à participer à la réunion, mais encore à remettre dans le délai qui leur est imparti un texte prêt à l'impression et qui puisse être reproduit dans la série de volumes qui, depuis bientôt cinquante ans, conservent pour la postérité la matière et les discussions des Entretiens. La Fondation compte sur la loyauté des invités et ne dispose bien évidemment d'aucun moyen de coercition. Si l'une des personnes invitées à présenter une communication à la Chandoleine, qui a participé aux discussions, lesquelles sont incluses dans le volume, renonce à transmettre un texte, elle ne peut que le déplorer. C'est ce à quoi elle est réduite dans le cas présent, le professeur Vincent Barras ayant déclaré forfait.

La Commune de Vandœuvres, sur le territoire de laquelle se situent les bâtiments de la Chandoleine, soutient depuis plusieurs années son activité par un substantiel subside. Celui-ci, d'entente avec les donateurs, est utilisé pour financer la publication du volume annuel d'Entretiens. Dans le contexte actuel, ce montant couvre approximativement les deux tiers des frais d'impression. Les organes de la Fondation Hardt expriment à la Commune de Vandœuvres l'expression de leur profonde gratitude pour ce soutien, qui allège quelque peu le lourd fardeau financier qui menace de plus en plus le fonctionnement de notre institution.

Grâce à l'efficace intercession du professeur Ernst A. Schmidt, président du Comité scientifique, les Entretiens 2002 ont bénéficié d'un appui généreux de la Fritz Thyssen Stiftung, qui a couvert non seulement les frais de voyage des participants, mais même une partie de leurs frais de séjour. La Fondation Hardt remercie chaleureusement les responsables de cette institution pour leur efficace soutien.

Une fois encore, la préparation des textes transmis en vue de leur impression a été assurée par notre bibliothécaire, Monsieur Bernard Grange, et la compilation des index réalisée par Madame Lavinia Galli Milić, assistante à la Faculté des Lettres de l'Université de Genève. C'est grâce au zèle et à l'amour du travail bien fait de ces deux personnes que le présent volume est l'égal en qualité de tous ceux qui le précèdent.

François Paschoud
Président du Conseil de la Fondation

TABLE DES MATIÈRES

I

JONATHAN BARNES

PROOFS AND SYLLOGISMS IN GALEN

At the beginning of Book 8 of the *Doctrines of Plato and Hippocrates* Galen recalls that his first aim in the work had been to determine whether "there is one power or several which govern men", and his second to determine what these powers are and where in the body they are situated. The outcome of the long discussion was a vindication of the Platonic view of the soul against various Stoic eccentricities. The vindication was achieved "in accordance with the laws of proof" (*PHP* V 648.6 K);[1] and it was, in principle, easily achieved. For the proofs which Galen rehearsed, and which Hippocrates and Plato had rehearsed before him, were simplicity itself; they had convinced all but the

[1] κατὰ τὸν ἀποδεικτικὸν νόμον: the phrase is repeated at *PHP* V 653.18; it is also found at *Loc.Aff.* VIII 201.6 and at *Adv.Jul.* XVIIIA 295-296, where Julian, "the sophist of the new dialectic" is mocked for his ignorance of ἀκολουθία — here the νόμος ἀποδείξεως is a rule of inference or principle of implication. I have not noticed the phrase outside Galen — but cf. Proclus, *In Ti.* I p.227 Diehl ("the law of the demonstrators requires us to inquire whether something is — where that is unknown — before we ask what it is"). At *Diff.Puls.* VIII 735.16 Galen talks of "dialectical laws" — which there prescribe the right way of constructing a definition. The same phrase is found again later: e.g. Proclus, *In Alc.* 334; *In Parm.* 651-652; Simplicius, *In Cael.* p.28.15-25 (on the right way of forming negations); Philoponus, *Aet.M.* 18, p.609 Rabe ("the dialectical laws say that the possible follows the possible" — i.e. if it is possible that P, and if P then Q, then it is possible that Q); and there is perhaps an ironical allusion in Sextus Empiricus, *M.* 8.108 (ἡ ... παρὰ τοῖς διαλεκτικοῖς νομοθεσία). The expression was known to Gellius, who latinizes it as *lex disciplinae dialecticae* (see 16.2.1-13). 'Logical law' in the sense of 'rule of dialectical debate' occurs at Asclepius, *In Metaph.* p.253.37-39 Hayduck. Note also, much earlier, Epictetus, *Diss.* 1.26.1 (νόμος ὑποθετικός).

philosophers; and if Galen's discussion had nevertheless run on and on, that was the fault of his asinine adversaries (*ibid.* 648-650).

The philosophers — Galen is thinking of the Stoics — produced anti-Platonic arguments by the bucketload. But even the most persuasive of them "were not constructed according to the demonstrative method" (*ibid.* 650). On the other hand,

> all those who have not yet touched on philosophy — geometers, arithmeticians, calculators, astronomers, architects, and even musicians and clock-makers and rhetoricians and grammarians, and in general anyone who has been trained in a rational art [ἐν τέχνῃ λογικῇ] —

will recognize that the view of Hippocrates and Plato is correct (*ibid.* 652). And Posidonius, "the most scientific of the Stoics because he had trained in geometry", felt obliged to reject the Stoic doctrine and side with the truth (*ibid.*).

> Not only was it not necessary for the account of the ruling part of the soul to fill five books — there was no need even for one entire book, at any rate for those who have learned what sort of thing a scientific proof is — something which, as I affirm, is appropriate to philosophers more than to geometers and arithmeticians and calculators and astronomers and architects, although the former have not practised it as the latter have. Thus Euclid, in a single theorem — the first in his book on *Phenomena* — showed in very few lines that the earth is in the middle of the universe and stands towards it as a point and a centre; and those who have learned the proof believe its conclusion as they believe that two twos are four. Yet some of the philosophers talk such nonsense about the magnitude and position of the earth that anyone would be ashamed of the whole profession. (*ibid.* 654)

The philosophers are "unwilling to use linear proofs [γραμμικαὶ ἀποδείξεις]", they "have not been trained to read linear proofs" (*ibid.* 656): *hinc illae lacrimae.*

A passage in *On my own Books* recounts how, as a young man, Galen recognized the importance of proof; how he therefore studied logic with the philosophers, both Peripatetics and Stoics; how he found them at loggerheads, disagreeing with one another and contradicting themselves — even though they too praised "linear proofs"; and how "I decided that I should distance myself from what they said and follow the character of linear proofs" (*Lib.Prop.* XIX 40-41).

Galen's main treatment of the subject, the fifteen youthful books *On Proof*, is lost; and although there are innumerable references to proof in the surviving works, there is no detailed discussion. But in outline his views are known. In particular, it is plain that proofs are syllogisms or formally valid deductions.

When Galen was a boy, two types of syllogism were taught in the schools: there was categorical syllogistic, historically associated with Aristotle and the Peripatetics; and there was hypothetical syllogistic, of which the Stoics were traditionally the patrons. The relation between the two syllogistics was disputed: in the *Introduction to Dialectic* Galen dismisses such disputes, maintaining that both types of syllogism are useful for proofs — categorical syllogisms especially for categorical propositions, hypothetical syllogisms especially for existential propositions (12.1-6; 14.1-2). The two syllogistics are thus complementary parts of logic.

But they do not exhaust the domain of logic:

> There is also another, third species of syllogism useful for proofs — I call them relational, although the Peripatetics insist on [βιάζονται][2] counting them among the categoricals. There is no small use of them by the arithmeticians and calculators. (*Inst.Log.* 16.1)

[2] βιάζονται: grammar (middle or passive?) and sense ('force', 'be forced', 'insist'?) are alike uncertain; but the drift of Galen's remark is not obscure. — I excise 'σκεπτικοῖς καὶ': cf 16.5.

The arguments which Galen goes on to mention were not new to logicians. On the contrary, the Peripatetics — as Galen notices — had rudely forced them into categorical form; and the Stoics — though Galen does not say so — had called them "non-methodically concluding [ἀμεθόδως περαίνοντες]". Against the orthodox logicians of the day, Galen claimed that these arguments were members of a separate species of syllogism, and hence that there were three rather than two types of syllogistic.[3]

Galen was impressed by the proofs which arithmeticians and geometers and other serious scientists advanced, and he was ashamed of the ways in which philosophers tried to prove their doctrines. Galen recognized a third species of syllogism, apart from the two species which were taught in the philosophical schools, and he observed that members of the third species were particularly common in mathematical and scientific work. It is natural to put these facts together: scientific and philosophical practice showed up the inadequacy of orthodox school logic and spurred Galen to the discovery of the third species of syllogism. And it is natural to congratulate Galen: was not the logic of the schools indeed inadequate, and do not scientific proofs indeed use relational syllogisms?

In *PHP* 8, Galen offers six exemplary proofs: one each for the location of the rational and the affective parts of the soul, and four for the desiderative part (V 655-660). The last four are presented in a disconcertingly nonchalant style, but the first two are set out with some formality, thus:

(I) Where the origin of the nerves is, there is the ruling part.
The origin of the nerves is in the brain.
Therefore the ruling part is there.

[3] Galen was always alive to the importance of distinguishing between what is relational and what is not — something which his opponents often failed to do (see e.g. *SMT* XI 569-570).

And:

(II) Where the affections of the soul more evidently move the parts of the body, there is the affective part of the soul.
But the heart clearly undergoes a considerable change of motion in anger and fear.
Therefore the affective part of the soul is in it. (*ibid.* V 655)

Strictly speaking — or so a modern reader might be tempted to object — neither argument is formally valid: to turn the proofs into formally valid arguments, we should have to change 'here' to 'in the brain' in the conclusion of the first proof, and to make several adjustments to the second. But this objection confuses formality with pedantry: the form of an argument is fixed not by its superficial linguistic expression but by its underlying semantic structure. Replace 'there' by 'in the brain' in the conclusion of the first proof and you change nothing: the new words present exactly the same argument as the old.

However that may be, it may well seem that the two proofs share the same logical structure, so that it will be enough to consider the first of them — which has already been announced at *PHP* V 587-588 and stated at 649. Then what is the structure of proof (I)? what sort of syllogism underlies it? To be sure, there need be no uniquely correct answer to this question. For just as a proposition may have any number of different formal structures, so an argument — which is a set of propositions — may have a multiplicity of valid forms. Galen perhaps recognized this: in a couple of passages, at *Sem.* IV 609 and *SMT* XI 499, he offers arguments which he says may be construed either categorically or hypothetically; and hence — or so it appears — he acknowledges that one and the same argument may exhibit two different and valid formal structures. In any event, Galen must have taken his paradigmatic proofs to be syllogisms, and hence he must have taken them to be categorical or hypothetical or relational — or any two, or all three.

In *PHP* Galen does not comment explicitly on the logic of the proofs. In general, although Galen is a stickler for demonstrative rigour, he rarely remarks upon the logical structure of the proofs which he commends. In particular, although he adverts to proofs a thousand times and more in his works, and although he must use the word 'syllogism' and its cognates several hundred times, the only texts outside *Inst.Log.* in which Galen characterizes an argument as categorical or hypothetical are the two from *Sem.* and *SMT*; and he never characterizes an argument as a relational syllogism.[4]

But perhaps the text of *PHP* points implicitly at the logical structure of the proofs? Three expressions which Galen uses have been or might be thought to advance the inquiry.

First, the adjective γραμμικός. Galen demands γραμμικαὶ ἀποδείξεις; and he surely took argument (I) to be one. Such proofs are especially associated with the geometers. Galen says that geometers make frequent use of relational syllogisms. Perhaps, then, γραμμικὴ ἀπόδειξις in Galen points to relational syllogisms.

Γραμμικός means 'to do with lines' or 'linear'. Ἡ γραμμικὴ θεωρία is the theory of lines (e.g. *UP* III 812.10; *Pecc.Dig.* V 86.16), γραμμικὰ θεωρήματα are theorems about lines (e.g. *UP* III 838.2; Nicomachus, *Intr.ar.* 2.21.1), and a πρώτη γραμμικὴ στοιχείωσις is an elementary treatise on lines (Theon Smyrnaeus, p.16.19-20 Hiller). Some arithmeticians distinguished three types of numbers — the linear, the planar, the solid;[5] but

[4] It has been found remarkable that, outside *Inst.Log.*, Galen nowhere mentions his relational syllogisms (they are not to be sought at *PHP* V 796-797, *pace* de Lacy, pp.707-708, nor in the parallel passage at *Nat.Fac.* II 28); and it is tempting to invent chronological hypotheses to account for the fact. But Galen recognized relational syllogistic early in his life (*Inst.Log.* 17.1); and in any event, what needs explanation is not Galen's silence about relational syllogisms but his general reticence about logical form.

[5] E.g. Nicomachus, *Intr.ar.* 2.6.1 (and often); [Iamblichus], *Theol.ar.* p.84.9-10 De Falco (= Speusippus, fr.2.4 Lang — but there is no reason to think that [Iamblichus] is quoting Speusippus); perhaps first — in adverbial form — at Anon. *In Tht.* 40, 19-23.

lines are also contrasted with numbers, so that Galen will refer to "numerical and linear theory which astronomy and architecture use as their base" (*Pecc.Dig.* V 80.4-6).

The adjective γραμμικός is often applied to arguments. In his discussion of Archimedes and the history of mechanics, Plutarch speaks of a λογικὴ καὶ γραμμικὴ ἀπόδειξις (*Marc.* 14 [305D]);[6] and Sextus says that Aratus proved something γραμμικῶς (*Math.* 1.304).[7] Sextus has in mind a geometrical proof — the proof of Euclid 4.15. Plutarch, too, is adverting to a geometrical argument. So perhaps a linear proof is a proof about lines, or a geometrical proof? But if Galen demands linear proofs for locating the parts of the soul, he is not looking for geometrical arguments.

When an Epicurean and a Stoic and a Peripatetic attempted to recommend their different views about the void, Galen found that "they possessed no demonstrative argument but only contingent and probable arguments — and sometimes not even those"; indeed "it was plainly evident to everyone present that none of them produced an argument which was compelling [ἀναγκαστικόν] or related to a linear proof [ἀποδείξεως γραμμικῆς ἐχόμενον] but only arguments made up of the sort of considerations which orators use" (*Pecc.Dig.* V 102-103).[8] Galen is chiding the philosophers not for their want of geometrical arguments but for their want of arguments which are like geometrical arguments.

In what way like? One of the Hippocratic commentaries remarks, in an aside, that

> linear proofs … not only persuade those who are learning a discipline, but also have a reputation among laymen as being

[6] The first surviving occurrence of γραμμικός in this, or any other, usage — though Plutarch surely was not the first have used the word. The occurrences of the phrase 'linear proofs' in Cleomedes (1.8, p.84.14; 1.11, p.104,20 Ziegler) should not be ascribed to Posidonius.

[7] Cf *Math.* 3.92; Nicomachus, *Intr.ar.* 2 ('linear and arithmetical proofs'); Ptolemy, *Harm.* 1.5 [p.12.8-9 Düring]; *Alm.* 1.1 [9.15-16, 142.6], and often.

[8] Cf *UP* IV 20.9-10; *Foet.Form.* IV 695.10, 701-702; *Aff.Dig.* V 42.7.

> very true — so they say that those who have shown something clearly and uncontroversially have used linear proofs [γραμμικαῖς οὖν ἀποδείξεσι κεχρῆσθαί φασι τοὺς ἐναργῶς τι καὶ ἀναμφιλέκτως δείξαντας]'. (*HVA* XV 439-440)

Laymen use the term 'linear proof' to commend an argument which they find compelling.There is a nice example of this use in Origen (*Cels.* 8.11).

To call a proof 'linear' is not to describe its logical form, and hence not to say that it is a relational syllogism. A linear proof is an argument, of any form, which meets the standards of the geometers — an argument which exhibits the rigour, the brevity and the demonstrative power which, or so Galen professes to think, typically mark the work of the Greek geometers.

The second of the three expressions is the noun πρόσληψις; for Galen so characterizes one of the premisses of his proof.[9] It is generally held that the term πρόσληψις was introduced by the Stoic logicians, and that it is a term of art in hypothetical syllogistic, where it designates the second or non-complex premiss of a mixed hypothetical syllogism. So perhaps the presence of the word πρόσληψις in the text signals that Galen takes argument (I) to have a hypothetical structure.

The term πρόσληψις was certainly used of Stoic syllogisms, and it was perhaps first used of hypothetical syllogisms by Stoic logicians. Thus Diogenes Laertius reports that

> an argument, as Crinis says, is something constituted from an assumption and an additional assumption and an inference [τὸ συνεστηκὸς ἐκ λήμματος καὶ προσλήψεως καὶ ἐπιφορᾶς]. (7.76)[10]

[9] See *PHP* V 649.16 and *PHP* V 654.1; and note ἡ προσληφθεῖσα at 588.4 — where Alexanderson's correction ἡ πρόσληψις commends itself.

[10] See also 7.80, 82. — 7.76 does not imply that Crinis was the first Stoic to use πρόσληψις in this way. No doubt it was so used by Chrysippus, if not by Zeno.

The Peripatetics had another use for the term πρόσληψις;[11] and that is no doubt why, to do the work of the Stoic πρόσληψις, they preferred μετάληψις.[12] But — as Philoponus noticed (*In APr.* 243.8) — it was πρόσληψις which caught on; and Galen uses it dozens of times to designate the non-complex premiss of a hypothetical syllogism.[13]

Nonetheless, the word πρόσληψις does not mean "non-complex premiss in a hypothetical syllogism": it means "additional assumption", or "supplementary premiss". You are trying to construct an argument for a given thesis. You take or are offered one pertinent proposition which may serve as an assumption or premiss; and then you hunt about for another — which will therefore be a further assumption or πρόσληψις. Nothing in the sense of the word πρόσληψις ties it to any particular syllogistic structure. At least once Galen calls the complex premiss of a hypothetical syllogism a πρόσληψις (*PHP* V 429). Alexander once or twice speaks of the πρόσληψις in a categorical syllogism (e.g. *In APr.* 22.9-10; 285.21-26); and Galen once implies that one premiss of a categorical syllogism will be a πρόσληψις (*Inst.Log.* 7.4).

Thus the occurrence of πρόσληψις at *PHP* V 649 does not demonstrate that Galen took argument (I) to be a hypothetical syllogism. Nonetheless, the fact that, in the vast majority of its

[11] See Alexander Aphrodisiensis, *In APr.* 378.12-18 Wallies, Galen, *Inst.Log.* 19.1 (syllogisms κατὰ πρόσληψιν).

[12] See Alexander Aphrodisiensis, *In APr.* 324.16-18; cf 19.3-5 Wallies; Philoponus, *In APr.* 242.22-243.8 Wallies.

[13] E.g. *Inst.Log.* 4.3, and often; *Ut.Resp.* IV 494.12; *SMT* XI 500.14; cf e.g. Sextus Empiricus, *PH* 2.234; *Math.* 8.233; 8.333; 8.450. — It is inexact to speak of the complex and non-complex premisses of a mixed hypothetical syllogism inasmuch as both premisses may be complex. It is worse to speak of major and minor premisses; for those terms are defined for categorical syllogisms and make no sense when applied to hypotheticals. Something along the following lines is needed. An argument has a mixed hypothetical structure if and only if it has two premisses, one of the form '$f(A_1, A_2, \ldots, A_n)$', where 'f' is an n-placed propositional connector and $n > 1$, and the other of the form '$f^*(B_1, B_2, \ldots, B_m)$', where '$f^*$' is an m-placed propositional connector and $1 \leq m < n$ and each B_i is either an A_i or else the negation of an A_i. (If $m = 1$, then 'f^*' is the empty operator 'It is the case that'.) The premiss containing the B_is is the πρόσληψις.

occurrences, πρόσληψις does indeed refer to the non-complex premiss of a hypothetical syllogism suggests that it might well have the same a reference at *PHP* V 649.[14]

The third of the three expressions is the adjective κυριώτατος. At *PHP* V 649 the first premiss of the proof is called ἡ τοῦ λόγου κυριωτάτη πρότασις.[15] The word is not explained; but it is tempting to take as a variant on ἡγεμονικός or 'guiding', which Galen uses at *Inst.Log.* 7.1-2 to designate the complex premiss of a mixed hypothetical syllogism. *Inst.Log.* 7.1-2 uses ἡγεμονικός without stopping to explain it, and it is not found in any other ancient logical text. But it is clear that it is a relational term, that premisses are ἡγεμονικαί of προσλήψεις; and it is clear, too, that a given proposition is ἡγεμονική of an additional assumption to the extent that it determines or limits the options for such items. Suppose that you are aiming at a hypothetical syllogism, and that you already possess a conditional premiss: then your additional premiss must be either the antecedent of the conditional or the negation of its consequent — the conditional in this way is ἡγεμονικός, it guides or controls its stable-mates.

[14] At V 649 Galen does not style his second premiss a πρόσληψις *simpliciter*: he says οἷον πρόσληψις. The turn of phrase seems to imply that the second premiss is not a πρόσληψις of the ordinary kind — and hence, perhaps, that the proof is not a hypothetical syllogism of the ordinary kind. But this argument carries little weight; for at V 588 there is no protective οἷον. The context at V 649 is this:

> This is the most authoritative premiss of the argument, being accepted by all doctors and philosophers; and its as it were additional assumption is, if true
>
> The origin of the nerves is in the brain
>
> and if false:
>
> The origin of the nerves is in the heart.

Perhaps, then, the qualifying 'as it were' is there on account of the second and false supplementary premiss, which Galen does not want to call a genuine πρόσληψις.

[15] Κυριώτατος also occurs at *PHP* V 25 and 260 (of λήμματα which the Stoics unaccountably omit from their arguments), and at 651 (of the first λῆμμα in Chrysippus' false proof). So far as I know, it is not used in any other text, Galenic or non-Galenic, of the premisses of hypothetical arguments.

Now at *Inst.Log.* 7.2 Galen contrasts "syllogisms from guiding assumptions" with "syllogisms from categorical propositions", so that he apparently takes guiding premisses to be restricted to hypothetical syllogistic. And at 7.4 he states that

> hypothetical syllogisms have the additional assumption determined, categorical syllogisms do not.

This implies that categorical syllogisms do not have guiding premisses. If 'guiding' and 'most authoritative' mean the same, then we may infer that Galen's proofs in *PHP* were not construed by him as categorical syllogisms.

Yet 'most authoritative' and 'guiding' are not synonyms, nor even equivalent expressions. At *PHP* V 260 Galen applies κυριώτατος to a premiss which is not complex. At *PHP* V 649 the first premiss is κυριωτάτη of the argument and not of the πρόσληψις. Similarly, at *PHP* V 261, Galen refers to premisses which are κυρίαι of the conclusion. Hence 'authoritative' and 'guiding' are expressions with quite different senses.

Philoponus speaks once or twice of "the most authoritative" premisses of a syllogism.[16] Here the superlative has no particular force: Philoponus uses it as a synonym of the positive form κύριος; and he uses it in a sense which Alexander had explained. The authoritative premisses of an argument are "the premisses which proximately [προσεχῶς] prove and syllogize the conclusion in question" (*In APr.* 281.32-282.1; cf 282.22-24). Alexander is commenting on *APr.* 42 b1, where Aristotle refers to the κυρίαι προτάσεις of an argument. Suppose that you infer C from A and B, having inferred A from D and E, and B from F and G. Then ABDEFG are all premisses for C;

[16] See Philoponus, *In APr.* 260.35; 263.19; *In Ph.* 773.17-19.

but A and B are the authoritative premisses.[17] Perhaps Galen took the term κύριος from the Peripatetics — and perhaps that suggests that he took argument (I) to be a categorical syllogism?

But in Galen κυριώτατος or κύριος does not mark a distinction between the premisses of a syllogism and the premisses of a prosyllogism. At *PHP* V 259, where Galen is discussing a Stoic argument which, from a structural point of view, is very similar to argument (I), the word κυριώτατος picks up a preceding ἀναγκαιότατος: the assumption in question is most authoritative inasmuch as it is an essential part of the argument. Presumably, then, a premiss is authoritative if it determines the conclusion — it is not an optional or redundant extra; and a premiss is most authoritative if it is indispensable to the argument — it cannot be replaced by anything else.[18]

Galen's Greek does not disclose the logical structure of his proofs. Perhaps considerations of a more abstract sort will do the trick.

First, then, is argument (I) in fact a categorical syllogism? Galen's formulation does not use the tell-tale words 'all' and 'some', and the argument certainly does not wear a categorical heart on its sleeve. But perhaps a categorical heart beats beneath the cloth?

If so, then the three constituent propositions of the proof must be construed as categorical, and we must discover three terms for the syllogism.[19] There are several ways of extracting suitable terms. One of them is this: let A be 'brain', B 'origin

[17] Note also e.g. Alexander Aphrodisiensis, *In APr.* 22.25-26; Proclus, *In Parm.* 696.18-21 Cousin (αἱ κυρίως προτάσεις).

[18] Alexander once remarks that a universal premiss is κυριωτέρα than a particular inasmuch as "it is proper to syllogistic justification to prove something on the basis of a universal" (*APr.* 48.12-16). But this is not pertinent to Galen, whose most authoritative premisses may be either universal or particular (*PHP* V 260).

[19] I assume, here and later, that the proofs do not rely on any unexpressed premisses: having criticized the Stoics for omitting premisses in their arguments (V 259-261), Galen can scarcely have offered an enthymeme as a paradigmatic proof.

of nerves', and C 'location of a ruling part'. Then construe the first premiss,

Where the origin of the nerves is, there is the ruling part,

as predicating B of every C; the second premiss,

The origin of the nerves is in the brain,

as predicating A of every B; and the conclusion,

The ruling part is there,

as predicating A of every C. Then build the following argument:

(IC) Every location of a ruling part is an origin of the nerves.
Every origin of the nerves is a brain.
Therefore, every location of a ruling part is a brain.

That is a perfect syllogism in Barbara.

Does Barbara therefore lie under Galen's proof? That is to say, is (IC) the same argument as (I)? Is the categorical structure overtly presented in (IC) also covertly present in (I)? Or rather, did Galen take (I) to be the same as (IC) or as some variant on (IC)? Aristotle had insisted that extracting the terms of a syllogism may be a subtle matter, the natural expression of an argument often hiding rather than exposing its logical structure.[20] Galen was no doubt aware of this; and the argument in *On Semen* which he explicitly states to be categorical is far from patently so. Nonetheless, it is far from plain that (IC) — or any categorical variant on (IC) — is the same argument as (I). Moreover, if Galen did think of (I) as a categorical syllogism, he did nothing to advertise the fact.

20 "You should not always try to set out terms in a single word — often there will be phrases for which there is no equivalent word. That is why it is difficult to analyse such syllogisms, and sometimes we fall into error ..." (Aristotle, *APr.* 48 a 29-32); cf Alexander Aprhodisiensis, *In APr.* 357.20-358.4.

What, next, of hypothetical syllogistic? Galen's proofs imitate, in their linguistic form, some pseudo-proofs which he ascribes to the Stoics. Thus Chrysippus argued as follows:

> Where the affections of the soul are, there too is the ruling part.
> The affections of the soul are in the heart.
> Therefore the ruling part too is in it. (*PHP* V 651)

Now an argument offered by a Stoic as a formal proof seems likely to be taken for a hypothetical syllogism. So perhaps argument (I), whether or not it is categorical, was intended to be construed as a hypothetical syllogism? (And the word πρόσληψις designates, as it usually does, the second premiss of such a syllogism.)

It is unlikely that Chrysippus presented the argument in the form which Galen gives it at *PHP* V 651. Galen had already alluded to it at V 271, 294 and 361. He found it in Book I of Chrysippus' *On the Soul*, which he quotes:

> Since anger arises there [i.e. in the heart], it is reasonable that the remaining desires too are there — and indeed the remaining affections and the reasonings and whatever is like them. (*PHP* V 294.9-11)

The argument which *PHP* ascribes to Chrysippus is something which Galen himself invented on the basis of this text. Still, it might be thought that if Galen invented an argument on Chrysippus' behalf, then he would give a Stoic structure.

If argument (I) is a hypothetical syllogism, then what sort of hypothetical is it? There is only one plausible answer: a hypothetical syllogism of the sort which the Stoics called 'first unproveds' (and which we call arguments in *modus ponens*). In that case, the first premiss of the proof,

> Where the origin of the nerves is, there is the ruling part,

must be construed as a conditional proposition. And it is, after all, equivalent to

> If the origin of the nerves is in a given place, then the ruling part is there

— and that has a conditional look to it.

Modern logicians will say that looks deceive: the proposition is not conditional, it does not have the form 'If P, then Q'. (It is a quantified conditional, of the form '(∀x)(if Fx, then Gx)'.) True; but why think that ancient συνημμένα must have the form 'If P, then Q'? There are important issues here; yet they are beside the present point. For whether or not the proposition

> If the origin of the nerves is in a given place, then the ruling part is there,

is a conditional, the argument

> If the origin of the nerves is in a given place, then the ruling part is there.
> The origin of the nerves is in the brain.
> Therefore the ruling part is there.

is not a first unproved. A first unproved is an argument "which infers the consequent from a conditional and the antecedent" (Sext.Emp. *PH* 2.157); or, as Galen puts it,

> in the case of a continuous hypothetical proposition — which the Chrysippeans call a connected principle — if we assume in addition the antecedent, we shall have the consequent as conclusion. (*Inst.Log.* 5.5)

The second premiss in the argument I have just constructed is not the antecedent of the first.

Argument (I) cannot be construed in this way as a first unproved. I find no other, more plausible, way of taking it as a first unproved — or as any other sort of hypothetical syllogism.

Is the argument a relational syllogism? What, after all, could be more appropriate than that Galen's paradigmatic proofs should show syllogisms which, in his view, were scientifically more important than either the categoricals or the hypotheticals?[21] But what is a relational syllogism? Galen offers no general characterization of the species; and the numerous examples which he produces in the third part of the *Introduction* do not invite an easy induction. Yet there appears to be a large hint towards a definition.

Having introduced a first group of relational syllogisms, Galen says that

> common to all these syllogisms is the fact that they have the same construction on the basis of certain axioms. (*Inst.Log.* 16.5)

Similar phrases, which have been alleged to express Galen's 'metatheorem', recur in the following pages.[22] Then is not a syllogism relational if and only if its construction, or its validity, or its probative power, depends on some axiom or axioms?

There are several difficulties here. First, the text in many of the relevant passages is peculiarly recalcitrant.[23] Secondly, the 'metatheorem' is expressed in several ways which are not evidently equivalent to one another. Thirdly, Galen never clearly explains exactly how axioms are supposed to underwrite relational syllogisms. Fourthly — and most pertinently —, he appears to hold that every syllogism, or at least every demonstrative syllogism, is underwritten by a universal axiom. At 16.10 he refers to "all the other demonstrative syllogisms". At 17.1 he says that

> pretty well all syllogisms gain their construction from the warranty of the universal axioms which are superordinate to them.

[21] The first illustrative argument in *Inst.Log.* is a relational syllogism — no casual choice.

[22] See 16.10, 11, 12; 17.1, 2, 3, 7, 9; 18.1, 6, 8; and note 1.2-3.

[23] Nowhere more so that at 16.5: the MS reading makes neither sense nor syntax; I read σύστασιν ὡς for συστάσεως — *alii alia*.

At 17.2 he affirms that

> it may be learned more clearly in the following way that all demonstrative syllogisms are such because of the warranty of universal axioms.

At 17.7 he remarks that

> most of the items which men syllogize and prove are said in virtue of an axiom.

In some of these passages, 'all syllogisms' or 'all demonstrative syllogisms' may be limited, by the context, to all relational syllogisms. But 17.7, at least, cannot be read with such a limitation; and it follows that the fact of being founded on an axiom does not define the class of relational syllogisms.

Perhaps relational syllogisms are underwritten by relational axioms, and that is what distinguishes them from other syllogisms? But the problem is thereby displaced, not resolved: instead of asking "What makes a syllogism relational?" we shall ask "What makes an axiom relational?".

If you want to know what makes a syllogism relational, then it is best to ask first what makes a syllogism categorical or hypothetical. Categorical syllogisms, according to Aristotle, reduce to Barbara and Celarent, the first two syllogisms of the first figure (*APr.* 29 b 15-25). Barbara and Celarent are 'perfect' or 'complete'; that is to say, their validity is 'evident' (*ibid.* 24 b 22-24). Their validity is evident inasmuch as it flows directly from the definition of 'hold of every' and 'hold of no' — inasmuch as it follows from what was later called the principle *de omni et nullo* (*ibid.* 25 b 39-40; 26 a 27-28). Thus, following Aristotle at one remove, we might say this:

> A syllogism is categorical if and only if its validity is guaranteed merely by the sense of the quantifiers ('of every', 'of no', 'of some', 'not of some').

Then for hypothetical syllogisms we might offer:

> A syllogism is hypothetical if and only if its validity is guaranteed merely by the sense of the propositional connectors ('if', 'or', 'and', 'not').

And so in the case of relational syllogisms we should be looking for something of the following form:

> A syllogism is relational if and only if its validity is guaranteed merely by the sense of Xs.

It seems reasonable to suppose that relational syllogisms must contain, in some essential fashion, relational terms — terms which fall in the Aristotelian class of τὰ πρός τι.[24] Hence:

> A syllogism is relational if and only if its validity is guaranteed merely by the sense of relational terms.[25]

It may then be imagined that the axioms which underwrite relational syllogisms are truths determined by the senses of the relational terms which the syllogisms contain.

At *Inst.Log.* 16.6 Galen remarks that with the aid of the axiom

> Items equal to the same item are equal to one another

we can prove the first theorem of Euclid's *Elements.* The proof took this shape:

> A is equal to C.

[24] There are two opposite objections to this supposition. On the one hand, some of the examples of relational syllogisms in *Inst.Log.* 16-17 do not essentially contain relational predicates — yet perhaps Galen thinks that they do. On the other hand, at 16.12 Galen perhaps mean to allow that some relational syllogisms do not contain πρός τι predicates — but the text is crucially uncertain, and in fact the examples in question do contain two-placed predicates. In any event, if relational syllogisms are not to be defined in terms of relational predicates, I do not know how they are to be defined.

[25] These definitions of the three types of syllogism (which deliberately leave open the possibility that an argument might belong to more than one type) require considerable refinement; nor do they purport to correspond to anything which an ancient logician may have thought or said. They are offered as a rough indication of how one might try to carve syllogisms into species.

B is equal to C.

A is equal to B.

It is a relational syllogism inasmuch as its validity is guaranteed merely by the sense of the relational term 'equal to'; and the pertinent aspect of the sense of 'equal to' is given by the axiom which underwrites the proof.[26]

Are the proofs at *PHP* V 649 relational syllogisms? Well, what are their relational terms? At this point argument (II) might be summoned into the box; for its first premiss contains the comparative adverb 'more evidently' [ἐπιφανέστερον], and comparatives generally express relations. But the second premiss contains no comparative — there the verb φαίνεται (which my translation turns into the adverb 'clearly') corresponds to and picks up ἐπιφανέστερον. Perhaps the text should be emended (say, by the addition of μᾶλλον), or perhaps some comparative notion should simply be 'understood'? Perhaps, on the other hand, the comparative form ἐπιφανέστερον here has no comparative force — Greek comparative adverbs are often 'positive' in sense.

However that may be, a modern logician will readily find a relational term in argument (I). For example, the second premiss —

The origin of the nerves is in the brain

— expresses a relation between the origin of the nerves and the brain, namely the relation of being located in. But perhaps Aristotle would have taken 'in the brain' to be not a relational term but a predicate in the category of 'where'; and perhaps Galen

[26] In the text of Euclid, 1.1, the axiom is used as a premiss of the argument, not as an external underwriting; and it must be admitted that some passages in *Inst.Log.* suggest that Galen too construed the axioms as supplementary premisses. But this cannot — or at any rate should not — have been Galen's considered view.

would have agreed.[27] However, the second premiss also contains the term 'origin' or ἀρχή which is indisputably relational and which Galen himself took to be relational (cf. *PHP* V 564).

The relationality emerges clearly if Galen's proof is rewritten as follows:

(IR) Where the nerves originate, there is the ruling part.
The nerves originate in the brain.
Therefore the ruling part is in the brain.

Is this argument relational? That is to say, does its validity depend merely on the sense of the relational term 'originate in'?

Suppose that we vary any or every term in the argument save only 'originate in': is the result always a valid argument? Or equivalently, if all the terms save 'originate in' are replaced by schematic letters, is every instance of the resulting schema a valid argument? Plainly, the answer is No. Replace 'there' in the first premiss by 'elsewhere' and the result is an invalid argument. Hence (IR) is not a relational syllogism. It does not follow that (I) is not a relational syllogism — still less that Galen did not take it to be one. But I can find nothing better than (IR), and (IR) will not wash.

Nor should we wish to find a relational syllogism in the text. For Galen's third species of syllogism is not a species at all. Consider again the Euclidean argument:

(A) A is equal to C.
B is equal to C.
———
A is equal to C.

Galen took that to be on the same logical level as,

(B) If something moves, something is void.

[27] See Aristotle, *Cat.* 2 a 1-2 ("in the market-place", "in the Lyceum"); and note Galen's curious examples of predicates in the category of 'where': "second in position from the earth" (*Inst.Log.* 2.1); "in the middle of the universe" (*ibid.* 13.7).

Something moves.

Something is void.

That is to say, in effect he construed the two-placed predicate 'is equal to' as a logical constant, just as in (B) 'if' may be construed as a logical constant. And Galen's relational logic is that system of logic which treats all and only two-placed predicates as logical constants.

Then take the following argument:

(C) Something runs.

Something moves.

It is valid in virtue of the sense of the one-placed predicates which it contains. So it belongs to another, fourth species of syllogism, which we may call predicative syllogisms. Predicative syllogistic is that system of logic which construes all and only one-placed predicates as logical constants. It is on all fours with Galen's relational syllogistic.

There are predicative syllogisms, and there are relational syllogisms — they are all arguments of the sort which the mediaeval logicians called "material consequences" and the Stoics "unmethodically concluding arguments". There are unsurveyably many of them; and although some of them come in little clusters or families — so that you may be tempted to talk of a 'logic of identity' or a 'logic of causality'[28] —, they are not systematizable and they do not form a species in the way in which categorical arguments and hypothetical arguments are systematizable and form species. You might say, crudely, that there is no such thing as predicative logic. In exactly the same sense, there is no such thing as relational logic.[29]

[28] But a modern logician who speaks of the 'logic of causality' will have in mind standard predicate logic afforced by some causal constants.

[29] "But modern textbooks usually contain a chapter called 'The Logic of Relations', so the subject must exist". Many textbooks contain such chapters; but the

Galen's paradigmatic proof is not a relational syllogism, it is not a hypothetical syllogism, it is scarcely a categorical syllogism. In other words, it is not caught in the net of Galen's logic — Galen is not equipped to elucidate its validity. But it is formally valid: how, then, is it best analysed?

Surely the connector 'Where ..., there — ' is the first item to think about. For any argument of the form

> Where X, there Y.
> X here.
> ———
> Y here.

is valid. Next, it seems clear that from the first premiss,

> Where the nerves originate, there is the ruling part,

there follows, by 'universal instantiation':

> If the nerves originate in the brain, then the ruling part is in the brain.

And from this conditional proposition and the second premiss of the argument,

> The nerves originate in the brain,

there follows, by *modus ponens*:

> The ruling part is in the brain.

Any modern reader with a smattering of formal logic will then be tempted to present the argument in a mixture of symbols and abbreviations, thus:

chapters have nothing to do with Galen's relational syllogistic: they do not describe a third sort of logic, after propositional logic and predicate logic. This is clear from the fact that they introduce no new rules of inference.

$(\forall x)(Oax \supset Lbx)$
Oac

Lbc

The validity of this argument can then be proved:

1	(1) $(\forall x)(Oax \supset Lbx)$	prem
2	(2) Oac	prem
1	(3) $Oac \supset Lbc$	1, UE
1, 2	(4) Lbc	2,3 MPP

The term 'originate in' or 'O' is not essential to the validity of the argument — it may be replaced by any other relational term and the result will be a valid argument. Moreover, the validity of the argument does not depend on the fact that it contains relational terms. For, as its proof indicates, it is an instance of the schema:

$(\forall x)(Fx \supset Gx)$
Fc

Gc

In short, the argument may be analysed as a hybrid of the categorical and the hypothetical: its validity depends both on the sense of the quantifiers (in the inference from (1) to (3)) and also on the sense of the connectors (in the inference from (2) and (3) to (4)).

This analysis of argument (I) is still hopelessly inadequate;[30] and there are, in any event, several other ways of devising an

[30] It treats 'the nerves', 'the ruling part' and 'the brain' as singular terms, which they are not; and it does not bring out the fact — which is not explicit in Galen's own formulation — that the nerves, ruling part and brain all belong to the same animal. A paraphrase of the first premiss which begins to do justice to these facts is this:

> In any animal, at whatever place all the nerves of that animal originate, at that place is located any ruling part of that animal.

analysis. But two things are, I think, clear: first, none of Galen's three syllogistics is capable of explaining the validity of the argument; and secondly, any adequate explanation will conjoin categorical and hypothetical features. Had Galen thought of uniting categorical and hypothetical syllogistic in some fashion, he would have been the third logician of history. Instead, he discovered a bogus third species of syllogism.

Any analysis of Galen's argument which takes this into account is formidably complex — and in fact exceeds the powers of standard predicate logic.

DISCUSSION

J. Jouanna: J'ai été très intéressé par votre étude du vocabulaire relatif au syllogisme. Je voudrais vous demander, à propos de γραμμικαὶ ἀποδείξεις, s'il existe des emplois antérieurs à Galien.

J. Barnes: One at least — in Plutarch's *Marcellus*; and probably another — assuming that Nicomachus wrote before Galen.

M. Frede: I wonder if the term γραμμικὴ ἀπόδειξις does not have roughly the force of 'proof *more geometrico*'. It might be worthwhile to look for more passages in which the expression is used. As for the use of γραμμικός, it might be relevant that διαγράμματα is used in the sense of 'geometrical proofs'. In any event, I think it is fairly clear that Galen did not think of the proofs as being linear in the sense in which Aristotelian proofs might be thought to be linear, proceeding from the prior to the posterior.

J. Barnes: I agree that 'linear' has nothing to do with priority and posteriority, and I agree that *more geometrico* is a rough equivalent — provided that the Latin tag is construed in a fairly generous fashion.

J. Jouanna: Concernant κυριώτατος, ce superlatif est employé chez Galien parfois aussi avec πρῶτος, ce qui ne fait que renforcer ce que vous avez dit sur la synonymie de κυριώτατος avec ἡγεμονικός. Mais bien entendu, dans l'histoire de la langue grecque, κυριώτατος est plus ancien que ἡγεμονικός. Enfin, quel est le rapport exact entre κυριώτατος et ἀναγκαιότατος?

J. Barnes: It is quite true that, in Galen, κυριώτατος often keeps company with πρῶτος; but in such cases Galen is alluding, consciously or not, to the 'to be or not to be' of ancient metaphysics: οὐσία ... ἡ κυριώτατά τε καὶ πρώτως καὶ μάλιστα λεγομένη (*Cat.* 2 a 11-12); and I am not sure that this encourages a *rapprochement* with ἡγεμονικός. As for ἀναγκαιότατος, I am inclined to think — although the evidence is admittedly tenuous — that, at least in *PHP*, it is equivalent to or even synonymous with κυριώτατος.

M. Frede: I wonder whether the term κυριωτάτη πρότασις at *PHP* V 649.15 refers to the contribution which the premiss makes not to the validity of the argument but to its probative character.

J. Barnes: In other words, without that premiss the argument might still be a syllogism but it would not be a proof? That sounds very plausible. But I suspect that it is something determined by the context rather than by the sense of the word κυριώτατος: the word means something like 'indispensable', and the context will answer the question 'indispensable for what'?

T. Tieleman: You argue persuasively that Galen's syllogisms on the location of the parts of the soul display both categorical and hypothetical elements. As you say, Galen himself does not comment on the logic of the proofs. But at *PHP* V 219-220 he does explain the construction and the sources of the proof concerning the regent part. He does so in an Aristotelian manner insofar as he starts from a definition in order to arrive at a major premiss; and in the near context he refers to Aristotle and Theophrastus as the philosophers who have offered the best accounts of scientific proof (*ibid.* 213; cf. 222). This makes it the more remarkable that he does not use strictly categorical syllogisms. Might Galen's logical education help to explain his attitude? Are there any examples from the later tradition which show a similar hospitality to hypothetical forms of inference?

J. Barnes: The text at *PHP* V 219-220 is indeed pertinent. In my paper I should have said that, although hypothetical syllogistic is associated primarily with the Stoics, certain hypothetical forms were discussed and accepted by the Peripatetic logicians (from Theophrastus onwards). So Galen might in principle have thought that his proofs were hypothetical in form and yet Peripatetic in spirit. But the fact remains that he says nothing about the logical structure of the proofs.

V. Barras: L'importance du syllogisme relationnel semble évidente dans le système de preuves que propose Galien. Tentant de relier — peut-être de façon artificielle — la logique de Galien à sa pratique d'anatomiste, je me demande si l'anatomie, qui peut être entendue comme l'art de mettre en lumière des relations cachées entre différents organes ou parties, n'a pas quelque affinité avec une logique 'relationnelle'. Votre exemple, "Where the nerves originate ...", abonde en termes relationnels qui sont à la fois ce que Galien anatomiste cherche à prouver.

J. Barnes: Je vous remercie pour votre suggestion, qui me paraît bien fondée: assurément Galien anatomiste aura remarqué l'importance des relations pour son étude. Il vaut pourtant la peine d'ajouter que la présence d'un terme relationnel dans un argument n'est pas une condition suffisante pour que l'argument soit relationnel: les syllogismes catégoriques et hypothétiques peuvent contenir de tels termes, pourvu que leur relationnalité ne soit pas pertinente à la validité de l'argument.

J. Jouanna: À propos du second texte que vous citez (*PHP* V 649) dans votre étude si suggestive sur les relations entre la logique et l'anatomie, je voudrais vous demander comment vous interpréter ταύτην τὴν πρότασιν. Pour ma part, je verrais une reprise de la πρόσληψις qui précède, à savoir la πρόσληψις ψευδής, "l'origine des nerfs est dans le cœur".

J. Barnes: The passage to which you refer contains several related difficulties. The transmitted text is this:

> ... ὅπου τῶν νεύρων ἡ ἀρχὴ ἐνταῦθα καὶ τὸ τῆς ψυχῆς ἡγεμονικόν.

> αὕτη μὲν ἡ τοῦ λόγου κυριωτάτη πρότασις ὡμολογημένη πᾶσιν ἰατροῖς τε καὶ φιλοσόφοις· ἡ δ' οἷον πρόσληψις αὐτῆς ἀληθὴς μὲν
>
> ἡ ἀρχὴ τῶν νεύρων ἐν τῷ ἐγκεφάλῳ,
>
> ψευδὴς δὲ
>
> ἡ ἀρχὴ τῶν νεύρων ἐν τῇ καρδίᾳ,
>
> γράφειν μὲν ταύτην τὴν πρότασιν ἢ καὶ λέγειν τοῖς ἀπείροις ἀνατομῆς δυναμένου τινός, οὐ μὴν δεῖξαί γε δυναμένου. πάντα γὰρ ἐν τοῖς ζῴοις τὰ μόρια νεύρων μετέχει, κτλ. (V 649.13-650.3)

Your question concerns the reference of ταύτην τὴν πρότασιν. In addition, one may wonder with what verbs the dative τοῖς ἀπείροις ἀνατομῆς should best be taken. And one may ask what is the sense of γράφειν. Each of these questions admits several answers which are, from a grammatical point of view, equally plausible. Different combinations of the different answers ascribe radically different doctrines to Galen. My own opinion, of which I am far from certain, is this. Galen wants, in this passage, to draw a contrast between the two premisses of the arguments by which he thinks the problem of the location of the parts of the soul is to be settled. One of those premisses will be a general truth — a truth of reason accepted by all doctors and philosophers. The other premiss, however, will be empirical, and in particular it will depend on anatomical knowledge — which is why the Stoic philosophers are incompetent in its regard. That being so, then, first, we should take ταύτην τὴν πρότασιν to refer neither to the false πρόσληψις nor to the true. Rather, it picks up ἡ … οἷον πρόσληψις αὐτῆς: Galen means that the second premiss of the argument, whatever it may be, is beyond the competence of those who are unskilled in anatomy. Secondly, τοῖς ἀπείροις ἀνατομῆς should be taken with all three infinitives — γράφειν, λέγειν, and δεῖξαι. Thirdly, γράφειν means 'draw', not 'write'. Hence the remark may be paraphrased as follows: "As for the second premiss of such arguments, if someone is ignorant of anatomy, you may draw it for them (they can understand a diagram showing the nerves all converging on the brain), and you may even state it to them (they can, in principle, understand the medical terms you use); but you cannot show them its truth (they have not done the practical work which that demands)". Other, very different interpretations of the passage are indeed possible; but I think that the following sentence πάντα γὰρ ... tells strongly in favour of my reading.

II

R.J. Hankinson

CAUSATION IN GALEN

Much of the disagreement between the later Greek schools of medicine, the Dogmatists, the Empiricists, and the Methodists, turned on the issue of the nature and discoverability of causal connections. Dogmatists, whatever else their differences, tended to agree that a causal understanding of the inner workings of the body, and of the progress of disease, was necessary for the latter's treatment.[1] They also were wont to essay precise distinctions in causal categorization, differentiating at the very least between the internal conditions responsible for (or predisposing towards) illness, and the external, antecedent occasions of those illnesses, their *aitia prokatarktika.* Empiricists refused to allow that the internal conditions were discoverable, or that even if they were an understanding of them would be of any use to therapy; but they took careful note of the antecedent circumstances that seemed relevant to particular conditions, in order to be able better to predict likely outcomes in future cases. The Methodists took no notice of such alleged *aitia prokatarktika*, supposing rather that all diseases were simply matters of excessive constriction or dilatation (or a combination of the two), and that the existence of such conditions was phenomenally obvious, at least to the trained eye, and dictated an allopathic therapeutic intervention.

[1] Partial, and controversial, exceptions to this rule are Herophilus (on whom see Hankinson 1990 and 1998, 2670-81) and Erasistratus (of whom more below; cf. Hankinson 1998, *passim*).

Galen is, on this score at least, a Dogmatist; and his rationalist rejection of Empiricist methodology as inadequate and Methodism as totally mistaken, a rejection to be found throughout his works, but most conveniently dealt with in *De sectis ingredientibus* (*SI*), presupposes a particular analysis of physiology, pathology, and their interrelations, as well as of the proper method of medical semiotics. At *De methodo medendi* (*MM*) 4.3, X 242-249 K, he takes issue with the Empiricist view that one may infer directly from the *aitia prokatarktika* of diseases to their proper treatment:

> None of the procatarctic causes of a disposition (*diathesis*) is indicative of therapy, but the indication (*endeixis*) of it [sc. therapy] begins from the disposition itself, while the individual activities (*energeiai*) are discovered both from the primary goal (*skopos*) and from the nature of the affected part, and of its ambient temperament (*krasis*), and what ever else are related to these things.[2] (1: *MM* X 242.16-243.3 K)

Thus for Galen it is crucial to be able to determine the state of the internal dispositions of the body, which themselves determine the functioning of its proper activities or *energeiai*. It is not enough simply to catalogue the external occasions of disfunction.

Earlier, at *MM* 1.8, X 63-67 K, in the course of a lengthy attack on the inadequacies of Erasistratean and Methodist pathology, Galen has offered his own account of the structure of proper (and deviant) bodily functioning. There are four elements: (1) the bodies themselves, or rather their dispositions; (2) their activities, what they characteristically do; (3) the causes of the bodily dispositions; and finally (4) "those which obtain in bodies both naturally and unnaturally, but which neither promote nor impede the activities" (64.11-13), the "symptoms

[2] All the technical terms of this passage are important and will be discussed further below.

which are necessarily consequent on the different alterations in bodies, whether they are in a natural state or not" (65.1-3).

A little later, at *MM* 2.4-5, X 97-115 K, Galen attacks both Methodists and Erasistrateans for their failure to attend to the proper causal structure of things. Galen's opponents are presented as treating what are simply concomitants or symptoms of the disease as though it were the disease itself (this is a charge distinct from, albeit obviously related to, that of the earlier passage in which he castigated their terminological confusions: *MM* 1.7-8, X 53-67 K). Galen posits someone who says

> That the reason why someone who has been fed exclusively on milk for several days is now unable to digest properly is the colour of his stomach has been altered, turned white instead of red: I think you would laugh, and rightly so. (2: *MM* 2.4, X 97.15-18 K)

This is a fictitious case, but no different, Galen says, from the practice of his opponents of holding various physiological conditions which they suppose to be concomitant with damage to natural activities responsible for the damage (97-98). But it is vital to distinguish the causal order of things. If the fictitious opponent persists in holding variations in gastric colour responsible for variations in digestive functioning, then

> I know of no way [sc. of refuting him] other than by demanding of the person making these claims to show first how it is that the stomach generally operates naturally as a result of its colour. (3: *MM* 2.4, X 98.10-13 K)

Galen's point is clear: even if it is true that variations of gastric function are attended by variations in colour, that is not enough to show that the latter are the cause of the former (although it may be good evidence for the supposition that they are causally connected in some way): causation is a matter of operational, and not merely functional, dependence.

Consider again elements (1)-(4) above. They are linked, Galen says in the following way:

> There are four different types of things that occur in bodies contrary to nature… one is the impaired activity itself [answering to (2)], the second is the disposition that brings it about [(1)], the third its causes [(3)], and the fourth the symptoms that necessarily follow it [(4)]. (4: *MM* 2.1, X 78.1-6 K)

Thus the underlying disposition (1), which is impaired or unnatural in the case of illness, brings about the damage to the activity itself (2), while in turn (1) itself has causes which are responsible for it (3); and finally the impaired activity (or perhaps the disposition responsible for it) bring further consequences (4), such as the gastric coloration of the man on the milk-diet, in their train. As regards (3), Galen writes:

> Something must stand in the same relation to the dispositions as the dispositions do to the activities, differing in one respect only, that the dispositions exist at the same time as the activities and it is never possible for an activity to be properly constituted unless the disposition of the bodies is natural, nor for it to be impaired without previous damage to the bodies [they are thus synectic causes of it: see further below]. The causes of the dispositions which impede the activities, however, may either have ceased to exist or still be in existence. (5: *MM* 1.8, X 63.18-64.8 K)

Why must something stand in the same relation to (1) as (1) does to (2)? The short answer is that Galen takes it to be axiomatic, and apprehensible *a priori*, that "nothing occurs without a cause" (*MM* 1.7, X 50.2-3 K; cf. 1.4, X 36-7; *De propriis placitis* [*Sent.Prop.*] 14.1, p.110 Nutton: n.32 below).[3] Hence the physical dispositions, whatever they are, which impair the natural activities must themselves in turn have been caused by

[3] On this and other causal axioms for Galen, and on their metaphysical and epistemological status, see HANKINSON 1998a, 376; 1991c; and 1991a, *ad loc.*

something. But by what? And what in any case are these dispositions? Answering those questions will takes us further into the terminological heart of Galen's theorizing.

In any event, Galen insists, typically, that, as long as one understands the basic schema of (1)-(4), and equally when one knows what as a matter of fact in each case fit into each of the schematic categories, it doesn't much matter which of (1) or (2) you choose to call the disease, as long as you do so consistently.[4] Reasonable fidelity to ordinary usage will rule out, he thinks, the candidacy of either (3) or (4), as well as the aggregate of all of them;[5] so, since

> It is essential that we assign names… clearly…; let us then call the disposition [(1)] that impedes the activity [(2)] the disease; whatever follows from it [(4)] a symptom; and whatever is responsible for it [(3)] a cause. (**6**: *MM* 2.1, X 81.12-16 K; cf. 1.8, X 65; and *CC* 8.10-12)

"Whatever follows from it" suggests that 'symptom' can be used more broadly than merely to cover the adventitious consequences of damage to activities (or the dispositions which cause them); and this is not a casual mistake. Earlier, Galen has suggested (although not necessarily in his own voice) calling the damage to the activity a "special symptom" of the disease (*MM* 1.8, X 65.9-10 K). Moreover, he will also on occasion treat symptoms as being dispositions (as indeed they are), although not of course dispositions in the sense of (1), those causally responsible for damage to activities. However that may be, the

[4] Cf. *De causis contentivis* 8.10-12, 10.7-8.

[5] See *MM* 2.1, X 78-79 K: if the aggregate of (1)-(4) is the disease, then the expressions "cause of disease" and "symptom of disease" become meaningless (since they imply distinctness from the disease, and yet on this conception of disease it comprehends them); and yet (Galen implies) they are not (his argument here is not wholly convincing: see HANKINSON 1991a, 161-2); and of course similar considerations will exclude (3) and (4) individually (and indeed collectively, although Galen doesn't canvas this possibility) as possible candidates for the referent of the term 'disease'.

broad outlines of the official position are summed up in a passage from *De symptomatum differentiis* (*Symp.Diff.*):

> A disease is a disposition of the body which is such as primarily[6] to impede one of its activities; those dispositions which precede (προηγοῦνται) it are not indeed diseases. And if some other dispositions happen along with them, following along with them like shadows,[7] we shall not call them diseases either, but symptoms, and so, on our account, not just anything which occurs in a body contrary to nature should immediately be labelled a disease, but rather only that which primarily harms an activity <should be called> a disease, while what precedes (προηγούμενον) it <should be called> a cause of the disease, but not indeed a disease. And if some other bodily disposition follows upon the disease, this will be called a symptom. Furthermore, the actual harm to the activity is a symptom of the animal, since everything unnatural in any way which occurs in the animal is a symptom: for this is how ordinary Greek usage regarding names has it. (7: *Symp.Diff.* 1, VII 50.4-17 K)

The taxonomy of unnatural conditions which we have been briefly analyzing presupposes, or at least is conditioned by, a particular theory of causation. In the domain (roughly) of what was for Aristotle and his followers efficient causation, the Stoics[8] distinguished between *aitia prokatarktika* and what they called *aitia sunektika* (or *sunechê*, or *sunechonta*: here as elsewhere the causal vocabulary is rich to the point of indigestibility with synonyms): containing causes.[9] This distinction was taken over

[6] The sense of 'primarily' (*prôtôs*) here is important: see below p. 50.

[7] Compare the famous Pyrrhonian image of ἀταραξία following on ἐποχή "as a shadow does a body": SEXT.EMP. *PH* 1.29; cf. DIOG.LAERT. 9.107, who attributes the image to Timon and Aenesidemus.

[8] See FREDE 1980; BOBZIEN 1998b, esp. ch. 6; HANKINSON 1999.

[9] The translations for these terms into English are equally varied. *Aition sunektikon* has been variously rendered as 'containing cause' (perhaps the most common, and my reluctant preference), 'cohesive cause' and 'sustaining cause', none of which gets it quite right; I had toyed with the translation 'comprehensive',

by the doctors, including Galen, although not without some refinements.

In what follows, I shall not say much about *aitia prokatarktika*, although the subject is important and I have dealt with it extensively elsewhere.[10] Suffice it to say that *aitia prokatarktika* are the evident, external occasions which set in train a pathogenic sequence of events. For such a set of events to unfold, conditions in the body of the patient must be propitious (or the reverse); which explains why not everybody is susceptible to the same antecedent causes (only if I am of an excessively hot and dry temperament, for example, will I develop heat-stroke after only mild exposure to sunlight: *CP* II 11-16), which in turn serves to defuse the objections of Erasistratus and others that they cannot be causes because they do not affect all equally. Thus, in fact, procatarctic causes serve to reveal those internal weaknesses — and as such are, for Galen, indicators of the internal conditions of individuals' bodies, internal conditions the knowledge of which is vital for successful therapy (*MM* 4.3, X 242-249 K).

By contrast, *aitia sunektika* are altogether more tightly linked to their purported outcomes. In its original Stoic sense, as Galen

which is a bit closer both to the literal meaning and to some of the implications of the term, but it too has unfortunate and misleading connotations; I shall adopt the convention (generally) of simply transliterating as 'synectic causes'. *Aition prokatarktikon* has fared no better, yielding 'antecedent cause', 'initial cause', 'salient cause' (via the Arabic); I was also tempted to seek a new rendering here too, but all the alternatives that suggested themselves ('pre-initiating', 'pre-arising', 'pre-originating') seemed too rebarbative; and so I will also adhere to the parallel convention of calling them 'procatarctic causes'.

[10] See HANKINSON 1987, 1988a, 1994a. Galen wrote a short text *De causis procatarcticis* [*CP*] vindicating their importance against the attacks of Erasistratus and others; it is edited with translation and commentary in HANKINSON 1998b. Erasistratus argued that antecedent causes, since they are not invariably followed by their purported effects, cannot properly be causes of them; thus he is committed — absurdly in Galen's view — to the position that all genuine causes must be sufficient for their effects. Galen agrees that *aitia prokatarktika* are not sufficient for their effects but denies that this means that they cannot have causal relevance to such outcomes as one of a number of contributory factors; equally, there is no reason to deny them the title of causes.

himself makes clear in his opusculum on the subject, *De causis contentivis* (*CC*),[11] a synectic cause was the cause of the existence of something;[12] they were identified with the subtle, volatile *pneuma* which, according to their physics, pervades everything (*CC* 1.1-5). Galen himself rejects this account, holding that in change it is the elements themselves which are directly affected and not some postulated *pneuma* which holds them together (3.1-5.5); but more importantly for our purposes he also rejects the view that it is an *a priori* causal axiom ("one indemonstrable and self-justifying") that "no body can exist in any state whatever without a synectic cause", holding that it leads to regress (since the Stoics themselves insist that causes are bodies: *CC* 6.1-3). In Galen's view, no cause of existence (or persistence) on the Stoic (or Neoplatonist, or Cartesian for that matter) model is required, and every genuine cause, on examination, will turn out to be one of generation and not one of being (*CC* 7.1-2; cf. *Adversus Julianum* XVIIIA 280 K; *De plenitudine* VII 524-528 K): "what has already been produced must necessarily have been so as a result of some cause, but is no longer in any need of a cause" (*CC* 7.3) — one might label this Galen's Principle of Causal Inertia, or PCI.[13]

[11] *CC* survives only in Latin and Arabic; the Latin text is edited in Kalbfleisch (1904); the Arabic in Lyons (1969).

[12] Hence Sedley's translation "sustaining causes": above, n.9.

[13] Jonathan Barnes asked whether this formulation was too strong — surely Galen allows that some types of persistent thing require causes of their persistence, his so-called *aitia phulaktika* (cf. e.g. *Ars Med.* I 365-366 K), and in that case should not PCI be weakened to the claim that some cases of persistent existence require no cause? I think it is better, however, to insist that for Galen existence properly so-called requires no preservative cause, although there are certain sorts of state, which involve the maintenance of a constant dynamic tension, which do require constantly active causes for their preservation — but such states are, precisely, better thought of as activities. Galen gives an example (*CC* 8.7-8): statues that are designed to lean forwards and would otherwise overbalance may be balanced in the rear with lead to prevent their toppling over. They seem to be at rest (i.e. in a state of continuous unchanging existence), but in fact their equilibrium is preserved by the constant dynamic tension of the opposing forces. In a similar vein, at *De motu musculorum* (*Mot.Musc.*) 1.8, IV 402-403 K, Galen argues that one should describe a hovering bird not as being at rest, but as rising

Galen diagnoses the source of this error (namely the rejection of PCI) in the mistaken belief that certain things which do have synectic causes (walking and talking) may be thought of as types of actual existence rather than of generation (certainly they are for Aristotle and others prime examples of *energeiai*): but in fact, properly understood, they are fundamentally processes, and as such can indeed have synectic causes (*CC* 8.1-2). The same is true of the pulse — in a sense it exists throughout one's life, but it is in fact a constant state of change (8.3-5). Even so, one may talk of synectic causes of the pulse metaphorically, as Galen himself has done:[14] the three synectic causes of the pulse being its function,[15] the vital capacity (*dunamis*) and the physical structure (heart and arteries) which produce it (8.6); we shall return to this claim shortly.

The main features of the Stoic synectic cause which are retained in the 'metaphorical' medical usage[16] are its co-temporality with its effect, and the functional dependence of the effect on the strength of the cause. Sextus (*PH* 3.15) gives as an example the dependence of the strangulation on the tightness of the noose (there is strangulation just as long as the noose is drawn

by its own muscular power at precisely the same rate at which it is falling due to its weight. Both of these cases, involving as they do an equipoise of constant dynamic tension, require continuously acting causes for their maintenance.

[14] The reference is to *De causis pulsuum* (*Caus.Puls.*), esp. 1.1-4, IX 1-7 K; see further text **10** below.

[15] *Chreia*: another word hopelessly difficult of translation, and variously rendered 'use', 'need', 'purpose', 'usefulness', 'utility', etc. At *De praesagitione ex pulsibus* (*Praes.Puls.*) 1.1, IX 210 K, Galen says that the *chreia* of the pulse is twofold: to preserve the innate heat, and to generate psychic *pneuma* (the instrument with which the soul effects purposive action); *Caus.Puls.* 1.3, IX 5-6 K concurs, adding the further function of expelling any smoky residue produced by combustion of the humours.

[16] And it should be pointed out that the Stoics themselves were perfectly happy to posit synectic causes of processes as well as of existence; in a famous example, Chrysippus compares human action with a rolling cylinder: it requires an external shove (analagous to the external impression need to move humans to action) to start it moving, but thereafter it moves under its own steam, as result of "its own force and nature" (CIC. *Fat.* 43), because of its "rollability"; on this, see HANKINSON 1999.

tight, and the tighter the noose the more severe the strangulation).[17] Synectic causes, then, are as one might say strongly, that is functionally, sufficient for their effects.[18]

Galen broadly accepts this account. In the course of discussing the reasons why the pupil dilates and contracts, he writes:

> The synectic cause, as one might say, of the generation of this [sc. dilation] is the tension of choroid membrane, just as its relaxation <is the synectic cause> of its contraction. (**8**: *Caus.Symp.* 1.2, VII 93 K)[19]

Just as in the case of the noose, there is a direct, indeed mechanical, connection between the tension of the membrane and the condition of the pupil. But of course this fact in itself is perfectly consistent with other causal factors being involved in particular cases of dilation or contraction (just as they may be in the case of the strangulation); we can ask about why it's a good (or in pathological cases a bad) thing for the pupil to be in the condition it's in; and we may refer to the action of the incidence of external light on the eye in bringing about alterations in the tension of the choroid membrane. That is to say, causal explanation will typically, and necessarily if it is to be complete, pay attention to a variety of different factors, all of which have an important role to play in the outcome. It is critical, in Galen's view, to be aware in general of the multiplicity of causal categories, and in particular cases correctly to assign to them the operative factors.

So far, then, the following picture has begun to emerge. Following the initial distinctions made by the Stoics, Galen distinguishes between *aitia sunektika*, present causes of present

[17] Cf. Ps.-Galen *Definitiones medicae* (*Def.Med.*) XIX 393 K: "Synectic causes are those which are such that when present the effect is present, when absent the effect is absent, when increased the effect is increased".

[18] Whether or not they are necessary for them depends on how the effects are to be individuated — and herein indeed lies one of Galen's substantial objections to the procedures of various other doctors; cf. text **14** below.

[19] And at *Caus.Symp.* 1.7, VII 132 K, he claims that heat is a synectic cause of not feeling hungry (just as cold is one of hunger).

effects whose intensity is directly correlated with that of the effects, and causal factors which precede their effects. And in so doing, he is of course answering to an absolutely general feature of ordinary causal assumptions, namely that we suppose sometimes that causes are co-temporal with their effects, but at the same time we want causation to be a temporally directional process involving the propagation of influence from earlier to later events; and this typically will involve causes which antedate their effects, and which may well no longer exist at later times when their effects are still felt. And these answer roughly to the Stoics' *aitia prokatarktika*.

But, at any rate in medical contexts, the situation is complicated by the appearance of a third category, *aitia proêgoumena* or preceding causes. These are by no means ubiquitous; and on occasion when Galen uses the verb *proêgeisthai* in causal contexts he does so non-technically, as an umbrella-term to cover any and every cause which precedes its effects (and hence to include procatarctic causes), as is apparently the case in text 7 above (indeed, if 'precede' is intended in an operational as opposed to a temporal sense, then it will cover synectic causes as well).[20] But on occasion he will also use the term *aition proêgoumenon* to refer to a stage of the causal process intermediate between procatarctic and synectic causes. On the other hand, he never deploys the distinction between causes *kath'hauta* and *kata sumbebêkos* as Aristotle does (*Ph.* 2.3, 195 a 26-b 4)[21] to distinguish between explanatorily lucid ways of picking out the appropriate

[20] And cf. *Praes.Puls.* 1.8, IX 267-268 K; *Caus.Puls.* 4.1, IX 156-157 K; *MM* 2.2, X 84-85; 11.13, 774 K; *De naturalibus facultatibus* (*Nat.Fac.*) 1.4, II 10.3-5 K; *De differentiis febrium* (*Diff.Feb.*) 1.8-9, VII 302-305 K; in some (but not all) these cases the non-technical nature of the terminology is signalled by the use of the aorist participle, προηγησαμένος, as for example in the phrase φανερᾶς προηγησαμένης αἰτίας (*Diff.Feb.* 1.8, VII 302.15 K), where the φανερά clearly indicates that the cause is external (in the appropriate sense: see HANKINSON 1987) and hence procatarctic.

[21] Although he does recommend replacing the name of a condition with its definition precisely in order to make its causal properties lucid: *MM* 1.5, X 39-40 K; see HANKINSON 1991a, *ad loc.*

causal factor and those which are not, which is of a piece with his later Greek emphasis on causation as a productive relation holding between types of events and dispositions, rather than on explanation as an intensional, referentially-opaque phenomenon. This terminology is also often ascribed to the Stoics, and I am less certain than I once was that this ascription is mistaken.[22] But it was certainly developed by doctors, in particular Athenaeus of Attaleia, founder of the Pneumatist school of medicine:

> (I) The distinctions [sc. in causal type], which Athenaeus held to be three, are these: first there are synectic causes, second preceding causes, and third procatarctic causes. They call the latter everything which exists outside the body and harms it, bringing on illness, while those which are of the kind that work within the body are called preceding causes, while the alterations of the innate *pneuma* which are brought about by them and even by externals such as the moistening, drying, cooling and heating of the body he calls synectic causes of diseases, since this *pneuma* permeates throughout the uniform parts, and alters them as it alters itself. (II) But frequently they say that synectic causes are produced directly by procatarctic causes. For example, when one is thoroughly heated by the sun, they say that our innate *pneuma* is of necessity made warmer in itself... (III) When these changes are small, then the disease is not yet established in the body; but when any part has its natural temperament altered to such an extent that its activities are harmed, a disease is produced in accordance with the distemper, which has as its synectic cause the immoderately warmed *pneuma*... (IV) The adherents of this school call the humours generated in the body when these are too hot or cold or moist or dry preceding causes; for they say that in time the solid parts are affected by them, which immediately leads to their activities being harmed. (**9**: *CC* 2.2-5)

[22] Compare HANKINSON 1987, with HANKINSON 1996, 1999.

Galen does not endorse the details of the pneumatic pathology here; but he does accept in its broad outlines the causal taxonomy it embodies, of internal changes to the constitution of the body being set in train by some external event and leading ultimately (if nothing is done about it) to an alteration of its internal physical structure which is sufficient to cause damage to some of its vital activities. Now, as we have seen, for Galen at least, the latter is not the disease itself but a consequence of it, the disease being the last stage in the causal chain, the distortion of the underlying dispositions which produce it; the disease, then, is itself for Galen a synectic cause (of functional damage); but this does not exclude the possibility of its also having synectic causes; and in any event, there may very well be stages in the process set in train by the procatarctic cause and culminating ultimately in the disease which damages the activity which are to be identified with neither of them, stages which may or may not be in some sense sufficient for their successors.

Here is Galen's most detailed account of the matter:

> (I) Of causes which bring about changes in pulses, some are causes of the generation of them while others are causes only of their alteration. Causes of their generation are the function (*chreia*) for the sake of which they are generated and the capacity (*dunamis*) by which and the instruments (*organa*) by means of which they are propagated, while all the rest are causes of their alteration, both those which are called preceding (*proêgoumena*) and those which are antecedent (*prokatarktika*) even to them. (II) So the genus of causes, not only in regard to pulses but in regard to everything else as well, is threefold: one, the primary and most important, which they call 'synectic', derives the name from its encompassing the essence of them [sc. the things it causes], and is a cause of generation, as we said earlier. (III) The other two classes are not responsible for the generation of pulses, but are rather causes which bring about changes

in pulses which have already been generated: thus thickness or abundance or viscosity or acridness of humours cannot produce pulses, but they can alter them. (IV) And equally cold and warm baths, winter and summer, and cold and heat in general, are causes of the alteration of pulses but not of their generation. And these latter are called 'procatarctic', being prior even to those in respect of the humours, which are preceding <causes>. (V) Speaking generally, things which are external to a body and alter it in some way are called procatarctic causes, because they precede the dispositions (*diatheseis*) of the body. Whenever these dispositions condition synectic causes, they are preceding causes of them. (VI) For instance, external cold brings about constriction of the skin, and as a result of that constriction normal exhalations are checked, which, being checked, form a mass, causing a fever to take hold, which alters the function of the pulse, which in turn changes the pulse itself. (VII) In this case the procatarctic cause is the external cold, while all the rest up to the alteration of the function of the pulse are preceding causes; and through the mediation of the preceding causes, the procatarctic cause alters the function of the pulse, which is one of the synectic causes, and this in turn brings about a change in the pulses themselves, (VIII) since it is not possible to bring about a change in some synectic cause and for what is brought to completion by it to remain unchanged. But unless an alteration is effected in one of the synectic causes, it is impossible to bring about a change in the pulses. (IX) For this reason these are the most important and most particular and primary causes of the pulses, and all the others are <causes> because of them. For it is on account of their effecting an externally generated alteration to the synectic causes that they are called causes, since in respect of their own particular substance and nature they are in no way capable of bringing about a change in them. (**10:** *Caus.Puls.* 1.1, IX 1-3.15 K)

That lengthy passage contains much of interest, and not a little to puzzle over. It is important to bear in mind that, although it embodies much of general import, it is still directed specifically towards the causal explanation of the pulses. Thus it should not be supposed on the strength of (I)-(IV) that no procatarctic or preceding cause can ever properly be described as a cause of something's generation, but only of its alteration, since in plenty of cases (in particular those having to do with the aetiology of disease), procatarctic causes, being in general necessary conditions of their outcomes, will indeed be causally implicated in the generation of things and not merely in changing them when they already exist. Equally, the sense of 'generation' at issue here is not that of 'create from scratch': the pulse, after all, as Galen himself emphasizes (*Caus.Puls.* 1,1, IX 4 K), is going to be there as long as the animal is alive, but it will require (in his view) a constantly active synectic cause (or set of synectic causes) to keep it going. But what is being generated, then, is the constant stream of activity; this is not a case to be rejected on the grounds of PCI.[23]

(II)-(IV) indicate that Galen is working with much the same general distinction between preceding and procatarctic causes as that which he attributes to Athenaeus of Attaleia; and this is confirmed by the example and analysis of (VI)-(VII). A Chill falling on the body from the outside is the procatarctic cause which brings about a sequence of events in the body, culminating in the alteration of the function of the pulse, which is the synectic cause (of the alteration in the pulse itself), all the intermediaries being preceding causes of it. It was, as we saw, a definitional feature of synectic causes that they are in a certain sense strongly sufficient for their effects, and are contemporaneous with them (although in quite what sense they are sufficient will require further specification). Thus as soon as the function of the pulse is changed, the pulse will alter in response (VIII). On the

[23] See n.13 above.

other hand, procatarctic causes are not sufficient for their effects (it is this which leads Erasistratus to deny that they are causes at all: *CP* I 6-10, VIII 96-114, XIII-XIV 162-186; Hankinson 1998b, 30-36; n.12 above). The case is less clear with the preceding causes; but the example of (VI) strongly suggests that preceding causes form a chain that will, in the normal run of things (i.e. if no extraordinary steps are taken to disrupt it), produce the synectic cause, and hence the disease; and this is consistent with the indications one finds elsewhere. Thus they will not be sufficient *tout court* for the synectic cause, but will be so other things being equal. And that is all to the good: the language of sufficiency (standardly indicating as it does a logical relation) is not ideally suited to capture the complexities of trans-temporal causation. On the other hand, it seems harmless enough in the case of the synectic cause: it is functionally co-variant with its effects, but, since it *is* their cause, the only way of altering the effects is by affecting the cause, which is precisely what (VIII) claims (note the directionality of the claim: it is not only that synectic causes and their effects are co-variant — it is that the relation of dependence runs from cause to effect and not *vice versa*).

However, things are not that simple. First of all, we need to ask what, precisely, is it to "alter the function of the pulse". And we need briefly to examine the notion of a function (*chreia*) here, and also to examine its relations with the other things described in this case as synectic causes, "the capacity by which and the instruments by means of which they are propagated" (**10** (I)).

That natural things have *chreiai* is a basic item of Galenic faith, and is at the core of his teleological view of the structure of the universe and its occupants.[24] His teleology is, as one might have expected, an amalgam of that of Plato and Aristotle. From Aristotle (and in particular *De partibus animalium*) he takes over the idea that animals are hierarchically organized

[24] For detailed accounts of Galen's teleology, see HANKINSON 1988b, 1989.

functional units, within which each part and its activities plays a subservient role directed towards the overall well-functioning of the whole. His monumental *De usu partium* (*UP*)[25] seeks to develop such a functional, teleological account in respect of the *chreiai* of all animal parts; and he does so explicitly by way of reference, in strikingly Platonic fashion, to the excellence of the design of the Demiurge. He takes issue particularly with Erasistratus and Asclepiades for not appreciating the fundamentally teleological nature of nature, and for having the temerity to suppose that some organs are without function (cf. *Nat.Fac.* 1.13, II 34-36 K; 2.4, II 91-92 K); and he refuses even to allow, with Aristotle, that some organs may be only indirectly teleologically explicable, as the necessary but in themselves purposeless consequences of other teleologically valuable processes.

So Galen stakes out a fairly extreme position in the pivotal ancient debate between teleology and mechanism: nature is a kingdom of ends, and you cannot understand it unless you understand its purposes. But that still leaves us with our initial question: what exactly are these *chreiai*? Galen distinguishes (*UP* 17.1, II p.437-8 Helmreich [= IV 346-348 K]) between the functions of the parts, and those of their *energeiai*, where the former subserve the latter: thus the function of the heart is to pump the blood, but that pumping itself is undertaken for some reason (to convey nutriment in the form of *pneuma* to the extremities, in Galen's view, and to regulate the body's internal heat: *Caus.Puls.* 1.3, IX 5.17-6.5 K; *De usu pulsuum* [*Us.Puls.*] 3, V 160-161; 8, 179 K).[26] Galen goes on to write "the *energeia* of a part differs from its *chreia* ... in that an *energeia* is an active

[25] Edited by G. HELMREICH (Leipzig 1907-1909).

[26] *Us.Puls.* is edited on D.J. FURLEY and J.S. WILKIE (Princeton 1984); it is devoted to showing that the *chreia* of the pulse and that of breathing are the same (regulation of innate heat and the expulsion of the "smoky residue": 3, V 161.11-12 K; cf. *De utilitate respirationis* [*Ut.Resp.*] 3, IV 491-492 K), in spite of differences in their modality of operation, and in spite of the fact that the stopping of breathing is immediately fatal, whereas the stopping of the pulse (at any rate in certain parts of the body) is not (*Us.Puls.* 1, V 149-153 K).

motion, whereas the *chreia* is what is commonly called utility (*euchrêstia*)". Moreover, an *energeia* is an internally-directed activity, something genuinely attributable to the part or structure itself, and simply some passive alteration induced by some external influence. Thus a *chreia* is what some activity, the normal functioning of the part in question, is for, what, in the overall economy of the animal, it seeks to accomplish;[27] and hence it serves to explain, teleologically, the existence of the activity in question.

Quite how such purposes come to be expressed is another matter. In *On the formation of the foetus* (*Foet.Form.*) Galen expresses puzzlement at how a structure as complex as the human embryo can arise from purely mechanical sources (clearly it can't just be chance, and it evidently involves design: 6, IV 687-689; 6, IV 693-6 K); the semen "contains the design of the craftsman" (5, IV 682 K), but it is not reasonable to suppose that first creative force simply disappears as soon as it has set things in motion: more probably it continues to work in some way until the parts are complete, when they are able to perform their own functions (5, IV 683-684 K). Finally (IV 700-702 K) Galen confesses himself at an *impasse* regarding the substance of the soul and how it operates, and as to how it comes to be formed in the first place — it seems unreasonable to suppose that the mere vegetative power of the seed can do the trick, and yet he finds the opinion of a Platonist that the artificing soul of the Demiurge extends throughout universe implausible: he cannot accept that scorpions and other noxious creatures could have been constructed by such a soul. So Galen is cautious about committing himself to the actual mechanisms

[27] As J.S. WILKIE ("'Use' and 'Activity'": Introduction, Section IV of D.J. FURLEY and J.S.WILKIE, 1984) notes, one may know the *chreia* of something without knowing its *energeia* (one may know what something is for without knowing how it does it) and *vice versa*: he instances the case of the circulation of the blood in the period immediately after William Harvey — it was known, on the basis of Harvey's elegant experiments and inferences, that the blood circulated, but not why it did so.

involved in particular types of generation; but that there are such mechanisms he thinks certain. Galen's Demiurge will require physical structures and their activities to carry out his designs, both on the large scale in the animal as a whole, and in the various sub-routines which go towards maintaining it.

Consider once again the beginning of *Caus.Puls.* Both the *chreia* and the capacity of the heart and the physical structures associated with it are synectic causes of the pulse, and not just of the pulse *tout court* but of its variations. For the *chreia* itself can vary, or perhaps rather require a varied response, according to circumstances. One of the functions of the pulse is to assist in regulating the body's natural heat (*Us.Puls.* 3, V 161 K), and obviously if the body is overheated, then it is going to need to work harder. This is the sense in which the pulse is responsive to the need, or *chreia*, and hence that in which the *chreia* is its synectic cause.

But matters are not quite as simple as that. As we have seen, Galen says that the *chreia* is only one of the synectic causes, along with the *dunamis* contributed by the heart and the physical structures of the heart and arteries themselves. The notion of there being more than one synectic cause of the same effect is at first sight surprising: synectic causes, after all, are supposed to be strongly sufficient for and co-temporal with their effects; so how could there be more than one of them? In one sense that question is easily enough answered: (a) the tension on the noose is the synectic cause of (b) the strangling, but (c) the pressure on the hands is the cause of (a), and perhaps (d) the intensity of the volition of the strangler is the cause of (c); here there is a sequence of distinct items, but distinct not in time but in analysis as events.[28]

[28] Note also that the items in this example meet another condition on genuine causality, namely that causes should be logically distinct from the things of which they are causes — and Galen is admirably sensitive to that Humean constraint. At *CC* 9.6-7, Galen rejects the view of those "who say that heating of the head by the sun is the synectic cause of the warmth that results in it, and that the cut is the synectic cause of the wound" on the grounds that the alleged causes here amount to no more than re-descriptions of the effects.

But in this case, it is perhaps better to speak of a sequence of synectic causes of one another, rather than of concurrent synectic causes of the same outcome: in other words, rather than treating (a), (c) and (d) all as synectic causes of (b), (d) causes (c) which causes (a) which causes (b). That distinction may appear somewhat scholastic: but there is a point to it, and it would probably have been endorsed by Galen. At all events, at *Symp.Diff.* 1, VII 47-48 K, Galen considers such a causal sequence (actually probably rather a temporal one — but that does not matter here) in which the first causes the second, the second the third, and so on; and he stipulates that while the first causes the second, and the second the third "primarily and essentially", the first causes the third "secondarily and incidentally (*kata sumbebêkos*)", although the second causes the third primarily and essentially (and cf. **11** below).[29] In other words, causal proximity is important: to be a remote cause is, for Galen, one of the ways of being an incidental cause (see below, p. 58). This in turn suggests that for something to be a synectic cause it must be proximate in this sense; and indeed at *Caus.Symp.* 5, VII 109 K, Galen says that it makes no difference whether you call the cause synectic, containing (*sunechon*) or proximate (*proseches*), which suggests that for him at least proximate (or direct) causes just are synectic causes (see also *MM* 2.4, X 97 K: certain doctors refer to the primary cause of an activity its proximate cause; and cf. 99; 2.6, X 116 K).[30]

[29] Galen actually suggests a further elaboration — the first causes the fourth "thirdly", etc. — but this need not detain us.

[30] This identification is by no means universal, however: if *aition proseches* lies behind Cicero's *causa proxima* at *Fat.* 41 (as seems very probable), then for Chrysippus a proximate cause is distinct from a synectic cause — indeed it is to be assimilated to an antecedent, procatarctic cause (however the case is complicated: at *ibid.* 44, Cicero seems to identify proximate and synectic causes). See HANKINSON 1996. The practice of Erasistratus seems different again; apparently for him nothing is properly a cause unless it is proximate, in the sense of being immediately precedent to, its effect: *CP* XIV 174-176; see HANKINSON 1998b, *ad loc.*

In fact, it seems that when Galen refers to the three factors being synectic causes of the condition of the pulse, he means that they are so taken together. The *chreia* on its own is not enough to condition the pulse — it requires the *dunamis* of the heart and the organic parts to be properly constituted too in order to be able to do its work; indeed, the *chreia* only gets properly expressed if these conditions are in place. This in turn indicates another important feature of Galen's conception of the synectic cause — such causes are sufficient for their effects only *ceteris paribus*: something may interfere with their having their customary effects. Thus we can say of the *chreia* that it is other things being equal sufficient for the alteration of the pulse; if everything else is as it should be, then an alteration in it will produce a functionally corresponding alteration in its effect, and will do so immediately. It is in this sense, then, that such causes can be considered to be synectic — but not of course that each of them is capable of inducing its effect in total isolation from everything else. Thus Galen seeks to sophisticate and deepen the methods and categories of causal analysis which he has inherited from the tradition. Indeed, in an important and little-discussed passage, Galen recognizes that in order to determine the specific effects of a particular causal factor, all others must be held constant and the item under investigation must be subjected to isolated alteration in order to determine its effects (*Caus.Puls.* 1.5, IX 10-11 K): thus Galen is well aware of a crucial feature of the experimental method in science, as well as anticipating Mill's canons of inductive inference.

The notion of a *dunamis* here requires further investigation. At *Caus.Puls.* 1.2, IX 4, Galen notes that the fact that the heart and the pulsative capacity operate continuously as long as an animal lives (and conversely that as soon as they cease it dies) makes it evident that they have some vital function, although it is much less clear (and much more controversial) what it actually is. As a result of this, some people choose to speak neutrally of an "incorporeal capacity" which makes use of these organs, whatever precisely it may seek to effect. A 'capacity' is thus a place-holder for a proper, full-blooded causal explanation, a useful form of words to be employed when such an explanation is not yet available, but by no means a substitute for it.

Elsewhere, Galen makes much use of this talk of capacities or faculties or powers; indeed, *Nat.Fac.* is written precisely to vindicate their postulation against the more naive (as he sees it) mechanism of the Epicureans in philosophy and Erasistratus and Asclepiades in medicine. Capacity-talk of this sort is intrinsically teleological: something has a *dunamis* just in case it has a tendency to promote some *energeia* (the Aristotelian vocabulary is not adventitious); and an *energeia*, as we have seen, is strongly tied to the idea of ends or goals (cf. *Nat.Fac.* 1.2, II 6-7 K; cf. 1.6, II 15 K, on the "formative" or "artistic" capacity). And one of Galen's principal criticisms of his opponents in *Nat.Fac.* is that they either reject teleological explanation altogether (Epicurus), or at best pay lip-service to it (Erasistratus), and that they try to account for everything by means of mechanical principles such as that of *horror vacui*, refusing to recognize the existence of the natural capacities of attraction, retention, propulsion, expulsion, and so on, which are, in Galen's view, peculiar to different organs of the body (*Nat.Fac.* 1.13, II 33; 1.16, II 60-63; 2.1, II 75; 2.3, II 83; 2.4, II 88; 91; 2.6, II 99; 2.9, II 132-134; 3.13, II 187 K). These capacities resist, then, any simple-minded and naïve reduction to simple mechanical principles; but for all that Galen, in the spirit of his agnosticism in regard to the internal causal principle of growth in the foetus, leaves open how they are precisely to be analyzed.

For, as Galen is well aware, assigning capacities to structures in this way is not itself a substitute for scientific investigation:

> All the... capacities fall under the category of relations: they are primarily the cause of the activities [sc. of the various organs] but incidentally of their effects. But given that the cause is relative to something, being the cause of what results from it alone, and of nothing else, it is obvious that the capacity also falls under the category of relation. And so long as we are ignorant of the essence of the activating cause

> we call it a capacity: thus we say that there is in the veins a blood-producing capacity, a digestive capacity in the stomach, a pulse-creating capacity in the heart, and in each of the other parts a specific capacity corresponding to its activity. So if we are to investigate methodically how many and what sort of capacity there are, we need to start from the effects — for each effect comes from a specific activity, and each activity from a specific cause. (**11**: *Nat.Fac.* 1.4, II 9-10 K)[31]

This is of a piece with his rejection of pseudo-synectic causes which are merely re-nominalizations of the effects:

> There are those who say that the heating of the head by the sun is the containing cause of the warmth that results in it, and the cut the containing cause of the wound. But they do so only because they do not realize that they are saying the same thing in different words. For the heating of the head is nothing more than the warmth produced in it… and the wound nothing more than the cut to the flesh. (**12**: *CC* 9.6)

Referring to things as *dunameis* is a preliminary to proper investigation as to their precise natures; and such capacities had better be genuinely separate causal factors. Such a thing is the heart's pulsative capacity. That is has such a capacity is evident; quite why, or indeed how, is controversial (although Galen believes that the pulse is transmitted through the coats of the arteries, and the flow of blood is caused by the expansion and contraction of the arteries rather than *vice versa*).

[31] Compare *Sent.Prop.* 14.1: "Everyone knows that we possess souls, since we plainly see the things that are activated through the body: walking, running, wrestling, the many varieties of perception; and we know on the basis of an axiom that commends itself naturally to all of us that there is some cause for these activities: for we know that nothing occurs without a cause. But because of our ignorance as to exactly what the cause of these things might be, we assign it a name on the basis of its capacity for doing what it does".

So it turns out that this *dunamis*, the physical constitution of the cardio-vascular system, and the *chreia* of the pulse, are all, taken together, the total synectic cause of the alterations of the pulse. At *Caus.Puls.* 1.5, IX 9.18-10.3 K, he writes that all three must "act together" (*sunergein*)[32] to produce swiftness and magnitude of the pulse, "the *chreia* urging on their generation, the *dunamis* being in a good condition, while the coats of the arteries are soft, or at any rate not hard". So the three factors must all co-operate in order to bring about the requisite effect, but the roles they play in it are analytically distinct and distinguishable; and at this point another feature of Galen's creative syncretism, his willingness to adopt a modified Aristotelian taxonomy of causes, comes to the fore.

At *Caus.Puls.* 1.2, IX 5 K, Galen assimilates the pulsative faculty to "the active (*drastikê*), productive (*poiêtikê*), and creative (*dêmiourgikê*) cause of the activity", having just said, echoing text **11**, that "we call this cause which creates (*dêmiourgousan*) the pulses, whatever it may be and even if we are ignorant of its essence, a *dunamis* because of its being capable of effecting the pulses" (*ibid.* 4-5). On the next page, he describes the condition

[32] *Sunergein* is cognate with *sunergon*, a word which has a technical sense in causal contexts, although that sense is quite distinct from any intended here. A *sunergon* is something that helps a synectic cause to achieve its result more easily than it would have done otherwise, but is not necessary for its effect (Ps.GAL. *Def.Med.* 160, XIX 393 K seems to imply that a *sunergon* may be individually sufficient for its effect, but this is highly aberrant). Michael Frede (1980, 237-243) argues that the Hellenistic schools know of two distinct causal triads: procatarctic, preceding and synectic causes on the one hand, and *sunaitia*, *sunerga*, and perfect causes (*aitia autotelê*) on the other; but this is over-schematic, and while Frede is himself aware of some of the problems involved in assimilating *sunerga*, or a sub-class of them, to procatarctic causes, I am not entirely convinced by his solution (*ibid.*, 242). CLEM.AL. *Str.* 8, 9, 25 mentions procatarctic and synectic causes, *sunerga* and "prerequisite causes" (αἴτια ὧν οὐκ ἄνευ: cf. PL. *Phd.* 99 b; CIC. *Fat.* 36). At *ibid.* 32, *sunaitia* take the place of the prerequisites, and while Platonic *sunaitia* might be fairly easily assimilable to the prerequisites (see HANKINSON 1998b, 10-13), prerequisites and Hellenistic co-operative causes are clearly different beasts. The upshot is that none of these divisions is systematic; but Galen never mentions *sunaitia* or perfect causes; and he uses the adjective *sunergon*, as he does the verb *sunergein* here, only in a general sense.

of the arteries themselves as being "instruments" (*organa*: *Caus.Puls.* 1.4, IX 6 K) of the outcome. *Aitia drastikê* or *poêtikê* is standard later Greek terminology for the Aristotelian efficient cause;[33] and the talk of instruments prefigures the later Platonists' addition of the instrumental cause (along with paradigmatic cause) to Aristotle's canonical four.[34]

Middle Platonists had already distinguished two categories of final cause, the paradigm and the end (*telos*) in order to make room in Aristotle's scheme for Platonic, hypostasized, independent Forms, as well as their immanent Aristotelian cousins (with the category of the end answering to Aristotle's non-hypostasized final cause).[35] I have found no earlier mention of instrumental causes (they do not feature in contemporary Peripatetic accounts: cf. Alexander Aphrodisiensis, *De fato* 2, Suppl.Arist. II 2, p.166.2ff. Bruns), but Galen does not claim to have invented the category (which in any case has Aristotelian antecedents: drugs are the *organa* by which the doctor effects his cures: *Ph.* 2.3, 195 a 1-3), and it is unlikely that he did so.

33 There are differences of emphasis, but the coincidences of meaning are more important; BARNES (1983) notes the proliferation of terms for efficient causation in later Greek philosophy (and he misses one or two); and Galen uses Aristotelian and Stoic terminology indiscriminately, frequently in the same context (cf. *CP* XVI 199), which suggests that he at least saw no important distinctions between them.

34 See SIMPL. *In Ph.* 1.1, CAG IX pp.10.35-11.2; 2.3, pp.309.2-324.4; PHLP. *In Ph.* 1.1, CAG XVI p.6.9ff.; 2.3, pp.241.3-247.18.

35 I have sometimes wondered whether Galen's occasional distinction between *telos* and *skopos* might be intended in part to mirror this Middle Platonist refinement, with the *telos* as the Aristotelian immanent end, and the *skopos* the goal towards which the individual (or the Demiurge) directs their attention. But Galen does not always make any such distinction (at *CP* VI 57, he explicitly says: "it makes no difference whether you call this [sc. the final cause] that because of which [δι' ὃ: although *CP* survives only in Latin, the Latin is so literal as to permit easy recovery of Galen's Greek] what comes to be comes to be, or its *chreia*, or its *telos*, or its *skopos*": see HANKINSON 1998b, *ad loc.*), and in any case, often when he does (e.g. at *SI* I 64: "The *skopos* of medicine is health; its *telos* is the achievement of it"), he seems to be far more influenced by the role the two terms play in Stoic action theory and ethics. Yet an important text (quoted below: **12**) does claim that the *chreia* and the *skopos* are different types of cause; and it may well be that Galen's syncretist desire to answer to a wide variety of different sources leads him into confusion here.

Thus we have the interesting result that the three co-operating synectic causes of the pulse can each be assimilated to elements within the sub-Aristotelian causal categories; and one of them is explicitly that of a final cause. It is often said that synectic causes represent a sub-class of the general category of efficient causation; that no longer seems to be quite the case. On the other hand, Galen himself insists that the distinction between instrumental and efficient causation may be a matter of perspective: at *UP* 17.1, IV 347 K, he remarks that a muscle may be thought of as an efficient cause of movement if we consider it from the point of view of the immediate effect, but when considered in regard to the origin of the action, the soul's volition, it turns out to be simply instrumental (cf. *CP* VII 73: a leg is an instrumental cause of a trampling, although in an obvious sense the leg is clearly *doing* something); thus the distinction is part of what allows the theorist to make analytical sense of sequences of causation which, as we have seen, Galen is particularly concerned to do (and as Aristotle, in general, was not); and instrumental causes (or at any rate some of them) may be thought of as intermediate efficient causes of their effects, but not as efficient causes in the strict Aristotelian sense of being origins of motion. Moreover, again at any rate in some cases, the action of these instrumental intermediaries may be supposed to be contemporaneous with the initial (initial in a causal rather than a temporal sense) efficient cause of the effect in question — and hence they too will meet the basic criteria for being *aitia sunektika*. Even so, instrumental causes are less important than the others: at *CP* VI 67, he describes the final and efficient causes as "primary and most important", with the instrumental and material as third and fourth respectively.[36] And this should

[36] There is no conflict between this claim and that made a couple of sentences later (VII 72) that efficient and material causes are the only ones essential to all cases of causation — it is of course a perfectly Aristotelian notion that some events lack final causes (*Ph.* 2.4-6), and one with which Galen concurs (VII 71); equally some sorts of production do not require instruments (or intermediate efficient causes: VII 71).

hardly be surprising given the scope and cast of his teleology, something made particularly evident by an important passage of *UP* (6.12-13, III 464-471 K), where he lays out his Aristotelian causal categories in their most complete form. Indeed this is the only passage (to my knowledge) where Galen acknowledges the existence of the formal cause at all, and here he does so only grudgingly.[37] Michael Frede (1980, 243) has noted that synectic causes are the Stoic analogue to the Aristotelian formal cause, while Galen held the original Stoic synectic causes to be pseudo-causes of being, not genuine causes of becoming, which in large part accounts for his coolness towards the concept of the formal cause (as also no doubt does his commitment to PCI).

But more important for our purposes is his diagnosis of what he takes to be Asclepiades' error in supposing that the coats of the pulmonary 'arteries' (actually the pulmonary veins) are thin because they work hard, whereas in fact the truth is the teleological opposite: they work hard because they are thin, and are thin in order to work hard (*UP* 6.12, III 464-465). He characterizes Asclepiades' mistake as one of mistaking "a most insignificant cause, one which is not a cause in the strict sense at all, but rather a cause only incidentally", i.e. the instrumental cause, with a proper (teleological) causal explanation. The point, presumably, is that they work hard in order to bring about something else (efficient movement of blood and *pneuma*); and to do that the machinery has been set up in the optimum possible manner — they can best fulfil their function if they're thin. Thus their thinness, which is a necessary condition of their efficiency, contributes to the functioning of the system by allowing them to work hard, and is as such an instrumental cause of its proper functioning.

Here another point of assimilation arises. In the causal sequences of texts **9-10**, the intermediate stages, those which lead from the initial impulse which disturbs the equilibrium of the system to the final synectic cause of the effect in which we

[37] See Hankinson 1998b, 14-18, 192-200.

are interested, the preceding causes in the terminology of these texts, will also turn out for Galen to be instrumental, although of course as they are neither cotemporal with the effects in question, nor (necessarily, at any rate) functionally correlated with them, they will not qualify as synectic causes of them. But there is another type of instrumental cause, the nature of which Galen discusses at some length in *CP* VI 63-5, VII 68-71 and 77: the instrument or tool in a more literal sense, the carpenter's saw and gimlet (although at *Caus.Puls.* 1.4, IX 6 K Galen appears to assimilate these two types of instrument). These too (or perhaps rather their actions) intervene between the original volition of the artisan and the finished product — but here the emphasis is not on the intermediate events with which they are associated (as in the earlier cases) but rather on the items themselves, and the ways in which their particular structures affect the nature of the outcome (a blunt chisel will produce shoddy carpentry, no matter what the skill of the artisan).

Moreover, while in the passage of *UP*, the instrumental cause is described as 'incidental', at *CP* it is enrolled among the genuine, *per se* causes, along with the final, material and the efficient, and as such contrasted with mere 'incidentals' such as "the location and the surrounding air" (*CP* VII 78-89).[38] The latter "have the status of prerequisites" (84, 89) but are not genuine causes. The language here clearly echoes Plato's at *Phaedo* 99 a-b; but the class of items so classified turns out to be quite different, which in turn emphasizes the distinctiveness of Galen's own conception of causation.

For something to be a genuine cause, for Galen, it must "a thing which of its own nature contributes to something's coming to be"[39]

[38] For a full discussion of the issues raised by this concept of incidentality, see HANKINSON 1998b, 203-206. Aristotle denied that place as such was properly speaking a cause (*Ph.* 4.1, 209 a 14 ff.), although that is hard at first sight to square with his doctrine of natural places. But others (such as the eclectic Potamo of Alexandria: DIOG.LAERT. 1.21) certainly allowed it.

[39] Compare CIC. *Fat.* 34-36: "We should not understand the term 'cause' in such a way as to make whatever precedes something a cause of it, but only what precedes it effectively: thus my going to down to the campus was not the cause

(VII 76; cf. 84).[40] This is not an easy notion to make precise, although intuitively it is clear enough: prerequisites are simply items which are needed, other things being equal, for the effect, but not for any particular properties they might have. Thus in Galen's example, a carpenter needs somewhere in which to work, but there is no particular place in which he needs to be; by contrast, the tools he uses will have a direct impact on the execution of his design (VII 76-80), and faults or inadequacies in them will result in imperfections in the finished products (VI 63-5).

It is evident from all of this that Galen is somewhat careless in his use of the term 'incidental'; but his position itself is not incoherent. In the *UP* passage, he means to devalue the importance of the structure of the arteries by comparison with other, as he sees it more important, causal factors, but he does not thereby impugn its status as a genuine cause, on the *CP* model (their thinness is directly contributory to their operation); while in the latter text he uses the distinction between essential and incidental in a more precise manner.[41]

of my playing ball, nor was Hecuba the cause of death for the Trojans because she gave birth to Paris… For in this account a well-dressed traveller will also be said to be the cause of his being robbed of them by the highwayman… But they [sc. the Stoics] say that there is difference between whether something is such that something else cannot be brought about without it, and whether it is such that something else must be brought about by it. Therefore none of those things is a cause, since none of them brings about the thing of which it is said to be a cause by its own force. Nor is that without which something cannot be a cause of it, but only that which is such that, when it is present, that of which it is the cause is necessarily brought about".

[40] Here as so often Galen appeals to ordinary Greek usage: this is what any ordinary person would choose to call a cause (cf. VI 55-56).

[41] It should be remembered that at *Symp.Diff.* 1, VII 47-48 K, he uses the distinction differently again, to differentiate between proximate and remote causes. But he never deploys the distinction between causes *kath'hauta* and *kata sumbebêkos* as Aristotle does (*Ph.* 2.3, 195 a 26-b 3) to distinguish between explanatorily lucid ways of picking out the appropriate causal factor and those which are not, which is of a piece with his later Greek emphasis on causation as a productive relation holding between types of events and dispositions, rather than on explanation as an intensional, referentially-opaque phenomenon.

Here we may quote from *Symp.Diff.* again, and in so doing return to our earlier theme of the proper analysis of disease:

> Health is a disposition (*diathesis*) productive of a natural activity (it makes no difference, as we have said, whether we say 'condition [*kataskeuê*]' or 'disposition', or 'productive of a natural activity' or 'cause of a natural activity')... In the same way a disease is an unnatural condition of the body which is the cause of the activity's having been harmed (or, more concisely, a disease is an unnatural disposition which impedes an activity). An affection (*pathos*) is a change (*kinêsis*) in the matter as a result of the agent; and this change as a result of the agent is an activity. And what contributes of its own nature some share of the generation for the thing generated is said to be its cause. And they are many in kind: for both the matter and the *chreia* and the *skopos* and the instrument and that whence comes the source of the change are causes. Each of these contributes to the completion of the thing generated. But those which, while contributing nothing, are still not to be separated from the things which do contribute, have the status of prerequisites. (**13:** *Symp. Diff.* 1, VII 47.4-48.4 K)

Here is another classification of causes, this time distinguishing *chreia* from *skopos*,[42] but making the same distinctions between essential and incidental causes (although not in the same language) which we have been noting, and also reinforcing Galen's unequivocal position that disease should be defined as the disposition which causes the damage to the activity, and not the actual damage itself. Moreover, the emphasis is again on the co-operative nature of causation. All of the causal types have something to contribute; and the effect will not come about (or at any rate will not come about in the same way or to the same extent: Galen is rightly tolerant of distinctions in the fineness

[42] See n.37 above.

of grain of causal ascription) if one or more of them is absent. But crucially, it is not only the various synectic components (*Caus.Puls.* IX 4-6) which have to be present in order for the effect to occur;[43] so too do their relevant antecedents, and equally the material in which the effect is to be produced must be in a suitable condition.

This latter contention is the cornerstone of Galen's causal theory.[44] By making the condition of the patient (in both senses) of equal causal importance to the action of the agent, he seeks to rehabilitate the notion of procatarctic causes against their detractors; indeed, this forms the bulk of the argument of *CP*. Procatarctic causes are at best necessary conditions of their effects (the diseases); but, 'the sophists' (paradigmatically Erasistratus) argue, if X is not invariably followed by Y, then X cannot properly (be called) a cause of Y (*CP* I 9-10, VI 46, VIII 96-114).[45]

That procatarctic causes do not necessitate their effects is readily conceded by Galen.[46] His opponents deny that antecedent heating can be a cause of fever because "only four out of a thousand spectators [at the theatre on a hot afternoon] develop a temperature, and of these only one, rather than all of them, becomes feverish" (II 11; cf. X 126-7); Galen accepts the validity of the case, but refuses to draw the same conclusions from it. The antecedent heating is certainly causally relevant, he thinks, and the fact that it does not affect everybody in the same way is readily explicable in terms of their differential *diatheseis*.

[43] At *Caus.Puls.* 1.5, IX 10.13-16 K, Galen remarks: "There is one method in all of these cases: varying only the cause under investigation, and maintaining all the others in the same state, to make the judgement regarding the alteration of the pulse".

[44] It is not, of course, proprietory to him: Sextus (*Math.* 9.242-243) tries to rebut an argument in favour of the coherence of causation which insists that causes will only affect suitable bodies, on the grounds that this makes the distinction between agent and patient incoherent; Galen's answer would be that the patient too has relevant causal properties that must be included in any complete causal picture.

[45] See HANKINSON 1998b, *ad locc.*, and 31-36.

[46] And also by Celsus, *Med.* Prooem. 58-60.

Some are simply more prone, because of the peculiarities of their internal constitutions, to be affected in such a way (cf. *Caus.Morb.* 2, VII 8-10 K). But the fact that only they are affected does not show that the heat had nothing to do with it, only that it was the heat in concert with something else, the suitability of the material, that brought about the result (*CP* VIII 98-101). This is of course precisely why Galen thinks that you don't infer directly from the procatarctic cause to the therapy (*MM* 4.3, X 242-249 K); you infer to the internal condition in virtue of which the procatarctic cause is able to exercise its effect in this case.

But of course this has no tendency to show that procatarctic causes do not have a genuine causal role to play in the production of diseased in those cases in which disease does in fact supervene. They do, indeed, contribute something 'from their own nature' — they are not merely prerequisites in the way in which place and opportunity are. Thus what unites all Galen's various types of *per se* (as opposed to incidental) cause is that they are all in some sense directly implicated in the outcome, either as being immediately (non-remotely) responsible for it, or as being genuinely (albeit perhaps mediately) contributory to it. And what is characteristic of synectic causes is that they are directly implicated in both senses.

We can now see why Galen calls the material and the efficient causes the only necessary ones: they are always required to make causal sense of any sequence of events (whereas some sequences will lack final causes). Moreover, Galen accepts that causation is a general, and generalizable, relation: properly understood, the whole cause of some effect will always be sufficient (other things being equal) to produce that effect. Thus he does not abandon the notion that causal sequences should be regular — he simply rejects the naive view that *anything* which may be legitimately viewed as a cause must be invariably correlated with its effects (this is where he parts company with Erasistratus); causing is co-operative.

But, crucially, this can even apply to items Galen will call synectic causes; and here he parts company, I think, with all of his predecessors, and at any rate feels his way towards an account of the causal relation of unprecedented sophistication. Distinguishing between items which are sure signs of some particular condition, and those which are not, but which are none the less proper to it, he writes:

> We have already clearly distinguished between those pulses which follow the synectic causes of necessity, and those which, while proper to them, do not follow them of necessity. Pulses for which there is a single cause of their generation invariably follow it; and such pulses will be perfect indicators of their cause, a vehement pulse of a powerful capacity, a faint pulse of a weak one. But in the case of the others where if many causes do not coincide the generation cannot be effected, we will say that these are proper to their causes, but not that they signify any one of them in particular. In the same way, if a pulse occurs from time to time from a single cause, but not always from the same one, it will be proper to all of its productive causes, but it will not reveal securely any one of them. For it is not the case that if the pulse is fast, then necessarily too will there be strength of the capacity, but sometimes it will be when the *chreia* of the generation of the psychic *pneuma* is greater, sometimes when there is an excess of heat, and sometimes when there is a softness of the instruments, or several of these, or all of them at once. (**14**: *Caus.Puls.* 1.7, IX 20.11-21.3 K)

Here Galen explicitly disavows the claim, central to all earlier accounts of the synectic cause, that such causes are invariably directly functionally correlated with their effects, or rather that they are so correlated independently of any other factor. Thus, it turns out, not only are procatarctic causes only causes in conjunction with other relevant factors: the same applies (although not in precisely the same way) to synectic causes too. They, too, at least some of the time, are only sufficient in the circumstances for their effects (to adopt the language of J.L.Mackie). And, of course, provided one sufficiently tightly specifies the 'circumstances', all causes will be, in a sense, so sufficient (at any rate in deterministic systems), which in turn suggests that such a characterization is less than helpful. I think that Galen implicitly at least recognized that fact; and for this reason allowed that synectic causes could be co-operative, and even that they might answer to different categories in the Aristotelian schema. What unites them, and makes them a coherent causal category, is that they are contemporaneous with their effects, and that (again, other things being equal), any alteration in one of the synectic causes is followed, and immediately, by a corresponding alteration in the effect of that cause. Alter the function of the pulse, and the pulse will alter in tandem with it — and similarly with its *dunamis* and with its necessary and immediate instruments. And of course this tightness of relation is true of neither procatarctic nor of preceding causes, no matter how they are to be characterized.[47]

BIBLIOGRAPHY

BARNES, J. (1991). "Galen on logic and therapy", in *Galen's Method of Healing*, ed. by F. KUDLIEN and R.J. DURLING (Leiden 1991), 50-102.

BOBZIEN, S. (1998a). "Chrysippus' theory of causes", in *Topics in Stoic Philosophy*, ed. by K. IERODIAKONOU (Oxford 1999), 196-242.

---- (1998b). *Determinism and Freedom in Stoic Philosophy* (Oxford 1998).

DE LACY, Ph. (1972). "Galen's Platonism", in *AJPh* 93 (1972), 27-39.

---- (Ed.) (1978-1984). *Galen. On the Doctrines of Hippocrates and Plato.* Edition, Transl. and Comm., CMG V 4.1.2, Parts I-III (Berlin 1978, 1980, 1984).

[47] This is a revised version of the paper presented at the *Entretiens*: in conformity with the prevailing conventions, I append a series of questions and answers. But I feel obliged to acknowledge the interventions of Jonathan Barnes, who did not submit a written question, for having forced me to clarify my position on a number of points, in particular in regard to the principle I label PCI.

DILLON, J. (Ed.) (1993). *Alcinous. The Handbook of Platonism.* Transl. with an Introd. and Commentary (Oxford 1993).

FREDE, M. (1980). "The Original Notion of Cause", in *Doubt and Dogmatism,* ed. by M. SCHOFIELD, M. BURNYEAT, J. BARNES (Oxford 1980), 217-249.

---- (1981). "On Galen's Epistemology", in *Galen. Problems and Prospects,* ed. by V. NUTTON (London 1981), 65-86.

---- (1982). "The method of the so-called Methodical school of medicine", in *Science and Speculation,* ed. by J. BARNES *et alii* (Cambridge 1982), 1-23.

---- (Ed.) (1985). *Galen. Three Treatises on the Nature of Science.* Transl. with an Introd. (Indianapolis 1985).

---- (1986). "Philosophy and medicine in Antiquity", in *Human Nature and Natural Knowledge.* Essays presented to M. Grene (Dordrecht 1986), 211-232.

---- (1987a). *Essays in Ancient Philosophy* (Minneapolis 1987: contains all previously cited articles).

---- (1987b). "The Ancient Empiricists", in FREDE 1987a.

---- (1988). "The Empiricist attitude towards reason and theory", in *Method, Medicine and Metaphysics,* ed. by R.J. HANKINSON, *Apeiron* Suppl.Vol. 21 (1988), 79-97.

---- (1990). "An Empiricist view of knowledge: memorism", in *Epistemology,* ed. by S. EVERSON, Companions to Ancient Thought 1 (Cambridge 1990), 225-250.

FURLEY, D.J. and WILKIE, J.S. (Eds.) (1984). *Galen on Respiration and the Arteries.* An edition with English transl. and comment. (Princeton 1984).

HANKINSON, R.J. (1987). "Causes and Empiricism", in *Phronesis* 32 (1987), 329-48.

---- (1988a). "Galien: la médecine et la philosophie antisceptique", in *Revue de philosophie ancienne* 6.2 (1988), 229-269.

---- (1988b). "Galen explains the elephant", in *Philosophy and Biology,* ed. by M. MATTHEN and B. LINSKY, *CJPh* Suppl.Vol. 14 (1988), 135-157.

---- (1989). "Galen and the best of all possible worlds", in *CQ* N.S. 39 (1989), 206-227.

---- (Ed.) (1991a). *Galen. On the Therapeutic Method Books I and II.* Transl. with an introd. and comm. (Oxford 1991).

---- (1991b). "Galen's Anatomy of the Soul", in *Phronesis* 36 (1991), 197-233.

---- (1991c). "Galen on the foundations of science", in *Galeno: obra, pensamiento e influencia*, ed. por J.A. López Férez (Madrid 1991), 15-29.

---- (1992). "Galen's Philosophical Eclecticism", in *ANRW* II 36.5 (Berlin 1992), 3505-22.

---- (1994a). "Galen's Theory of Causation", in *ANRW* II 37.2 (Berlin 1994), 1757-74.

---- (1994b). "Galen's Anatomical Procedures", in *ANRW* II 37.2 (Berlin 1994), 1834-55.

---- (1994c). "Usage and abusage: Galen on language", in *Language*, ed. by S. Everson, Companions to Ancient Thought 3 (Cambridge 1994), 166-187.

---- (1996). "Cicero's Rope", in *Polyhistor. Studies in the History and Historiography of Ancient Philosophy*. Presented to Jaap Mansfeld, ed. by K. Algra *et alii* (Leiden 1996), 185-205.

---- (1998a). *Cause and Explanation in Ancient Greek Thought* (Oxford 1998).

---- (Ed.) (1998b). *Galen on Antecedent Causes.* Edited with an Introd., Transl. and Comm., Cambridge Classical Texts and Commentaries 35 (Cambridge 1998).

---- (1999). "Explanation and causation", in *The Cambridge History of Hellenistic Philosophy*, ed. by K. Algra *et alii* (Cambridge 1999), 479-512.

Helmreich, G. (ed.) (1907-1909). *Galeni De usu partium libri XVII*, Vol. I-II (Leipzig1907-1909).

Kalbfleisch, K. (ed.) (1904); repr. in Lyons 1968.

Lyons, M. (ed.) (1968). CMG Suppl.Orient. II (contains *CC* in both Arabic and Latin translation) (Berlin 1968).

Nutton, V. (Ed.) (1999). *Galen On my own Opinions.* Edition, Transl. and Comm., CMG V 3.2 (Berlin 1999).

Siegel, R.E. (1968). *Galen's System of Physiology and Medicine* (Basel 1968).

DISCUSSION

V. Barras: Le passage du traité *Caus.Puls.* 1,1, IX 1-3 K, sur lequel vous attirez notre attention, paraît en effet exemplaire non seulement pour l'analyse de la chaîne causale relativement à l'altération du pouls (cas paradigmatique si l'on considère l'importance de l'examen du pouls dans la pratique médicale), mais aussi dans les différentes situations cliniques. Pensez-vous qu'un 'schéma' similaire, bien que peu ou pas explicité par Galien à ma connaissance, soit également opératoire dans ses expériences de vivisection?

R.J. Hankinson: It's possible; at any rate, everything he does in such cases should be compatible with such an analysis. However, in the cases I think you have in mind, involving neural ligature and section and so on, the point is to discover what immediate results follow from particular interventions — the idea is that if you intervene in the causal process which delivers voluntary motion, say, at any point, then that motion will be affected. Now you can intervene in a number of places, but standardly you will do so at some point in the conduits that carry neural impulses from the brain to the affected parts; those conduits would be, in Galen's terminology, instrumental in supplying neural impulses, and are certainly genuine causes. But I don't see the other items in the scheme (in particular procatarctic and preceding causes) as being of any relevance here. Of course, a lot turns on just how you characterize the effect you're interested in.

T. Tieleman: You say that Galen was aware of a crucial feature of the experimental method, namely the requirement that the item under investigation must be subjected to *isolated* alteration in order to determine its intended effects (cf. *Caus.Puls.* 1.5, IX 10-11 K). It would be useful to have some corroboration on this point. Do you know of any experimental reports that illustrate this requirement? I myself think of the successive interception of the nerves, arteries and veins connecting the heart and brain, described at *PHP* 2.6, p.148 ff. De Lacy (= V 262-267 K). Here each type of vessel, Galen explains, has to be blocked *in isolation* so as not to spoil the experiment which aims at establishing the function of each vessel. Is this an example of the point you made?

R.J. Hankinson: Yes, I think it is — thank you very much. I'm not sure quite how explicitly Galen signals the methodology in this passage, but at the very least it is implicit there.

V. Boudon: À propos de la définition de la maladie citée notamment dans votre texte n.7 (*Symp.Diff.* 1, VII 50.4-17 K) comme "lésion d'une fonction", je m'interroge sur le fait que cette même définition est donnée ailleurs par Galien avec une dimension supplémentaire, celle de lésion *sensible* d'une fonction (*Ars Med.* 27, I 379.13 K). Convient-il de voir une volonté manifeste d'évacuer la sensibilité dans le passage de *Symp.Diff.*, et si tel est le cas, quelle conclusion peut-on tirer sur le statut de la cause προήγουμενον?

R.J. Hankinson: I hadn't noticed that divergence in definition, but as you say it is there. I'm not sure whether to suppose that Galen means deliberately to suppress the criterion of sensible apprehensibility in this passage, although I cannot see why he should have supposed in the first place that a disease must be manifest to its sufferer; surely it would make better analytic sense to suppose that there could be such diseases, although of course if they manifest no discernible ill effects then there will probably not be much point in treating them (except possibly prophylactically, to prevent them declining to a condition where they are manifest to the sufferer). I'm inclined, weakly, to think that the criterion of apprehensibility answers to the ordinary language sense of disease, what 'all Greeks think', but that it needn't necessarily be an integral part of the proper analysis. And I'm not sure in any case what difference it would make to the status of the preceding cause, which after all covers a variety of internal conditions, not all of which need be apparent to the patient — but since the preceding cause is not itself the disease, unless I'm missing something here I don't really see why this matters.

J. Jouanna: Puis-je revenir sur la définition de la maladie du texte n.7, et de la distinction entre 'empêcher' et 'léser'? Il ne semble pas que cette distinction soit opérante ici, car la maladie est définie comme ce qui empêche ou lèse *primarily*. C'est cette notion qui importe. À propos de ce texte, je voudrais revenir sur la notion de symptôme. La formation du terme permet de rendre compte de ce que Galien entend: c'est un évènement qui tombe (πίπτειν) avec, en même temps, sans qu'il y ait une relation de cause à effet, mais simplement de concomitance. À ce propos, il me semble que *sun*, qui a dans σύμπτωμα le sens d'accompagnement, prend un sens différent dans *sunektikos*, où *sun* signifie 'ensemble'. Qu'en pensez-vous? Si la cause synectique est celle qui fait 'se tenir ensemble', on comprend qu'elle soit, comme vous le dites, "the cause of the existence of things".

R.J. Hankinson: I had supposed that there was, at least implicitly, a difference between impediment and lesion, in that the latter seems to suggest damage of a permanent, or at any rate of a serious sort, as the former does not. But you are of course right that the significant feature, at least from the causal point of view, of the definition consists in the idea that it is what is primarily responsible for the damage, where 'primarily' of course means 'directly, immediately', and not just 'principally'. As regards the etymology of σύμπτωμα, again you are obviously right, although it should be stressed, as I tried to do in the body of my paper, that while a σύμπτωμα is defined purely in terms of temporal concomitance, that does not *preclude* there being a causal relation between a symptom and what it is a symptom of — and indeed standardly there will, at any rate for Galen, be just such a relation. Again, you are right about the different sense of the prefix *sun* in the case of *sunektikon* — and this is exactly why the term had the sense it had for the early Stoics, of being a cause of something's continued existence, something which literally holds something together. But again, as I tried to make clear, Galen rejects this sense, and thinks of 'cohesion' is a metaphorical way, as involving the functional dependence, in the ways I specified, of the effect on the cause.

M. Frede: If I understand you correctly, what is interesting about the beginning of *De causis pulsuum* is a development of the notion of a *causa contentiva* as applied to items like the pulse, more particularly to the pulse of a patient in a particular circumstance. The suggestion is that the *aition sunektikon* is constituted by three factors, (i) the *chreia*, (ii) the relevant *dunamis*, (iii) the instrumental cause, but also that the *chreia*, since we are dealing with a particular case, has to be the *chreia* not of the pulse in general, but of the pulse of the particular patient in particular circumstances. One advantage of thinking of the *causa contentiva* in that way is that, thus conceived, it gains in explanatory power. Against this background I have two questions: (i) I wonder to what extent the three constituents (use, power, instrument) at the abstract level are independent explanatory factors, whether, for instance, they can be identified independently of each other; (ii) I wonder to what extent, even when applied to a particular case, they gain sufficient independence from each other to make an explanation in terms of the *causa contentiva*, thus conceived of, more explanatory.

R.J. Hankinson: This is absolutely the crux of the matter. Your questions are tightly linked, and I shall try and answer them together. Of course, there is an obvious sense in which the *chreia*, perhaps here best rendered as 'need', is conceptually, and indeed actually, distinct from the other factors, and hence *a fortiori* can be identified as such. After all, one function of the pulse is to expel smoky residues. If your temperature is elevated for whatever reason you produce more of them, and consequently there is a greater need, other things being equal, for their expulsion. But evidently the body can have such needs and yet be unable to satisfy them, in this case either because the heart's *dunamis* isn't up to it, or because the mediating mechanism of the arterial system is damaged in some way. It surely isn't the case that, in some viciously circular manner, we can only identify the need in terms of the *dunamis* and *vice versa*. But of course this isn't the whole story, and what matters here I think is whether the need, so identified, can fulfil any genuinely explanatory role, much less one which we would be inclined to recognize as causal. And this of course takes us to the heart of the question of teleological explanation. Galen's teleology, as I stressed, is an amalgam of Plato's and Aristotle's, but crucially he takes over from the former the idea that the structures and organizations of animals' bodies literally reflect the design of a designer. Thus it will be non-trivial for him to say that the reason why the cardiovascular system is constructed the way it is is in order to accomplish such-and-such a goal in the overall running of the animal's body. And if it needs to get rid of smoky residues in order to survive, or at least to function in the optimum manner, then the designer will have seen to it that the animal will have been constructed in such a way as to accomplish this subsidiary task. And this 'fact' — if of course it is one — explains, in a perfectly straightforward sense, why the animal is made the way it is, and why also (which is what matters to us), its functions vary as they do according to variant ambient circumstances. Now, I think conceived this way the goal, or need, or whatever, really can function as a fully-independent, non-reducible element in explanation, and one which moreover *implies* the existence of further facts which are causal in our sense (at any rate if reasons can be causes). This seems to be a distinct advantage of adopting this sort of teleology over that of Aristotle, where, notoriously, it is hard to make genuine independent room for the final cause. So I think, at least at the conceptual level, the schema is vindicated, and does indeed, as you suggest, potentially at least gain in explanatory power (I say 'potentially', since such styles of explanation will ultimately be acceptable only to the extent to which the background assumptions they rely upon, in this case crucially that of the existence of benevolent, intelligent designer, turn out to be true — which is obviously an empirical question). In sum, then, Galen is aware of the danger of vacuous pseudo-explanation in which the explanans is merely a restatement of the explanandum; and I do not see that in this case he runs the risk of falling foul of his own strictures on the matter.

III

Michael Frede

GALEN'S THEOLOGY[1]

Galen already in his life-time acquired a great reputation as a physician and a medical writer. He soon was to acquire the status of an authority in questions of medicine. But Galen thought of himself not just as a physician, but also as a philosopher. When he had turned fourteen, his father sent him to study with four philosophers in his native town, Pergamum, a Stoic who had been a student of Philopator, a Platonist who had been a student of Gaius, a Peripatetic who had studied with Aspasius, and finally an Epicurean who had come from Athens (*Aff.Dig.* 8, V 41,10-42,2 K). It was only when he had become sixteen that Galen's father, himself an architect with a strong interest in the mathematical sciences, prompted in this by "evident dreams" had him take up the study of medicine (*Ord.Lib.Prop.* 4, *Scripta min.* II p.88,13-17 Mueller = XIX 59,7-11 K; *MM* 9, 4, X 609,10 K). But it is clear from the wording in both of the passages just referred to that Galen, when he took up medicine, continued to study philosophy and that this was an interest which he actively pursued throughout his life. Thus he tells us that when he went to study in Smyrna (in 149, after the death of his father), he did so to follow the lectures of Pelops in medicine and those of the Platonist Albinus (another student of

[1] In writing this I have been greatly helped by the work of Pierluigi Donini, in particular his article "Motivi filosofici in Galeno", in *PP* 35 (1980), 333-370. I would also like to thank Elaine Matthews for her generous help with the evidence from inscriptions concerning Galen's father Nico.

Gaius) in philosophy (*Lib.Prop.* 2, *Scripta min.* II p.97,9-11 = XIX 16,8-10 K). Indeed, he wrote a great number of treatises on philosophical questions, most of which, unfortunately, have been lost. But we get a good idea of the extent and the scope of Galen's philosophical writing from his *De libris propriis*, in which chapters 11 to 16 are devoted to his philosophical works. He even managed to acquire a certain reputation as a philosopher. Already Alexander of Aphrodisias, his younger contemporary, refers to him (*In Top.* 8, 5, CAG II 2, p.549,23 Wallies), and so do Themistius, Simplicius (cf. *In Ph.* 7, 1, CAG X, p.1039,13 ff.), and Philoponus (cf., in particular, the latter's *De aeternitate mundi* 17, 5, p.599,23 ff. Rabe).

In trying to characterize Galen's philosophical position in general, we should start from the fact that Galen, following the advice of his father, refuses to commit himself to the whole of the doctrine of any one philosopher or philosophical school (*Aff.Dig.* 8, V 42,6-43,8 K). This, presumably, is why his father made him attend the lectures of representatives of all four major philosophical schools. It seems to be in important ways the same attitude which he adopts in medicine and which in *De libris propriis* 1 (*Scripta min.* II p.95,2-10 Mueller = XIX 13,12-14,1 K) he characterizes in the following way: he does not regard himself as a Hippocratean or a Praxagorean or as a member of any sect (αἵρεσις). He rather selects (ἐκλέγειν) from each group what seems to him to be fitting. But, he says, this selective or eclectic attitude does not prevent one from having particular admiration for some ancient author or authors. At this point, unfortunately, the text becomes corrupt; but we will hardly go amiss if we assume that Galen is saying something to the effect that he regards Hippocrates as a classical paradigm of a physician. Analogously, then, Galen also in philosophy, to use his own language, is eclectic, rather than an unwavering and unquestioning partisan of any one philosopher or any one philosophical school. But this does not prevent Galen from regarding some ancient philosopher or other as deserving our particular attention or admiration, just as Galen's eclecticism in medicine does not prevent him from regarding Hippocrates as a model.

It seems to me to be obvious that it is Plato who for Galen plays the role in philosophy which Hippocrates plays for him in medicine. This is why he writes the *De placitis Hippocratis et Platonis*. Indeed, he speaks of the philosopher as "the most divine Plato" (*PHP* 9, 9, 3, p.598,9 De Lacy = V 792,4 K; *UP* 16, 1, II p.377,14-15 Helmreich = IV 266,3-4 K). Very clearly Galen also is much indebted to Aristotle, but Aristotle for him does not seem to have the status he attributes to Plato. In general his philosophical views are along Platonist lines. In his indebtedness to Aristotle he does not differ from most Platonists of late antiquity who integrate a good deal of Aristotelian doctrine into their Platonism. His relation to Stoicism is more complex. Again, there is no doubt that Galen in fact is very much indebted to Stoicism, but the degree of his indebtedness is obscured by the fact that as a rule he refers to the Stoics in a critical manner. Also in this regard, though, Galen does not differ from many Platonists of late antiquity, for instance from Plotinus. But it would be a mistake to think that Galen, in spite of his claim not to belong to any philosophical school, in fact just is some kind of Platonist. What stands in the way of thinking this is his refusal to address and to answer a number of questions a Platonist in his day was expected to have an answer to. He, for instance, not only refuses to claim that the soul is immortal, as a Platonist is expected to do, he refuses to answer the question concerning the soul's immortality one way or the other.

This brings us to a second feature of Galen's philosophical position in general. Galen not only is eclectic in his philosophical views, he also is rather selective as to which questions he is prepared to express a view about. When Galen first studied philosophy, he reports *Lib.Prop.* 11 (*Scripta min.* II p.116,20 ff. = XIX 40,3 ff. K), he, as far as this had depended on his teachers, would have become a Pyrrhonean, given the disagreements between the different schools, but often even among philosophers of the same school. What prevented him from becoming a Pyrrhonean was the conviction he had acquired when being taught geometry and arithmetic, mainly by his father, who in this followed a family tradition, that there is such a thing as conclusive proof, the sort of proof geometers support their claims by. In another place, *Aff.Dig.* 8 (V 42,4 ff. K), Galen tells us, again in connection with his father's sending him to attend the lectures of different philosophers, that his father, having himself been trained in geometry, arithmetic, architecture, and astronomy, was looking for teachers who supported their claims with proofs; he took the failure to do so to be the source of disagreement and controversy. Galen, then, is also looking for proof in philosophy. But when it comes to questions of which Galen thinks that there is no evident answer to them, he becomes very hesitant. Even here, though, he is making a distinction. In *Foet.Form.* 6 (IV 699,7-700,6 K) he states that he is unable to say what the οὐσία of that soul is which might be thought to be the cause of the formation of the foetus, and that he hence also is unable to identify the cause which is responsible for giving the foetus the form which will be so marvellously suited to the needs of the animal. It is not only that he has not been able to find a scientific proof as to what the οὐσία of the soul consists in, he has not even been able to arrive at a plausible (πιθανόν) answer (700,2-5). For the answers which are on offer there not only is no proof, they are not even plausible. Some lines further down in the same text (700,17-701,6) Galen criticizes the view of one of his Platonist teachers. He had claimed that it is the world-soul which is responsible for the formation of the foetus of animals. Galen finds this not even plausible, because it borders on blasphemy to assume that the world-soul would concern itself with the formation of creatures like scorpions.

Earlier in the same chapter of the treatise (695,3 ff.) Galen reports how he turned to philosophers, who make it their business to discuss the world-order and the coming into being of things, to find out from them what it is that causes the artful formation of the organism. He was expecting to get an answer in the form of a proof *more geometrico*, but got conflicting accounts, none of which even met the demands of rhetorical plausibility (695,10-11). These answers often not only are not definitive, they do not even seem to be possible answers, given that there is something which seems to rule them out (696,14 ff.). So Galen does distinguish between definitive answers, backed up by conclusive proof, and answers which, though not supported by proof, are supported by reasonable argument and are not ruled out by considerations to the contrary. Galen allows himself such plausible views, but is hesitant to express them.

Galen also seems to think that all philosophical inquiry should serve a practical end (*PHP* 9, 7, 11, p.588,18-20 De Lacy = V 780,13-16 K: πρακτικὸν ... τὸ τέλος), this is to say that it should aim at gaining a better understanding of things which will allow us to live a better life. I infer this, for instance, from the fact that in the passage from *PHP* referred to, Galen seems to distinguish between philosophers who pursue theoretical knowledge for its own sake and those who pursue it to the extent that it is necessary for a good life, to then criticize some of the latter for sliding from the pursuit of useful questions into pursuing useless questions. The primary objection in the latter case does not seem to be that they are inconsistent in claiming that philosophy serves a practical end and in, at the same time, pursuing practically useless questions, but rather that they have allowed themselves to pursue useless questions at all, having been taken in by the similarity between certain useful questions they were pursuing and certain related, but useless questions. It is only thus deceived by similarity that they pursue questions of a kind such that we are no better off for knowing the answer to them.

If we now look at Galen's extant philosophical writings and at what we can find out about his lost writings in philosophy, for instance on the basis of his own *De libris propriis*, it is clear that his interest in philosophy was very much focussed on logic and on ethics. Thus his account of his philosophical writings in *De libris propriis* is divided into a long section on logic or dialectic dealing with books useful for learning how to demonstrate things (chap. 11), a section on ethics (chap.12), and chapters (13-16) dealing with writings pertaining to Platonic, Aristotelian, Stoic, and Epicurean philosophy. The writings in this last section, too, are almost all devoted to logic or to ethics. Galen seems to have written almost nothing on physics or theoretical philosophy. This is particularly striking, if one has any temptation to think, not just that Galen believed that medical practice should be based, as far as possible, on a solid scientific medical theory, but also would like to think that a solid medical theory has to be firmly based on natural science, i.e. physics in the ancient sense. But I take it that the reason why Galen is hesitant to write about physics or theoretical philosophy is at least twofold: he thinks that for the most part physics is useless, and that for the most part it is theoretical in the sense of 'speculative', since the available evidence does not suffice to settle many of the questions raised in a definitive way. But I will later also want to suggest that part of Galen's hesitation about theoretical philosophy or physics is religious in nature. It is not just that Galen, as we saw a moment ago, criticizes a view about the formation of the foetus as almost blasphemous, because it conflicts with his elated view of the world-soul. He also seems to think that the way the world is ordered, including the way living beings come into being and pass away and the way they are formed, reveals a divine power or divine powers at work, though we do not know how they are involved in bringing about the effects we observe, for instance an organism with a certain structure. It is as if they were hidden from us, some kind of mystery. There is at least one passage in Galen, in the *De usu partium* 15, 1, in which Galen talks as if it were impious to inquire into how certain bodily parts actually come to be formed the way we can perceive them to be formed. In this text Galen turns to the discussion of the penis. Given its function, it has to satisfy certain requirements: it must be hollow, and it must, at the appropriate time, be hard, but should not always be hard. He explains in some detail the construction problems involved. Parts like arteries, veins, sinews, nerves, bones, flesh would not serve the purpose. Galen argues that the penis is a bodily part without parallel in its construction. What it is like we find out by anatomy. Hence we can see how the Demiurge wanted it to be so that it would fulfil its function (II p.342,4-5 Helmreich). But then Galen continues "do not try, do not dare to inquire how it came to be this way. For, of what you would not even know that it was this way, if you had not learnt it from anatomy, how could you reasonably dare to inquire how it came about. It is sufficient for you to have found out that every part has been formed in such a way as its use demands. But if you try to inquire how it came to be this way, you will be found to be not only insensitive to your own weakness, but also to the power of the Demiurge". Here, it seems that what is in question is not so much that the art of medicine would not be served by finding out how a bodily part comes to be formed with a certain structure, or that we for some trivial reason would not be able to find out what the answer is. There clearly is some suggestion of the inscrutability of nature's or the Demiurge's ways, of the impropriety of daring (τολμᾶν, II p.342,6 and 8) to inquire into things which it is not for human beings to know.

It is clear why he thinks that ethics or practical philosophy is useful. As to logic or dialectic it is mainly useful because it teaches us how proofs have to be constructed; and we have already seen what importance Galen attributes to proof, in the mathematical sciences, in medicine, or in philosophy. But he also thinks that a lot of logical inquiry is useless. In *Lib.Prop.* 11 (*Scripta min.* II p.116,12-18 = XIX 39,14-40,1 K) he complains that many of the theorems in Stoic or Peripatetic logic he later found to be of no use for demonstration. Similarly in *PHP* 9, 7, 16-18 (p.588,29-590,4 De Lacy = V 781,10-782,6 K) he complains that, though logic is needed and necessary, many have extended their logical inquiries into areas the study of which is pointless. The same is even more true of physics or theoretical philosophy. A certain amount of physics is needed, for instance for medicine and for practical philosophy or ethics and politics (*PHP* 9, 7, 17). Thus, for instance, we do need to know in medicine that, as Plato says, the human body is a composite of earth, fire, air, and water, and that diseases are due to a deficiency or an excess of one or more of these or to their displacement (*PHP* 8, 2, 21, p.494,22-25 De Lacy = V 667,3-6 K). Now Hippocrates, according to Galen, thinks that there is no need to inquire further, for instance into the nature of these elements and how they come to have their observable powers of, say, heating and cooling. For this art, medicine, is a practical art, and the pursuit of such questions is irrelevant to the practice of medicine. But Plato, as if he believed that theoretical philosophy was eminently worthwhile, insists on pursuing these questions, for instance questions about the constitution of the so-called elements (*PHP* 8, 3, 2-5, p.494,28-496,10 De Lacy = V 667,10-668,13 K). Galen goes on to point out that it is irrelevant for the present discussion whether or not Plato was right in his view about the constitution of the elements (*ibid.* 6), but does not refrain from finally quoting Plato himself to the effect that his account of fire is only a likely (εἰκῶς) account (*ibid.* 11). Galen clearly does think that physics in the sense in which it is pursued by philosophers for the most part is useless, and for the most part advances at best to likely or plausible conclusions. In *PHP* 9, 7, 9-16 (p.588,7-33 = V 779,16-781,15 K) Galen gives us a long list of questions pursued by natural or theoretical philosophers which are idle: whether there is something beyond this world, and if so, what sort of thing it is, whether the world is self-contained, whether there is more than one world, perhaps even a great number of them, whether this world is generated or ungenerated, whether, in case it has come into being, it was brought into being by a demiurgic God or by blind chance (*ibid.* 9-11). Or there are such questions as what the οὐσία of the gods is, whether they are altogether incorporeal or whether, like us, they have bodies (*ibid.* 13). Not only does Galen think that there is no need to know the answer to such questions, he also thinks that in this view he is just following the position of Socrates and his followers like Xenophon and, indeed, Plato himself, who for this reason attributes the account of nature given in the *Timaeus* not to Socrates, but to Timaeus (*ibid.* 15-16). Not only is it not worthwhile to pursue such questions, but there is no definitive, accurate answer to them which everybody will agree on. The most one can hope to achieve in such matters is a plausible or probable account. This is how far Plato extends his account of *physiologia* in the *Timaeus*, and this is why he makes Timaeus in the dialogue at the beginning of his account (*Tim.* 29 c-d) say that we should not expect, when it comes to the gods and the generation of the universe, to get more than plausible answers to many of our questions (*PHP* 9, 9, 3-5, p.598,5-19 De Lacy = V 791,17-792,17 K). Somewhat earlier, in *PHP* 9, 6, 21-22 (p.576,27-578,4 De Lacy = V 766,7-767,3 K), Galen had explained why there is such widespread disagreement among philosophers. Many of the questions they deal with, and he explicitly refers to some of the questions listed above, cannot be settled by empirical evidence, the way medical questions can be. And Galen obviously also assumes that we cannot settle them *a priori*.

Galen, then, seems to take a rather dim view of what we can expect of physics as a science. In this view he believes himself to be just following Socrates and Plato. And when it comes to the probable account Plato offers in the *Timaeus*, it is clear from many passages in Galen that he is rather hesitant to even accept as probable some of the views Plato sets forth in his account.

With this we can, finally, turn to the task I have been allotted, namely to say something about Galen's theology. Theology, the way the term is understood in antiquity, is a matter of giving an account of God or the gods. But antiquity knew and distinguished various sorts of account of the gods, and thus various sorts or senses of 'theology'. One distinction, which suits our purposes well, seems to have been common and is well-known through Augustine's report of Varro's version of it in *Civ.* 6, 5 (cf. 8, 1), namely the distinction into mythical, civic, and natural theology. There are the traditional myths or legends about the gods; there are the accounts of the gods which are presupposed by one's following the πάτριος νόμος, the established cults of one's community (cf. e.g., Sextus Empiricus, *PH* 1, 17 and 24; 3, 218; *Math.* 11, 49) and there are the accounts of God or the gods given by philosophers which are supposed to meet the standards of rationality any philosophical account is supposed to satisfy, accounts of a kind which will also be adopted, in some form or other, by a wider educated public, and in terms of which educated persons will try to understand the traditional myths, but also the public cults they participate in. It is in this last sense that philosophers like Aristotle (cf. *Met.* 5, 1, 1026 a 19), Cleanthes (Diog.Laert. 7, 41) or Proclus (cf. his *Elementatio theologica*) talk of theology as a philosophical discipline. And it is in this sense that I want to talk about Galen's theology. But I will also have something to say about Galen's religious beliefs, at least to the extent that this has some bearing on his theological views.

Galen's theology is not a subject scholars have had much to say about. There are many reasons for this. One simply is that at least the extant writings do not offer more than scattered remarks on theological questions. Galen did write a hypomnema on Aristotle's first unmoved mover (*Lib.Prop.* 14, *Scripta min.* II p.123,4-5 = XIX 47,6 K). But unfortunately this treatise, though translated into Syriac and into Arabic (cf. R. Degen, "Galen im Syrischen", in *Galen. Problems and Prospects*, ed. by V. Nutton [London 1981], 158, Nr.118) has been lost. There seems to be at least one fragment of it preserved in Arabic, though. In it Galen talks about the followers of Moses and Christ who are taught to accept everything on faith (cf. R. Walzer, *Galen on Jews and Christians* [Oxford 1949], 15). There is a question as to whether, as has been suggested, this can be the treatise attacked in a writing attributed to Alexander of Aphrodisias and edited by N. Rescher and M. Marmura (*The Refutation by Alexander of Aphrodisias of Galen's Treatise on the Theory of Motion* [Islamabad, s.d. (1966)]). For in this text the author criticizes Galen for attacking, in an essay sent to Herminus, Aristotle's claim at the beginning of *Ph.* 7, 1, 241 b 34-242 a 49, that everything which is in motion is moved by something. Now Aristotle's claim seems to be directed against Plato's assumption that the soul is self-moving (cf. *Phaedr.* 245 d 7-8). Having produced an argument for this claim, Aristotle proceeds (242 a 49 ff.) to argue that if something is in motion there ultimately must be some first mover which is not itself in motion. So Galen in the lost treatise on Aristotle's first unmoved mover may have been attacking this argument for a first unmoved mover by criticizing the claim that everything which is in motion is moved by something, and Alexander's response would be a response to this criticism. If, then, the treatise attributed to Alexander were a response to Galen's *On the first unmoved mover*, we would have a number of further fragments and would know a good deal more about Galen's treatise. But, given at least the focus of Alexander's criticism, this further information does little to help us to understand Galen's theology. What we would learn from it would just be that Galen thinks that Aristotle does not have a proof for his doctrine of a first unmoved mover. And so I am not going to pursue this text any further. We might, though, in passing take note of the fact that the author, perhaps Alexander, characterizes (p.16) Galen as somebody who in general inclines towards Plato (rather than Aristotle, we have to understand), but also as somebody who, at least in this context, was prepared to make abusive remarks about Aristotle's argument (p.18).

As things stand, then, all we have to go on to reconstruct Galen's theology are some remarks here and there in his extant writings, remarks moreover which are not easily fitted into a reasonably detailed, systematic view of Galen's theology. In fact given what we have said earlier about Galen's attitude towards theoretical philosophy or physics in general and certain theological questions, like the question concerning the nature of the gods, one might easily come to think that in the sense we are looking for there is no such thing as Galen's theology, that Galen rests content with the religious attitudes he has been raised in.

But this clearly is not the case. For if we again look at *PHP* 9, 7 we see that among the many questions pursued in theoretical philosophy or physics and which Galen regards as pointless, there is one which Galen exempts from this criticism, the question concerning providence and the gods (9, 7, 12, p.588,20-22 De Lacy = V 780,16-17 K). I take it that Galen has in mind that it really does matter whether we believe that there are gods and that they are provident. For he immediately goes on to say (*ibid.* 13) that it is better for all of us to inquire whether in the world there is something superior to man in power and wisdom, apparently presupposing that such a being would deserve to be called 'divine' or a 'god'. So inquiry into the existence of gods and their providence, according to Galen, is not useless. And obviously he also thinks that it does yield an answer, if properly pursued. Indeed, as we can see from *Plac.Prop.* 2, Galen believes himself to have not just a plausible or probable view concerning God's existence, but firm knowledge of it, though in the same chapter he again gocs through a catalogue of questions concerning God or the gods to which he has no answer. For instance, he, here again, does not know what the οὐσία of God or the gods is, but also remarks that he cannot see what harm is supposed to arise from the fact that human beings do not know the answer to this question. As we will see later, Galen also believes himself to know that God is provident.

So Galen does have a view on some theological questions. Yet, one might still wonder whether Galen thinks that there is such a discipline as 'theology' and whether Galen himself has a detailed theological position which we could try to reconstruct. There seems to be only one passage in the whole of Galen's work in which he uses the word 'theology', namely in *UP* 17, 1 (II p.447,23 Helmreich = IV 360,13 K). Galen says that what might at first seem to be a small matter, namely the study of the use of the parts, will turn out to be a true starting point (ἀρχή) for an accurate theology (θεολογίας ἀκριβοῦς), a matter much weightier and much worthier than the whole of the art of medicine. He goes on to say (II p.447,25-448,3 = IV 360,15-361,1 K) that the study of the use of the parts not only is helpful for the doctor, but much more so for the philosopher who, after all, is trying to gain knowledge of the whole of nature, as opposed to the doctor who is concerned with just the human body. Here Galen does seem to think of theology as a philosophical discipline, a discipline one will pursue if one tries to understand the whole of nature. After all, whether we follow Plato, Aristotle, or the Stoics, God is a principle of nature. It also is clear from this passage that Galen does not think of theology as an entirely speculative enterprise. For he talks of an accurate (ἀκριβής) theology. We can gather at least part of the force of the characterization as 'accurate' by comparing *PHP* 9, 9, 5 (p.598,14-19 De Lacy = V 792,10-17 K). There Galen quotes Timaeus in the dialogue as saying that it is unreasonable to expect him to provide accurate (ἀπηκριβωμένους) accounts on all matters concerning the gods and the generation of the universe, if all he can give is an overall plausible account. So part of the point here in *UP* must be that theology, properly pursued, can provide definitive answers to at least some questions. To be properly pursued it needs to have the right starting-points, unquestionable truths. Such truths, Galen obviously thinks, are provided by the study of the use of the parts of the human body. The facts ascertained in this study show that there must be a Demiurge and that he is provident, but also a number of other things about God. So we do have firmly established theorems about the Demiurge. How they can be derived, Galen tries to show, or at least to indicate, in the course of the *UP*, but in particular in *UP* 17, 1 where he explicitly talks about theology. But earlier in this same chapter Galen also expresses some views which he himself qualifies as only plausible or probable. So in this sense there clearly is such a thing as Galen's theology, though some of his theological views are qualified by himself as merely plausible or reasonable.

In what follows I will try to work out what this Galenic theology amounts to. But before I turn to this, I want to return in considerable detail to *Plac.Prop.* 2. I hope that this will help us to get a firm grasp of the background and of some of the details of Galen's theology.

In the *De placitis propriis* Galen tells us what his position on various controversial questions is. To some questions Galen believes himself to have a definitive answer, to other questions he does not know the answer, though in some of these cases he is willing to make a conjecture (14, 4). After a prefatory first chapter he in chapter 2 begins with questions concerning the world, to then mainly deal with questions concerning God or the gods. Chapter 3 deals with questions concerning the soul, chapter 4, after an initial sentence about celestial bodies, treats of questions concerning the constitution of terrestrial bodies. From chapter 5 onwards we deal with more specific questions concerning the body, the way it functions, and hence also about the soul. There is a certain pattern to chapters 2, 3, and 4 which deal with, as it were, global questions. In chapter 2 Galen claims to know that there are gods, or at least that there is a Demiurge. He knows this on the basis of experience, his own and that of others. For what can be observed by us unequivocally indicates a Demiurge at work. But he disclaims any knowledge of the οὐσία of God or the gods. By this he means, I take it, that he does not know who or what sort of thing God is, what is constitutive of God, what it is that reveals itself in its operations or effects which we can observe. In chapter 3 Galen claims to know that there are souls. We know this because we observe animals to move in a certain characteristic way and to perceive things. And we just call that which makes them move in this way and perceive things, whatever it is, 'soul'. So there are souls. But Galen disclaims any knowledge of what the soul really is, of what it is that makes animals move in this way and perceive things. When in chapter 4 Galen turns to terrestrial bodies, by contrast, he claims that he does know what they are: they are mixtures of fire, earth, water, and air. It is not just that we can observe the effect a terrestrial body has on another body, for instance the effect a drug has on a patient. In this case we also are not entirely at a loss as to what it really is which has this effect. It is a body which is produced by the mixture of the four elements with their characteristic observable qualities.

But before Galen turns to terrestrial bodies, he in the first sentence of the chapter, in a subordinate clause, explains why he passes over the celestial bodies: he disclaims any knowledge of them. This is a rather summary and at least in one regard surprising claim. It is rather summary because surely Galen does know something about the celestial bodies, for instance that they do exist. For we plainly see them. It is somewhat surprising, given that Galen had a particular interest in the mathematical sciences, that his father had had a special interest in astronomy, and that, hence, Galen must have known something about astronomy. We will have reason to return to his astronomy later. For the moment I am interested in what Galen may have thought he did not know about the stars. Given the way the clause about the celestial bodies is incorporated into the sentence about terrestrial bodies, it is tempting to think that one thing he claims ignorance about is their constitution, their οὐσία; whereas he does know that terrestrial bodies are formed by a mixture of the four elements and he thus, to some extent, can understand the effect they have, he does not know what the constitution of the stars is, what their οὐσία is. There is, e.g., the question whether their body is immaterial in the sense that it is not constituted by the four elements, from which all mortal, sublunary bodies are formed, but by a substance *sui generis*. In the latter case they are perhaps eternal, since they do not decompose into the four elements. Whereas the formation of mortal terrestrial bodies is part of the διακόσμησις for which the Demiurge is responsible, it emerges from a passage in *UP* 3, 10 (I p.176,21-24 Helmreich = III 241,1-3 K) that Galen assumes that celestial bodies like the sun are precosmic in the sense that they themselves, as opposed to their position, are not part of the way the world is ordered by the Demiurge. That is to say, they are the bodies they are, with a certain shape and size, independently of the order imposed by the Demiurge. There are all sorts of questions Galen may have about the stars and their motion, for instance whether they have a soul, what the origin of their soul is, and what the role of their soul in their motion is. But what matters for the moment is that Galen, though he does not explicitly say so, seems to think also of the stars as beings of whose existence we do know by observation, but whose οὐσία we are unable to determine, as a result of which we also cannot definitively answer certain questions about them. We only seem to begin to be on safe ground cognitively once we deal with the terrestrial objects surrounding us. But even here our understanding is severely limited. We know that terrestrial bodies are formed from a complete mixture of earth, fire, air, and water. But, when it comes to the question what earth, fire, air, and water really are, whether they are really elements or whether they, as Plato suggested in the *Timaeus* 48 b 3-e 1, can be reduced to more basic items. Galen avoids answering it (*PHP* 8, 3). Galen also claims not to know what total mixture amounts to, whether it only involves the mixture of the qualities or also of the matter. He sometimes claims that human beings are unable to effect a total mixture, since this requires a divine power (*Temp.* 1, 9, p.34,5-15 Helmreich = I 562,15-563,9 K).

With this we can turn to the details of chapter 2 of the *De placitis propriis*. Unfortunately this text is only extant in a Latin and in a Hebrew version. Each of them depends on an Arab version. So in both cases we are at least twice removed from a Greek copy of the original text. Correspondingly there are important divergences between the two extant versions. In a crucial place the Latin text clearly is corrupt (2, 2, p.58,8-9 Nutton).

The text, as it stands, does refer to God, the creator or demiurge of all the things in this world (cf. 2, 1, p.56,17 & 23; 2, 2, p.58,8), the power of God (cf. 2, 1, p.56,20; 2, 2, p.58,9 & 15), the powers of God (cf. 2, 1, p.56,21), and certain workings or works of God or his powers, referred to as *operationes* (God: 2, 2, p.58,7; his powers: 2, 1, p.56,22; 2, 2, p.58,5). The original text also may have referred to gods. The text on either version says something like this (2, 2, p.58,1-2): "I will not talk the way Protagoras did who denied that he had any knowledge about them (*de ipsis*)". The plural pronoun could refer back to the divine powers mentioned in 56,21 or the workings of these powers mentioned in the same line. The pronoun also seems to be taken up by the feminine plural pronouns *earum*, *ipsae*, *earum*, *ipsis* in 2, 2, p.58,4-5. Since the text in 58,5 talks of "the workings of them (*earum*)", the reference of *ipsis* in 58,2 should be, not to the workings, but to the powers. But Protagoras did not talk about divine powers, let alone about their workings. What Protagoras notoriously said, as Galen must have known, was that he did not know anything about the gods, neither that they exist, nor that they do not exist, nor what sort of beings they are, and this is what Galen must be referring to here. Thus Nutton, in his comments on 2, 2, p.58,1-5 (p.135), rightly calls into question the use of the feminine pronouns in 58,2-5. As Nutton puts it, they seem to be "another example of the tendency of Arabic translators to avoid suspicions of polytheism". So we have to reckon with the possibility that Galen in 2, 2, p.58,1-2 had said "I will not talk the way Protagoras did when he denied any knowledge about the gods" and that in 58,4-5 he had used the appropriate masculine pronouns to refer back to the gods Protagoras had disclaimed any knowledge of. If we adopt this view, the text not only talks of God whose οὐσία Galen does not know, but also of gods whose οὐσία he has no knowledge of, though he recognises their existence. That Galen believes in gods, but claims not to know their οὐσία we already know from *PHP* 9, 7, 13 (p.588,22-25 De Lacy = V 781,1-5 K). If we follow this suggestion, the references to divine powers in 2, 2, p.58,1-5 will disappear, but the change will leave the reference to divine powers in 2, 1, p.56,21 intact.

Now, one thing we would like to get clearer about is how God, the gods, the power of God, the divine powers, and the works or workings of God or the divine powers which we can observe are related to each other. This question arises, even if we do not follow the suggestion that Galen in the original text explicitly did refer to gods. It arises in the following way. Though there are serious problems with the text, it is clear that in 2, 2, p.58,7-11 Galen refers to the workings of God (58,8), the God referred to in 2, 1, p.56,23 and thus God, the Demiurge, referred to in 56,17 and 23. In the sentence in question Galen refers to the fact that he once was cured from a disease (2, 2, p.58,9-11). This, whatever the difficulties with the sentence may be, clearly is one of the works of God mentioned at the beginning of the sentence, something Galen himself has experienced. It is natural to assume, as also Nutton does, that Galen here is referring to the life-threatening illness he also talks about in *De libris propriis* 2 (*Scripta min.* II p.99,9-11 Mueller = XIX 19,1-3 K). There Galen is reporting how Marcus Aurelius asked him to accompany him on his campaign against the Marcomanni, but Galen managed to persuade the emperor to excuse him. Galen informed him that Asclepius, his πάτριος θεός, had told him not to join the emperor on his campaign, and that he had been a worshipper (θεραπευτής) of Asclepius, ever since the god had saved him (διέσωσε) from a terrible disease. The emperor, out of respect for the god (προσκυνήσας τὸν θεόν), ceded to Galen's request. Presumably the disease in question is the one Galen also is referring to in *Cur.Rat.Ven.Sect.* 23

(XI 314,18-315,7 K). There Galen tells us how he treated a condition he was suffering from, following two clear dreams sent by Asclepius, by arteriotomy. So Galen does seem to believe in gods like Asclepius.

What, then, is the relation between God and Asclepius, given that our sentence seems to ascribe Galen's cure, which he elsewhere attributes to Asclepius, to God. One possible answer would be that Galen just identifies Asclepius with God. As we learn from Aelius Aristides (*Or.* 42, 4), some Pergamenes did think that Asclepius was the ruler and saviour of the world. We will return to this later. But Galen in this text also seems to be talking about the gods in the plural. In any case he does so in other texts, for instance in *PHP* 9, 7, 12 (p.588,20-22 De Lacy = V 780,16-17 K). We naturally would assume that Galen distinguishes between God who is responsible for the ordering of the world and its governance and lesser gods or divine beings, and that Asclepius is one of these lesser gods.

Now it is obviously the case that the supporters of the cult of Asclepius over time managed to promote Asclepius to an ever more elevated status, first from a hero, the son of Apollo and a woman, to a god; he then came to be identified with Apollo himself; and now we see him promoted to be the ruler of the world, set over the lesser gods. It is somewhat difficult to believe that Galen, whatever his devotion to Asclepius and Pergamum, would accept such a view except as part of a more comprehensive view about the relation between God and the many gods. Such a comprehensive view we find, for instance, in a letter by Maximus, presumably one of Augustine's old teachers in Madaura, to Augustine, preserved among Augustine's letters (*Epist.* 16). Maximus thinks that all reasonable, educated persons should be able to agree that we all worship one God and Father whose powers pervade the world and who is invoked by many names referring to different aspects or, as it were, parts of him. This is a view on which all the lesser gods are somehow aspects of the one God, such that in worshipping them we are worshipping God under one of his many names. Galen's view presumably is along these lines. But we would expect it to be more articulate.

There are two possibilities which come to mind. The simpler one is this: our text also refers to the power of God (2, 2, p.58,9) through which Galen was cured (cf. also the next sentence, 2, 2, p.58,14-16, which seems to refer to the same event or similar events). It obviously is part of the power of God to be able to cure persons and thus to save them, and more generally to save them from calamity or impending disaster. Thus Galen may identify Asclepius with God insofar as he has the power to cure and to save persons.

Analogously other gods might be identified with God insofar as it is part of his power to be able to bring about other things, insofar as he has other powers. But there also is a more complicated possibility: God has, as it were, agents who act in his name, under his authority, according to his will, with a power he has given them and which they exercise in his name. In this case Asclepius and other gods would be such agents of God. It still would be true that God cured Galen through his power, but it would be through an agent of God who effected the cure exercising the power given to him by God, namely Asclepius. At least for the time being we will have to leave open the question which of these possible views Galen might espouse, and hence how he sees the relation between God and the gods.

But whichever of these views we take to be Galen's, it seems clear that the marvellous power referred to in 58,15 is the power of God mentioned in 58,9 (cf. 58,8), and hence it seems plausible that the divine powers are the powers associated with, or even identified, with the gods. In fact, as the text of the Latin version stands, Galen in 2, 1, p.56,21 explicitly identifies the power of God with the powers we become aware of in our experience, for instance the power Galen became aware of when he was cured. The Hebrew version in this place just talks of God and his powers (rather than his power) and identifies these powers as those we become aware of in observing the effects of their exercise. But it, too, later (cf. 2, 2, p.59,14 and 24-25) speaks of God's power, and hence it, too, implicitly seems to identify the power of God with these divine powers. Now the expression "God's power" is ambiguous. It might refer to God's overwhelming powerfulness, but it also might refer to his ability to do whatever it is that he does, that is to say to a specific, but unspecified, ability or power, the power which goes with being God, the power such that if something has this power it must be God, just as one might think that the soul has a particular, specific power. But whether "the power of God" refers to his powerfulness or to a specific power he has, we in either case would want to know what it is that he can do which makes him so powerful. Yet it might be the case that if we try to specify the power or the ability of God, we do not succeed, since we do not know how he actually goes about providing the world with its order. What we can do is to look for the effects of what he does in providing the world with its order. These are the works or workings of God. He, for instance, does cure persons from disease or saves them from ship-wreck (2, 2, p.58,7-14). Thus we attribute to him the power to heal and the power to save persons in calamity. The way we proceed is rather similar to the procedure Galen describes in chapter 14 of our treatise: we know that scammony produces purging and that medlar produces constipation. But we do not know how scammony and medlar produce these effects; we do not know what they do which has this effect, what causes the effect. And since we do not know the cause, we talk of the purgative power of scammony and the constipative power of medlar, after the effect they have. But what it is about scammony and medlar which has this effect we do not know (14, 1, p.110,19-22). Galen uses these examples to explain how we specify the powers of the soul. His explanation is not as straightforward as we might wish, because in giving it he is mindful of the uncertainty as to what the soul is. We know that there is a soul, because the soul makes us do the things we as living beings do, like walk or run. But we do not know what it is, and hence also do not know what it does such that as a result of it we walk and run and do all the other things living beings do. Hence we introduce powers named after the observable effects of its activity, of its exercise of its power, for instance the natural powers associated with the vegetative soul: the attractive, the expulsive, the retentive, and the transformative powers (cf. *Plac.Prop.* 13, 7). In that sense, then, God's power is these divine powers.

A problem is raised by the phrase *scilicet deitas, id est virtus deitatis* in 2, 1, p.56,20. The Hebrew version has, in Nutton's translation, "namely God and the divine powers". The problem is threefold. To begin with, it is puzzling why Galen would need something like a *scilicet* clause at all, let alone one in this clumsy position. For it is perfectly clear without the clause that the subject of the two preceding indirect questions is God: Galen does not know whether he is corporeal or incorporeal and where he is located. So why should he add *scilicet deitas*? Secondly, there is the related question why the Latin version here uses *deitas* rather than *deus* (*deus* in 56,23 and 58,8). Are the two terms here used interchangeably, as they often are, or does *deitas* here have a special meaning? Thirdly, the Latin, but not the Hebrew version seems to identify God with his power. Nutton rightly notes that Galen never identifies God with his power or, for that matter, with the divine powers. Hence he considers deleting the reference to the divine power or the divine powers as being due to the familiar phenomenon of expansion in the process of translation (p.134; cf. also p.31). But it hardly solves the problem to consider *id est virtus deitatis* as due to expansion in translation. For now *illa* in the next sentence (56,21) will refer to *deitas*, and thus God again will be identified with his powers. Thus, if we assume that *id est virtus deitatis* does not correspond to anything in Galen's original text, we will also have to assume that Galen's next sentence originally started like this "his are the powers whose …", (*et illius sunt virtutes*), assuming a corruption of a pronoun in the genitive singular. Nutton himself in his translation deals with the problem by rendering *id est virtus deitatis* by "or rather the power of the deity". The force of the *id est* clause now would not be to identify God with the power of God, but rather to clarify or modify the question raised concerning God's location, explaining that this might be rather a question concerning God's power. Perhaps we could achieve the same result by translating "that is to say the power of God" or by translating "or, to be more precise, the power of God". Galen had said that he does not know whether God is corporeal or incorporeal. If God were a body, we could ask for his location. If God is incorporeal, there is a question as to whether he can have a location. But even in this case there might be a question as to the location of God's power.

Galen here in *Plac.Prop.* 7, 1 (p.76,25-78,5) expresses the view that, even if the soul were immortal and incorporeal, this would not rule out its inhabiting a body. In this sense it would have a location. And Galen certainly locates the faculties or powers of the soul in different parts of the body, for instance the natural faculty, that is the natural powers, in the liver. But it is far from clear whether what he considers as a possibility for the human soul, namely that it inhabits a body, though incorporeal, he also considers as a possibility for God, if he is incorporeal. And in any case, Galen, by parity of reasoning, must assume that, if the soul is incorporeal, it is not ruled out that it itself is not located in the body, though the faculties and powers he distinguishes are. Plotinus, indeed, in *Enn.* 4, 8, seems to take the view that the soul is not located in the body. He certainly says of the world-soul that it is not in the world, but governs the world by the presence in it of its least power (4, 8, 2, 33). It is clear, also from the language and the imagery, that Plotinus in this text is heavily influenced by Ps.Aristotle's *De mundo* or a closely related text, just as Alexander of Aphrodisias is in *Quaestiones* 2, 3, a text to which we will return later. The author of *De mundo* in 398 b 1 ff. argues that just as it would not be fitting for the Great King to leave his palace to involve himself in the actual details of the διοίκησις of his realm, it would be all the more unfitting for God to leave his place on high. He, instead, lets his power pervade the whole world and make the sun and the moon and the heaven move in the appropriate way. Here God himself is not in the world (and thus presumably incorporeal), but his power is in the whole of the world. Thus, to return to Galen, if God is incorporeal, the question of his location might turn into the question of the location of his power.

Now, even if Galen nowhere else does identify God with his power, it still remains a question whether Galen could identify God with his power. The answer, obviously, is that he could, if he had a certain conception of God, namely as something absolutely simple. In fact, some in antiquity took the view that the soul is the same with its powers, because its οὐσία is incomposite. This is the view Iamblichus ascribed to Plato (*ap.* Stob. *Ecl.* I p.367,11-14 W.). By contrast Iamblichus ascribed to the Stoics the view that the soul is a corporeal οὐσία to be distinguished from its powers which are qualities of this οὐσία (*ibid.* 17-21). Also for Galen the question arises in the case of the soul. But since he does not know what the οὐσία of the soul is, and hence does not know whether the soul is corporeal or incorporeal, but does specify the powers of the soul, he at least cannot have a definitive view as to whether the soul just is its powers. *A fortiori*, it seems to me, as long as it is a question for Galen whether God is corporeal or not, it cannot be his definitive view that God just is his power. In any case, just as Galen insists that we are aware of the power of the soul and hence know that there is a soul, though he does not know what the οὐσία of the soul is, what it really is that has this power, so he in our chapter also insists that he is aware of the power of God, but does not know what the οὐσία of God is, what it really is that has this power. Now it might be the case that God's οὐσία is such that he just is his power. But as long as we do not know what his οὐσία is, we are not in a position to say that God is his power. Hence it would be strange, if Galen here identified God with his power.

With this we can turn to the second problem raised by the *scilicet* — clause, its use of *deitas*. *Deitas* in principle could be the translation of an Arabic word, distinct from the word for God, which would be used to render θειότης. Θειότης is extremely rare in pagan Greek, but it does occur, for instance, in Plutarch, *Quaest.conviv.* 4, 2, 2, 665 A, in Alcinous, *Didasc.* 10, p.164,33 Hermann, and in the *Corpus Hermeticum* 9, 1. The meaning is somewhat of a puzzle, but the Hermetic text sheds some light on it: God differs from the activity of the intellect. So 'divinity' or 'deity' would refer to what God does. This would also fit the Plutarch passage and a number of other texts. So 'deity' in this sense could be identified with the exercise of God's power or even the power itself, especially if we assume that it is always exercised. The point of the *scilicet* clause now would be to modify the question about the location of God; it is supposed to be understood, if necessary, as a question as to the location of God's activity in ordering the world. But there are three more occurrences of *deitas* in our text (2, 1, p.56,20; 2, 3, p.58,17 & 20). The three passages can all be given more or less tolerable sense, given this meaning of *deitas*, but in all of them we would rather expect Galen to talk of God. This leaves us with the first problem, as to why he used a *scilicet* clause at all. The answer, given the preceding discussion, should be that Galen is trying to make room for the possible answer that though God himself has no location, his power does.

There is one further point worth drawing attention to. Galen clearly and explicitly in this text talks of God's power. But the Hebrew version, precisely in the place in which the Latin version is corrupt, explicitly talks of "his power and his providence" (2, 2, p.59,14). Even if Galen did not explicitly talk of providence in this passage, he clearly implicitly does. For he does talk about the purposeful structure of animals, the help we receive in divination or through dreams, the signs God sends, his cures, his saving persons. All this clearly comes under the heading of providence. Now there is a question as to the nature of the providence Galen ascribes to the Demiurge, for instance in *UP*. This question has been caught up in the controversy as to whether Galen basically is a Platonist or a Peripatetic. Paul Moraux in particular has taken the latter view. Correspondingly he argues (for instance in *Der Aristotelismus bei den Griechen* II [Berlin 1984], 771 ff.) that Galen in his conception of providence follows a Peripatetic line, according to which divine providence only extends down to the sublunary sphere to the extent that it is responsible for the features living beings have in virtue of belonging to a species, that Galen nowhere indicates that God takes an interest in, say, the welfare of particular human beings. But it does seem to me that according to our passage God does take an interest in the welfare of particular human beings in particular circumstances. And this still is true, if it should turn out that God leaves it to divine agents to make the particular provisions his providence demands. In *UP* 10, 14 Galen explains how our visual apparatus is arranged in such a way that, though we have two eyes, we do not as a result see double; to the contrary, our visual power thus is doubled. To show the first requires some mathematics, and Galen here, afraid to put off his readers, as often also in other writings, had decided to pass the matter over. But a god (θεὸς δέ τις) told him to give an account also of this fact with all the mathematical apparatus required, as he then did (II p.110,7 Helmreich = III 837,5 K). Surely this god was concerned with what Galen was doing and made him do the right thing, thus showing providence for Galen and those who might read his work who would now encounter another impressive piece of evidence for the consummate art with which the body is constructed. And given that *Plac.Prop.* 2 seems to count such activities of the gods among the workings of God, it would seem clear that the providence of Galen's God does extend to individual human beings. Galen's view in this matter seems to be rather along Platonist lines.

In spite of all these difficulties the basic thought in chapter 2 of the *De placitis propriis* down to p.58,17 is reasonably clear. Galen does know that there is God. He does know this because of the workings of God which we can observe. They reveal a marvellous power which must be the power of God. But Galen does not know what the answer to some other questions about God is, to begin with the question what God really is, what it is that has this power. But, according to Galen we are none the worse off for not knowing what God's substance is.

Now this agnosticism (as it has been called) about God, and similarly about the world as a whole, about the soul, and about the celestial bodies, has been diagnosed by Moraux and others as revealing Galen's sound sense of the limitations of human knowledge and his aversion to idle speculation. I have no inclination to question this diagnosis. But if it is taken a step further by claiming that this agnosticism reveals scientistic leanings on Galen's part who would rather give a natural explanation for everything than to have to refer to God, the soul, and the divine celestial bodies, I would disagree. It seems to me that the final lines of our chapter, 2, 3, p.58,17-21, reveal that Galen's preceding remarks, and in particular the agnostic remarks, do not just reflect a robust awareness of our cognitive limitations, but are equally a reflection of a religious attitude on Galen's part. Galen here says that he sees that in matters divine he should follow the law and accept Socrates' teaching. The reference to Socrates parallels the reference to Socrates in *PHP* 9, 7, 16 (p.588,29-33 De Lacy = V 781,10-15 K) at the end of a list of questions concerning the world and God almost all of which according to Galen it is useless to pursue.

For Socrates Galen gives Xenophon as his source. De Lacy in the *apparatus fontium* to *PHP* 9, 7, 16 refers to the *Memorabilia* 1, 1, 11-16. This reference is appropriate enough for the passage in *PHP*. But Nutton (*app.font.*) thinks that also our text refers to this passage. This seems doubtful since *Mem.* 1, 1, 11-16 does not explain the reference to a law in the Latin version and the corresponding "as ordained by religion" in the Hebrew. But there is another passage in the *Memorabilia*, 4, 3, 13 ff., in which Xenophon does have Socrates talk about a law and gives advice as to how one should treat the gods. The whole chapter 4, 3 is of such interest for our purposes that I summarise it in some detail. According to Xenophon Socrates tried to persuade people that what mattered most was soundness of mind, but in particular soundness of mind in regard to the gods. How Socrates went about this we are supposed to see from a discussion Socrates had with Euthydemus. It begins with a long catalogue of the ways in which the gods provide for us, indeed an account of how the whole world is arranged in such a way as to benefit us and to provide us with what we need. Part of this providential endowment is that we have been given perception, reason and language; and, if with all this we sometimes still do not know what prudence requires, the gods are prepared to assist us by means of divination (4, 3, 11-12). At the outset Euthydemus had confessed that so far he had given all this no thought, but as Socrates goes on to spell out how the gods care for us, Euthydemus quickly catches on, makes remarks to the effect that we should be thankful to the gods, but also points out that Socrates seems to be particularly dear to the gods, since they tell him what to do and what not to do (12). Socrates passes this remark over; instead he now exhorts Euthydemus not to wait till he sees the gods in their actual shape and form, but to venerate and to honour them just on the basis of seeing their works (ἔργα). The gods themselves seem to indicate that this is their will. For not just the other gods distribute their benefits without showing themselves in the open, even the god who orders and preserves the whole world, in his administering the world and doing the greatest deeds remains himself invisible; all we see is what he is doing. Even the sun does not allow people to see it precisely, but deprives those who shamelessly try to do so of their eye-sight. Even the servants of the gods, like thunder bolts and winds, are themselves invisible. And so is the soul, which is divine, if anything about us is. She rules in us, but remains herself invisible. The conclusion Socrates draws is this (14): we ought to realize the power of the gods on the basis of what we see happening, and to honour the divine. At this point Euthydemus anxiously asks how he can appropriately thank the gods for all their care. Socrates assures him that the Delphic Apollo gives the answer: by following the law of the city. Socrates explains: the law of the city everywhere is to honour the gods as well as one can by ἱερά.

Now, I think, there can be little doubt that this is the passage Galen has in mind. Here is the law, and here is the precept Socrates gives as us to how one should be pious, to be sound of mind in regard to the gods. There are a great number of parallels in detail, for instance the detail that we have to content ourselves with seeing the works of the gods and worshipping them on the basis of this, without seeing the gods themselves, or the reference to the great power of the gods revealed to us in their works, or the reference to their boundless providence, the reference to divination, but also the reference to the god who rules the world and is responsible for its order. Galen's claim to know that God exists, but not to know his οὐσία, clearly is in the spirit of Xenophon's remarks. In fact, Galen in claiming this is giving expression to a religious view which must have been widespread among the educated in late antiquity and which we encounter in more or less the same words in Flavius Josephus, *Contra Apionem* 2, 117. According to Josephus Moses has taught the Jews to believe that God is one, known to us by his power, while it is unknown (or unknowable, ἄγνωστον) what he is like in his οὐσία. It would be a mistake to think that Josephus is referring to a specifically Jewish belief. This would undermine his purpose. He is responding to Apion's polemical attack on Jews and Judaism. Josephus' remark is meant to show that what Moses taught the Jews is what many, if not most, educated pagans in his day believed.

In fact, as we can even see in this very text, Galen himself tries to follow the law and Socrates' precept, though this here is slightly obscured by Nutton's translation. Socrates teaches that we should honour the gods of the city as well as we can by ἱερά. In the Latin version the final lines of the chapter are introduced by *et video quod debeam praedicare*, rendered by Nutton as "and I see that I should declare… the law…". But what Galen seems to be saying is that he sees that he should praise God. Correspondingly the Hebrew version says "Therefore I thought that I should exalt and praise them <sc. the divine powers>" (p.59,28-29). If we turn to the *De usu partium*, we find Galen telling us in 3, 10 (I p.174,5-17 = III 237,9-238,3 K) that he is composing a true hymn on our creator. True piety, he says, does not consist in the sacrifice of many oxen or the burning of a fortune's worth of incense, but in grasping first oneself, and then expounding to others, the wisdom and the power and the goodness of the Demiurge. He characterises his treatise as a ἱερὸς λόγος. Galen presents the last book of *UP*, 17, as an epode, to be compared to the hymns to the gods the worshippers sing in front of the altar (17, 3, II p.451,19-27 = IV 365,13-366 K). Obviously Galen understands the injunction to honour the gods as well as one can by ἱερά as amounting in his case to writing something like the *De usu partium*. He tells us in *UP* 17, 1 (II p.448,3-8 = IV 361,1-5 K) that being introduced to the use of the parts constitutes an initiation into mysteries everybody should be introduced to, far superior to the Eleusinian or Samothracian mysteries. Obviously Galen has a certain understanding of what it is to be pious as well as one can, but there is no reason to doubt that he is serious in what he is saying, to suspect that all this is just literary form. Galen must have thought that those who expressed their piety in more conventional ways did so because in this way they honoured the gods as well as they could.

Now the injunction was more specifically to follow the law of the city, to worship the gods of the city according to established custom. And we have already seen that Galen refers to Asclepius as ὁ πάτριος θεός and declares himself a worshipper of the god (*Lib.Prop.* 2, *Scripta min.* II p.99,11 = XIX 19,3 K). So he also follows the injunction in this regard. But just as Galen has a conception of his own of what true piety consists in, what the appropriate sacrifice is, what the mysteries are which one should be initiated into, we might also wonder whether Galen had a conception of his own of Asclepius and of the worship appropriate for him. There has been a discussion as to what Galen is referring to when he calls himself a θεραπευτής of the god. Is this referring to a function of the cult of Asclepius, or to Galen's participation in the cult, or to worship in the sense in which the practice of medicine and the writing of medical books might be conceived of as worship (cf. F. Kudlien, "Galen's Religious Belief", in *Galen. Problems and Prospects,* ed. by V. Nutton [London 1981], 120-121)?

But, before we turn to this, I want to briefly look at a passage in Macrobius' *Saturnalia*, the speech of Praetextatus. It sheds some light on the talk of powers in *Plac.Prop.* 2; though considerably later than Galen (around 430 A.D.), it reflects on how already in Galen's time educated persons may have thought of Asclepius and his relation to God. In this speech all gods are said to stand in a certain relation to Zeus who is identified with the sun (*Sat.* 1, 17, 2; 23, 1). This claim at the very outset (1, 17, 2) is qualified: it only holds for the gods within the world, thus leaving room for a God or gods who transcend this world. The unique position of the sun within this world is supposed to be due to the fact that the sun governs the stars which regulate our affairs here on earth, such that what happens around us down here is due to the sun (1, 17, 3). What precisely the relation between the gods and the sun is remains somewhat unclear, except that it is not outright identity. What is clear is that the different gods are associated with the different effects the sun has, directly or through the stars, on our affairs. These different effects are ascribed to different powers (*virtutes*) of the sun (1, 17, 4). Accordingly Asclepius is introduced in 1, 20, 1 as the power (*vis*) of the sun to heal. Already in 1, 17, 5 Apollo had been presented as the power of the sun which is responsible for divination and healing. Hence in 1, 20, 4 Asclepius and Apollo are identified.

There are a good number of other late ancient texts which reveal a similar religious or theological view, associating the different gods with the various powers of the god who rules this world, powers we are aware of through their effects. But the immediate relevance of this text to Galen's *Plac.Prop.* 2 and his view of Asclepius should be clear. It clearly is not Galen's considered view that the Demiurge is the sun. Otherwise he could not say in *Plac.Prop.* 2 that he cannot answer the question whether the Creator is corporeal or not. We will later see that in *UP* it is his tentative view that the sun is not the Demiurge, but rather an instrument in his creation.

But it does look, as if Galen has to somehow identify Asclepius with the Divine power to heal and to send us signs or with that which has this power. This leaves open a considerable number of possibilities. One is that Galen identifies Asclepius with God insofar as he has this power. Another is that he identifies Asclepius with an instrument or an agent through whom God exercises this power or to whom God has given this power. Another is that Galen hypostasises this power, as Philo is tempted to hypostasize the power of God. But whichever possibility we choose, it will be the case that if Asclepius heals somebody, it will ultimately be God who heals the person.

Now there is no doubt that Asclepius played an important role in Galen's life. If we are right in assuming that Galen at the end of *Plac.Prop.* 2 refers to Xenophon's *Memorabilia* 4, 3, the law referred to in *Plac.Prop.* is the law of one's city which enjoins one in the first instance to worship the gods of the city, the ancestral gods. In the case of Pergamum, by Galen's time, Asclepius is one of the ancestral gods, perhaps the most important one in the life of the city. Galen, as we saw, refers to Asclepius as ὁ πάτριος θεός. And we know from various passages in Galen himself what an important role the god played in Galen's life. Galen's father had made him study medicine prompted by a dream. Galen thought that his life had been saved by a dream sent by the god. And Galen was willing to be guided by evident dreams not just in his life, but also in his medical practice.

But the question here is how Galen thought of Asclepius and what attitude he took towards him. F. Kudlien in his article "Galen's Religious Belief" (in *Galen. Problems and Prospects*, ed. by V. Nutton [London 1981], 117-130) on p.117 claims: "But I think that Galen's feelings towards at least one of the Greek gods — Asclepius — were more intimate, more personal ones. The demiurge god, as one may say with Grant, 'is nature', which in fact means a certain degree of abstraction. To state, however, that 'for Galen nature has taken the religious meaning that the gods formerly had' (Grant), is in my opinion an over-generalization". I am inclined to think that both Kudlien and Grant are wrong.

It is true, as we can see from *UP*, that Galen identified the Demiurge with nature. It is also true, as we can see from *UP*, that Galen thinks that many talk of nature in a vague, unreflected way as being responsible for natural phenomena. But it is not true that Galen himself has this vague, somewhat abstract notion of nature. It rather is the case that Galen thinks that what happens naturally or in nature is ultimately the work of the Demiurge. And this Demiurge is not some abstract principle. Though Galen cannot say what it is that is the Demiurge, it is the Demiurge of Plato's *Timaeus* who is responsible for the order of the world and for what happens in the world naturally, things we can observe and only explain by recourse to a Demiurge who, for instance, is good, just, wise, provident. It is this Demiurge whom Galen took to be the God worshipped, for instance, by the Jews, as we see in a famous passage in *UP* 11, 14, though Galen thinks that God is misconceived by the Jews. But there is not the slightest suggestion that he is misconceived by them, because they think of him as a person. It is rather that they fail to acknowledge the rationality and the providence involved in the creation. As to Asclepius, it seems to me to be clear on the basis of the part of *Plac.Prop.* 2 which we have considered so far that Galen must think that he owes his cure by Asclepius to the Demiurge.

This becomes even clearer, if we are right in our interpretation of *Plac.Prop.* 2, 3 (p.58,17-18) *et video quod debeam praedicare*. This means something like "and I see that I should sing the praise of God". Galen obviously does think of God as the object of his praise and hence his worship. And he seems to think that in worshipping Asclepius, he is worshipping God, though it remains somewhat unclear how he understands the relation between Asclepius and God, except that the power of healing has its origins in God.

At this point it may be relevant to refer to the fact that at least some of Galen's fellow citizens in his life-time, and among them some of the more educated citizens, also had their own views about the relation between Asclepius and Jupiter, and thus perhaps about the relation between Asclepius and God, the ruler of the world. For the new sanctuary of Asclepius which was built in Pergamum in Galen's youth was dedicated to Zeus Asklepios or to Zeus Soter Asklepios. It was erected by Rufinus who had become a Roman senator and then had retired in his home town after having served as consul. After him the new complex was called Ῥουφίνιον ἄλσος. Now Galen was not only perfectly aware of the fact that the new temple was dedicated to Zeus Asklepios, as we can see from *AA* 1, 2 (II 224,15 ff. K). Here Galen refers to Rufinus as the man who was building the new temple of Zeus Asklepios for the Pergamenes. Galen also must have known why the temple was dedicated to Zeus Asklepios. For it is likely that he knew Rufinus anyway. And he tells us that his teacher in medicine, Satyrus, was spending his fourth year in Pergamum staying with Rufinus. In any case, Aelius Aristides, a friend of Rufinus and somebody Galen also will have known, tells us (*Or.* 42, 4): "The powers of Asklepios are great and many; or rather all powers are his... And it is precisely because of this that the people here [*sc.* in Pergamum] erected a temple for Zeus Asklepios". Aristides adds that if his teacher is to be relied upon in this regard, Asclepius is the ruler and the saviour (σωτήρ) of the world. He notes, though, that some say that Asklepios is the son of Apollon and hence the grandson of Zeus. This will have been a traditional view in Pergamum. But if we follow Aelius Aristides Rufinus and his friends not just identified Asklepios with Zeus insofar as he has, or is the source of, the power of healing or of sending signs, but took the further step of simply identifying Asklepios with Zeus by attributing all power and the rule over this world to Asklepios. We can only speculate whether some of them identified Zeus in turn with the sun. In this context it should be noted that of the large number of votive inscriptions found in Pergamum there is at least one (nr.63, *Altertümer von Pergamon*, VIII 3: C. Habicht, *Die Inschriften des Asklepieions* [Berlin 1969], p.103) which is dedicated to Zeus Soter Asklepios. An Aemilius Sabinus and an Aemilius Herennianus offer thanks for having been saved in the Atlantic and from the barbarians. We also find three votive inscriptions dedicated to Zeus Asklepios in Epidaurus (*IG* IV^2 1, 399, 470, 481) and one in Hermione (*IG* IV 692).

With this we can turn to the details of Galen's theology. Galen's talk in *UP* 17, 1 of an accurate theology makes it natural to proceed by discussing first those things Galen claims to know about God, to then turn to his more speculative views about God's ordering of the world. Galen in *UP* 17, 1 asserts that the study of the use of the parts will constitute a true or proper starting point for an accurate theology. What he seems to have in mind is this. If we study the use of the parts of human beings or of animals, especially of we advance to an anatomical study of the parts, we by observation ascertain certain facts. And from these facts we can safely infer certain theological truths. We have a true or proper starting-point, because we base our inferences not on speculative assumptions or hypotheses, but on what we can observe to be the case, and hence on something that is evident. The sort of evidence Galen relies on is this. If we study a part of the body we can determine what use it serves. When we study the part more closely we see that it is constructed in such a way as not just to serve this use, but to serve it, all things considered, optimally. We may wonder whether this is manifest. But Galen believes he is able to show this. On the basis of this sort of evidence, and certainly on the basis of the evidence accumulated from the study of all the different parts, Galen thinks he can make certain inferences about God. For these inferences to yield conclusions which constitute an accurate theology, it also must be the case that the facts observed unequivocally indicate certain theological truths. It is not clear how, formally speaking, Galen thinks of these inferences. They seem to be a matter of indication (ἔνδειξις, cf. *UP* 17, 1, II p.447,20 = IV 360,10-11 K): we make an inference from something manifest to what we need to assume to explain it. In any case, Galen seems to assume that the manifest facts, either taken severally or jointly, allow for no other explanation than that there is a God and that there are certain things true about him. But Galen, of course, realizes that not everybody will grant him this. And so Galen, to judge from remarks he makes repeatedly, for instance in *UP* 17, 1, II p.446,3-7 (= IV 358,8-11 K), seems to think that any right-minded, reasonable, unbiased person in view of the stated facts about the use and the construction of the parts, will come to the conclusions he wants to draw. If, for instance, a person dogmatically clings to an atomist view of the world and with it to the claim that this world has come about by chance, this person will also resist Galen's theological views. But such a person, in Galen's opinion, is unreasonable. And Galen in *UP* goes out of his way to show in detail that it is quite unreasonable to assume that animals of the design we encounter could be the product of chance, but also to argue that an atomist does not have the resources to explain the structure of animals, because atomism does not allow for the complete mixture of substances. Hence Galen feels entitled to draw his conclusions, because he believes he can show that those who resist them do so, because they make assumptions which are unfounded or even patently mistaken. Hence Galen has no qualms to speak of these theological conclusions as a matter of evident cognition (*UP* 15, 7, II p.364,22 = IV 248,9-10 K).

Galen does not say that the study of the use of the parts is the starting point, but a starting point, because, as we can see from *Plac.Prop.* 2, observations about the design of animals are not the only evidence available to us on which to base theological conclusions. There is also the order of the world in general, there are the cures, there is divination, there are persons saved from death. But Galen clearly thinks that the study of the parts provides particularly striking and uncontroversial evidence for the desired conclusions. Take the case of the young man in Smyrna, described in *UP* 8, 10 (I p.481,22-482,1 = III 664,3-8 K). The anterior ventricle of his heart was badly wounded, but he survived, by the will of God, it was thought. This, according to Galen, turns out to be right, but not quite in the way people will have thought. For Galen points out that the young man would not have had a chance to survive, if both ventricles had been wounded. On the other hand, it is the providential function of double organs that one continues to serve, if the other is affected. So in this sense the young man's survival was due to God's providence.

As we have seen already in *Plac.Prop.* 2, one inference Galen believes to be able to draw from the observable evidence is that of the existence of a Demiurge or God. This is an indirect inference from the overwhelming power and wisdom revealed, for instance, in the design of animals. There hence must be something, even if we cannot say what it is, which has this power or wisdom. What is presupposed by this argument, as I already indicated, is another argument. Galen relies on the assumption that there are just two possibilities: either the world we live in is a world of atoms of some kind or another which by chance have come to form a world like ours, or it is a world formed by an agent of unimaginable wisdom and power. One reason why we can reject the former view is that material living beings presuppose the complete mixture of the elements, that is, as we might say, chemical compounds. Such compounds presuppose that the elements permeate each other completely, or that at least their characteristic qualities mix, in such a way as to give rise to a new kind of body with new properties of its own. This presupposes that the elements are continuous and hence infinitely divisible bodies, rather than discrete minimal bodies of some kind or other without any quality. Such discrete minimal bodies by definition cannot form a genuine mixture (κρᾶσις or μῖξις) or a compound with new qualities; they can only be juxtaposed to each other (παράθεσις), the way different kinds of flour when mixed will still not form a genuine compound, but a mass in which the small particles will be merely juxtaposed, but remain identifiable as particles of wheat, rye, or barley, however finely we grind them. Now Galen in *Temp.* 1, 9 (p.34,5-15 Helmreich = I 562,15-563,9 K) claims that only God or nature can produce a genuine complete mixture, whereas human beings can only produce something which looks like a mixture of the eye, but is not (for instance, in our terms, a suspension which looks like a solution). We can only act on things by contact from the outside, whereas God or nature can pervade matter and bring about from the inside a total change (*De causis procatarcticis* VII 81). This is not to deny that we can produce alloys, but just to say that the most we can do is to juxtapose two or more substances in such a way that they, under the appropriate conditions, because of a divine force in them, will form a genuine compound. Atoms, needless to say, can only act on each other by touch. They cannot pervade each other. Thus bodies cannot be formed from atoms, and their formation involves a power which is God's or comes from God.

This presupposed, Galen thinks that the evidence unequivocally shows that there is a God, that he is of an enormous power, that he is perfectly wise, that he is good, that he is just, that he is provident. I will not go into the details of how Galen thinks that all this is borne out by the evidence. I just want to note that, if Galen were right, his theology, though so far only consisting of a relatively short list of propositions, would be a considerable achievement. A measure of this is the fact that we learn from Sextus Empiricus (*PH* 3, 2-12) that the major issues among philosophers were the question whether God or gods exist and whether there is Divine providence. Galen would at least have settled these questions. Granting this, we might want to know how, on the basis of this list of propositions, we are going to proceed further in theology. Galen makes no suggestions about this. One has to wonder whether, given Galen's views, he would have been able to proceed much beyond such a list of propositions. This will become clearer, if we now turn to his theological speculations.

According to Galen we do know that there is a Demiurge who is responsible for the order of things in the world, for instance for the way human beings are constructed. We might find the claim that the construction of human beings is unequivocal evidence for the existence of God more persuasive, if it came accompanied by an explanation of how it is that God accounts for the structure of human beings, of how he brings it about that human beings have this structure. Given what has been said, it should be clear that Galen would not have much sympathy with this complaint, in fact may find it blasphemous. Nevertheless, he in the course of *UP*, but in particular in *UP* 17, 1 does make some tantalizingly vague remarks about what might be involved in such an account. Not surprisingly he tends to qualify these remarks with terms like "probable" (cf., e.g. 17, 1, II p.446,16 = IV 359,3 K).

Given the tradition in which Galen stands, it is not astonishing that Galen attributes a crucial role to the sun (*UP* 17, 1,

II p.446,15 and 447,8 ff. = IV 359,1-2 and 15 ff. K). After all the sun is responsible for the seasons, the seasonal changes, growth and decay, periodic generation and corruption. There would be no life on earth without the sun. In religious thought in late antiquity the sun increasingly takes a central place and tends to become the god which rules the world. But P.L. Donini ("Motivi filosofici in Galeno", in *PP* 35 [1980], 354) has drawn attention to a very important passage in *UP* 3, 10 (I p.176,13-177,23 = III 240,10-242,8 K) which rules out the possibility that Galen identifies the Demiurge with the planet. The passage is interesting for two reasons: it involves the claim that the sun does not have its position relative to the other planets, and thus to the earth, of its own, but receives is as part of the ordering of the world, and it gives the sun an astronomically 'unorthodox' position, namely as the middle or fourth planet. Galen says that the sun's being of the size and the sort (τοιούτῳ ... οἷος ...) it is is due to itself, but its being positioned in this place of the world is the work of him who gives the world its order (τοῦ διακοσμοῦντος ἔργον). For the place the sun has is the best place for it in the world (I p.176,21-177,1 = III 241,1-5 K). For if it were placed lower, say in the place of the moon, everything around here would go up in flames. If it were placed in the place of some higher planet, the earth equally would be uninhabitable (I p.176,17-21 = III 240,14-17 K). So the orbit of the sun is not determined by the sun, but by the Demiurge. The Demiurge places it in an orbit with a view to the effects of the course of the sun on life on earth.

One implication of Galen's distinction between the two kinds of truths about the sun is that, when the sun is put on its orbit as part of the ordering of the world, it already exists as a body of a certain sort and size. Hence it, as a body of a certain kind, is not the result of God's ordering. In this sense it is precosmic. Hence, presumably, it is eternal. Now, what is true of the sun in this regard also is true of the stars in general. But it is rather more difficult to imagine that the Demiurge reduces a chaos to order which already involves well-formed bodies like the stars than to envisage him giving shape to a pre-existing chaotic matter. So this is a further reason to think that Galen in fact must be thinking of the world and its order as eternal and correspondingly of the Demiurge as eternally creating and maintaining the order of things, by, for instance, creating ever new specimens of the various kinds of mortal things. And Galen also must be thinking that it is not literally true that the sun is put on its orbit by the Demiurge. It always has been on this orbit. But that it is on this orbit is, in a way not explained, due to the rule of the Demiurge.

But the passage is also interesting for another reason, because of the place it attributes to the sun in the order of the planets; it is placed in the middle, that is as the fourth of the seven planets. This is of significance in two regards. This is not the classical order we find in Plato, Eudoxus, or Aristotle, where the sequence is Moon, Sun, Venus, Mercury, Mars, Jupiter, Saturn, but one that did become the standard order later, namely Moon, Mercury, Venus, Sun, Mars, Jupiter, Saturn. This is attested first for Diogenes of Babylon, a student of Chrysippus (Cicero, *Div.* 2, 91). This order apparently is of Babylonian origin and presumably came to Greece before Diogenes. In thinking about this rather dramatic change in the order of the planets, it might be of some use to take account of a passage in Simplicius' *Commentary on Aristotle's Physics* 2, 2, CAG IX p.291,21-292,31 Diels (= Posidonius, Fr.18 Edelstein-Kidd). It quotes a text Simplicius has taken from Alexander's lost commentary in which Alexander quotes Geminus' *Epitome* of Posidonius' work or works on celestial phenomena. The point made is this. The phenomena of stellar, in particular planetary motion are compatible with any number of mathematical models or sets of hypotheses of the kind astronomers develop. In order to decide which of them is true one has to be a natural philosopher who knows about the οὐσία and the δύναμις of things, why it is better for things to be this way, and various other things which are not the concern of the mathematical astronomer. So, if one has some view of the οὐσία of the sun, or at least of its δύναμις, and of why it is better for the sun to have the middle position, one might opt for the corresponding mathematical model. Now it seems that those who chose the middle position for the sun did so to do justice to what they thought was the elated position of the sun not just relative to what happens to things on earth, but also relative to the stars. The sun is the leader of the planets who accompany it on both sides. At least sometimes it seems to be thought that it governs or controls their motions. In any case the central position attributed to the sun now clearly reflects the crucial role attributed to it in the functioning of the kosmos as a whole.

We already vaguely begin to see how Galen imagines things to be. The Demiurge creates living bodies of a certain kind. But he does not directly involve himself in this. He rather brings it about that the sun moves in a certain way. And the sun controls the motion of the other planets. And the stars by their joint motion have an effect on life here on earth which is profound. In fact some would think that life here on earth is controlled by the motion of the planets. In fact Alexander of Aphrodisias (*Quaest.* 2, 3, *Suppl.Arist.* II 2, p.48,15 ff. Bruns) presents it as a common view that the divine body, that is the sun or more generally the heaven, by its motion communicates a power to the body adjacent to it, which is propagated all the way down to earth and is responsible not just for there being living beings, but even rational beings. It is something along these lines that also Galen seems to be thinking.

There is an intriguing parallel to this passage in Galen's *UP* 3, 10 about the way the Demiurge accounts for the path the sun takes in the hymn to the sun to be found on another inscription in Pergamum, published by H. Hepding (*MDAI* [*A*] 32 [1907], 356-360, inscription nr.115).[2] It is a votive offering by one "Aelius Nico, architect". It is of particular interest, since we

[2] Cf. on this also *Steinepigramme aus dem griechischen Osten* I, hrsg. von R. Merkelbach und J. Stauber (Stuttgart 1998), 605-607.

know from the *Suda* (*s.v.* Galenos) that Galen's father's name was "Nico". Moreover we know that Galen's father was an architect. Unfortunately we know from Pergamene inscriptions of two persons called "Nico", both architects, the other a "Julius Nicodemus, also called Nico". For both of them we have several inscriptions, and in both cases the date of the inscriptions would fit Galen's father; Aelius Nico has a slight edge, because, like Galen's father, he obviously is interested in numbers, in geometry, in fact stereometry, and in astronomy. But whether or not he is Galen's father, the hymn is of interest, since it reflects the view of an educated Pergamene citizen contemporary with Galen. Lines 2-4 are a somewhat unfortunate adaptation of Euripides' *Phoenissae* 3-5. They address Helios who sends his rays to mortal beings, fixes the course of the sun, but also (lines 5-6) sees to the orderly motion of earth, water, air, and fire. Obviously "Helios" in these lines does double duty. It once refers to the celestial visible body, but then also to something else which puts the sun on its orbit, very much like Galen's Demiurge. We are also reminded of the distinction Praetextatus makes between the sun and something higher than even the sun.

There are then two issues which we need to get clearer about. The first is how, according to Galen, the sun is crucially involved in maintaining the order of the world, in particular the sublunary world of generation and corruption. The second issue is what sort of thing, in Galen's mind, the Demiurge could possibly be and how he manages to make the sun move in the way it has to move, if it is to maintain the desirable order of the world. The first problem is very much like the problem Alexander of Aphrodisias is trying to deal with in *Quaest.* 2, 3. The treatise begins with the question what the power is which the divine and hence immortal body communicates by its motion to the body contiguous with it which is subject to generation and mortal. The question is pressing because it is thought that it is this power which is the cause of there being bodies with a soul, that is living beings, and thus also of human beings having a rational soul. It is in this way that divine providence is thought to, for instance, have provided us with reason and an intellect (p.48,15-22 Bruns). The problem arises because we do not know whether this power communicated to the contiguous body is the very nature of this contiguous body, or, as it were, a second nature of it. It cannot be its very nature, because for there to be a contiguous body to which the heavenly body communicates this power, it already has to have its own nature to be an actual body. But if it is another nature added on to it, it does not seem to contribute anything to the perfection of the body, for instance the human being, because it as such already is rational (p.47,31-48,15 Bruns). Alexander then considers two views as to how the problem might be solved, of which presumably he favours the second. The first view is that the divine power is communicated to the simple bodies, the elements, but does not perfect them. They remain just what they are. But the power shows up in the composite bodies which result from the mixture of the elements. Their natures are the product not just of the natures of the elements, but also of the power communicated to them to different degrees, depending on their purity. It is thus that we get bodies which are alive or even intelligent (p.48,22-49,27 Bruns). On the second view we challenge the initial assumption that there already is an actual contiguous body to which a divine power is communicated. We assume that the power originating in the divine body is involved in the very formation of the elements and that it is the cause of their natures and powers. It is due to ever more complex mixtures of these bodies that we get bodies with highly complex and sophisticated powers which have, though, their source in the power which originates in the heavenly body (p.49,28-50,27 Bruns). There are several ideas Alexander here refers to, or even avails himself of, which seem to be widespread in his day, some of which also in some form or other are to be found in Ps. Aristotle's *De mundo*. There is the idea that living beings, including intelligent beings, are to be explained by appealing to a power, originating in a divine being, which spreads throughout the world. There is a chain of propagation of this power. It is handed down by contact with the next link in the chain. As it is handed down it diminishes. Thus, if it is communicated to fire, fire hands it on to air, air to water, water to earth, but earth will have very little of it or will have it in a very attenuated form, because it is gross, while fire is pure and subtle.

It clearly is against this background that we have to look at Galen's very sketchy account in *UP* 17, 1. If we do, it becomes clear that Galen thinks that the crucial power which is handed down is the power of understanding, the intellect, or, as we might want to say later, the power of cognition. He has an argument to the effect that an intellect of enormous power resides in the heavenly bodies, that is the stars and in particular the sun. And then he tries to explain how this cognitive power is communicated downwards so as to be found also on earth. The reason why he tries to do this is only partly apparent from our text here; it will explain why there are intelligent beings here on earth, namely human beings. But I assume that Galen also is thinking of the fact that there are perceptive beings on earth, namely animals, and that the formation of living beings quite generally requires a certain understanding.

Galen, then, makes the assumption, which he takes to be plausible (εἰκός), that a much better and sharper intellect resides in the sun, in the moon, and in the stars quite generally than in bodies on earth (17, 1, II p.446,16-19 = IV 359,2-6 K). His reason for thinking this is the following. Even in the filth down here on earth ("For what else shall we call what is composed of flesh, blood, phlegm, black and yellow bile?") we find beings which are highly rational with plenty of understanding, if we think of Plato, Aristotle, Hipparchus, or Archimedes (II p.446,23-447,7 = IV 359,9-17 K). But it is plausible to assume that the purer the material constitution of the body is, the more powerful the intellect will be which dwells in the body. But the material constitution of the celestial bodies, in particular the sun, is a marvel in its beauty and hence, presumably, in its purity (II p.446,13-16 = IV 358,17-359,3 K). Hence the celestial bodies, in the first instance the sun, must have an extremely powerful intellect. Galen here is presupposing that the elements themselves are ranked according to purity in the following order: fire, air, water, earth, and that accordingly the bodies mixed from them are, depending on the proportion of the different elements in the mixture, more or less pure, terrestrial bodies being the most impure because of the large proportion of water and earth they contain. He may also assume that the elements themselves come in purer or less pure forms. In any case, the heavenly bodies will consist of particularly pure fire and hence will be the purest, first among them the sun. Thus the sun will be the most intelligent.

Galen's next task then is to explain how this power of understanding which the sun and the stars have is communicated to what is below and contiguous with them. This he tries to do in II p.447,8-12 (= IV 359,17-360,4 K). It seems to him (δοκεῖ) that a rather remarkable intellect also is to be found in the air which is between us and the celestial bodies and which envelops us. Galen tries to explain this in the following way: it cannot be the case that the air participates in the bright light (αὐγή) of the sun, but not its power. By "its power" Galen must be referring to the powerful intellect of the sun. For he is trying to explain why one should believe that there is an intellect in the air. Thus the thought must be that the air also must share in the intellectual power of the sun, though it receives it in a diminished form. This is why the intellect in the air is called only "not inconsiderable". This is in accord with the principle that the power of the intellect depends on the purity of the matter of the body in which the intellect dwells. Presumably there is a connection between the air's sharing in the light of the sun and its receiving from the sun a not inconsiderable power of understanding. For the air, due to the light of the sun, itself becomes light-like (αὐγοειδές), and this makes it, or allows it to be, intelligent. We will pursue this further in a moment. So the sun due to its light fills the contiguous air with intellect or understanding. But the air which envelops us (II p.447,9-10 = IV 360,1-2 K) will pass this on to the terrestrial sphere. So an intellect of some power arrives even here on earth from the bodies above, though this is the impurest part of the world (II p.446,11-13; p.446,7-9 = IV 358,14-17; 358,11-13 K). One effect of this is that we get intelligent beings even here on earth (II p.446,23-447,7 = IV 359,9-15 K). But Galen also suggests that the intellect which arrives in the terrestrial sphere and spreads through it is responsible for the formation of animals quite generally (II p.446,7-11; 446,19-22 = IV 358,11-14; 359,6-9 K). He does this while saying at the same time that the formation of plants and animals in this filth reveals the power of the demiurgic intellect. So his view clearly is that the Demiurge does not directly create these plants and animals in this filth, but via a power which in a diminished form arrives on earth and which even in this diminished form produces such marvels. This, too, we need to pursue further by looking at other texts.

But before we do so, we have to assure ourselves that we are right in assuming that Galen wants to suggest that the power of the intellect quite literally is communicated to the terrestrial sphere via the air which is filled with the light of the sun. The way Moraux (*Der Aristotelismus bei den Griechen*, II 766) understands Galen's account, it involves a mere analogy. He says: "The activity of the celestial intellect extends down to the terrestrial world in such a way that this world participates in its power in a manner analogous to that in which the air surrounding us participates in the light of the sun." But it seems to me that Galen is trying to do more than merely to offer us an analogy. He is trying to explain why he thinks that the air is filled with intellect, and thus to explain how the terrestrial world shares in the power of the celestial intellect by sharing in the power of the intellect in the air. And there is an intellect in the air, because the air shares in the light of the sun. This is why

Galen says that it could not be the case that air shared in the light of the sun, but not in its intellectual power. That Galen assumes a close connection between intelligence or, more generally, cognition, and light, becomes clear if we look at the role light plays in Galen's doctrine of cognition.

Notoriously from Plato onwards down to late antiquity the αὐγή of the sun or of fire is referred to again and again in discussions of the soul and in particular of the cognitive powers of the soul. Thus Chrysippus, for instance, thought that the final state of total conflagration of the world consisted in a state of even distribution of fire in the form of αὐγή and that in this state the world had become a pure contemplative intellect. Platonists like Porphyry saw in the union of the sun's light and air an analogy to the union of soul and body. There is one place in Galen's doctrine in which a light-like substance plays a conspicuous role, namely in his theory of vision. This involves appeal to a certain kind of pneuma which Galen in *UP* sometimes calls "psychic" (7, 8, I p.394,6 = III 542,2 K), but more often αὐγοειδές or also φωτοειδές (8, 6, I p.464,14-19 = III 640,16-641,4 K; 10, 3, II p.66,2-5 = III 774,9-13 K; 16, 3, II p.384,16 = IV 275,12 K). It is produced in the ventricles of the brain, runs through the nerves which connect the eyes with the brain, and fills the eyes (*UP* 7, 8, I p.394,4-5 = III 541,18-542,1 K; 16, 3, II p.384,16-17 = IV 275,12-13 K). Hence also the eye is called αὐγοειδές (8, 6, I p.465,20 = III 642,10 K) or "the most light-like and the most sun-like" part of the body (*UP* 3, 10, I p.177,19-20 = III 242,3-5 K). Galen explains in *UP* 8, 6 (I 464,17-21 = III 641,2-6 K) why the organ of sight cannot be airy (ἀερῶδες), but must be pure and light-like, since otherwise we could not discriminate colours properly. It is in virtue of this psychic pneuma that we have the ability to see. Quite generally it seems to be his view that cognition presupposes psychic pneuma. It is then this pneuma which allows things to have cognition and some kind of understanding.

Against this background we can look at a passage in *PHP* 7, 7, 24-26 (p.474,20-29 De Lacy = V 643,9-644,3 K). Galen is criticizing the Stoic, the Epicurean, and, to some extent, the Aristotelian theory of vision. In his view the air surrounding us, when lit by the sun, is of the same character as the pneuma produced in the brain which allows the eyes to see (7, 7, 19, p.474,4-5 De Lacy = V 642,7-9 K). He claims that there is no difficulty in hypothesizing that the light (αὐγή) of the sun itself is perceptive, just as the pneuma in the eyes, which comes from the brain, being light-like (φωτοειδές), is perceptive. I note in passing that it now should be clear why the air contiguous with the sun becomes intelligent, because it becomes light-like.

But to return to the *PHP* 7, 7 passage, at this point Galen brings in the soul. According to Galen there are two possibilities: either the soul is corporeal, in which case it is to be identified with this, as it were, light-like and ethereal (αἰθερῶδες) pneuma, which is the position, he thinks, the Stoics and Aristotle are driven to; or the soul is incorporeal, and in this case this light-like pneuma constitutes the vehicle (ὄχημα) of the soul which it uses to communicate with the body. This, obviously, is a Platonist position. But Galen himself, notoriously, cannot make up his mind whether the soul is corporeal or incorporeal (cf. *Plac.Prop.* 3, 2, p.60,10-11).

With this in hand we can return to the account in *UP* 17, 1. We now understand how the sun by its light makes the air be endowed with a rational soul or an intellect. Air by itself, as we saw, according to Galen is not cognitive, not even perceptive. But by the light of the sun it becomes light-like. And now there are two possibilities, given that Galen does not want to commit himself to a view about the nature of the soul. If the soul is corporeal, the view will be that the sun by its light turns part of the air into light-like air and thus a soul in virtue of which the air has understanding. Or the soul is incorporeal. In this case the sun by its light turns part of the air into the appropriate vehicle for a soul. Hence an incorporeal soul will enter it, and it will become intelligent in this way. Correspondingly the contiguity with this intelligent air must bring it about that on earth bodies are formed which contain or even also produce a lower grade psychic pneuma. In this way we get animals and human beings. And again the question arises whether the soul just is this psychic pneuma or whether it just is the vehicle, in which case an incorporeal soul will enter the body and make it have some understanding.

With this we can turn to the other question concerning *UP* 17, 1 which we had set aside. In this text Galen seems to me, as I said, not just to try to explain how even on earth we do have intelligent beings, but how quite generally animals are formed in such an intelligent way. What is more, even in slime and rotten plants and fruit animals are formed which reveal the intellect of the Demiurge (II p.446,19-22 = IV 359,6-9 K). It has been thought that this remark is in conflict with Galen's rejection later, in *Foet.Form.* 6 (IV 700,17-701,6 K), of the view of his Platonist teachers that it is the world-soul which is responsible for the formation of living beings. Galen rejects this view, because, though the world-soul clearly would dispose of the art and the power to do so, it would be blasphemous to think that the world-soul is concerned with the formation of such base creatures as scorpions, snakes, worms, and the like. I have already explained that there is no conflict, because, though it is the Demiurge who creates all these creatures, he does this through the power of understanding of something down here on earth. After all, we do have to remember that the Demiurge of the *Timaeus*, too, does not himself fashion the bodies of mortal creatures, but leaves this to the younger gods. An architect or master-builder who builds a house is not expected to get his own hands dirty, and the image of the Demiurge in the *Timaeus* clearly is that of a master-builder.

There must then be something down here on earth which has the understanding required for the formation of a foetus, in part precisely to avoid the perceived blasphemy. At the same time this understanding must ultimately derive from the Demiurge, if the Demiurge is to be the creator of everything. Hence in *Foet.Form.* Galen considers the question whether the soul which is going to govern and to use the finished body is the very soul which forms the foetus, without being able to decide the question. But it is exactly because he, as we can see from *Foet.Form.*, is very concerned with the question whose understanding it is that is involved in the formation of animals, that in *UP* 17, 1 he wants to explain how an intellect, something with cognition, arrives on earth to take on this responsibility. Given that Galen, even in *Foet.Form.*, sees himself utterly unable to decide what it is that is responsible for the formation of a foetus, we should not expect more clarity or enlightenment from our brief sketch in *UP* 17, 1.

With this we can finally turn to the question what the Demiurge is who through the sun administers and maintains the world. It seems a hopeless task to even try to answer the question, given that Galen explicitly insists that he does not know what the Demiurge, or what the soul is, and hence presumably what the intellect is, nor whether they are corporeal or incorporeal. On the basis of *UP* we only have two clues: the Demiurge is not the sun, and the Demiurge is an intellect (II p.447,21 and 446,22 = IV 360,11-12 and 359,8-9 K). The number of possibilities is enormous. But I will let myself be guided by the fact that Galen clearly countenances that there is such a thing as the world-soul. It is an intellectual soul or an intellect. Like of any soul Galen can think of it as being either corporeal or incorporeal. If it is corporeal, it will be just a particularly pure form of fire, like Chrysippus' αὐγή. And, if it is incorporeal, it might be outside the body, riding, as it were, on it like a vehicle, the way Plato in the *Timaeus*, 41 d-e, explains how the Demiurge fashions rational souls, equal in number to the stars which he then places (ἐμβιβάσας) one on each star as on a vehicle. So, if one assumed that Galen's Demiurge was the world-soul, this would leave open the possibility that it is an intellect which governs the world from the outside, riding on it, as it were. Now there is one passage in Plato *Laws* 10, 895 e–899 d, which may be relevant to our purposes.

Galen knew the *Laws*. He wrote a *compendium* of them, presumably one of his eight *compendia* of Platonic dialogues he refers to in *Lib.Prop.* 13 (*Scripta min.* II p.122,13 Mueller = XIX 46,15 K). A fragment of it is extant in Maimonides (cf. *Galeni Compendium Timaei Platonis*, edd. P. Kraus et R. Walzer [London 1951], 100-101). The relevant part of the text of *Leg.* 10 must have been well known in late antiquity. It is, for instance, excerpted at length in Eusebius (*PE* 12, 51, 4-34). Plato argues that all motion in the world has its source in the self-motion of some soul or other. There is one best soul, but the motions in the world presuppose a number of souls. The best and most perfect soul must be the one which moves the heaven with care and in perfect order (10, 898 c). We then turn to the motion of the sun, the moon, and the other stars (10, 898 d). We focus on the sun and ask how the soul moves it. There are three possibilities: (i) there is a soul inside the sun which moves it the way our soul moves us; (ii) the soul provides itself with a body of fire or some sort of air and, as some say, pushes with this body the body of the sun from the outside; or (iii) the soul remains without a body, but manages to lead the sun by some extraordinarily marvellous powers (898 e 8–899 a 4). We then are told that the soul, whichever of the three ways it moves the sun, brings light to all things and thus should be called a god (899 a 7-10). On the basis of this Plato goes on to argue that there are gods and that they are provident.

The way this text seems to me to be relevant is this. The most perfect soul which moves the heaven in the most perfect way, making it rotate around its axis, traditionally is identified with the world soul. And so this is also what Galen may be assuming. And he might identify it with the Demiurge. Now the soul of the sun makes it rotate around itself. But we also know from the *Timaeus* that the sun by the world-soul is made to move in a circle along the ecliptic. It is in this way that she brings light to all. Thus Galen, identifying the world-soul with the Demiurge, can say in *UP* 3, 10 (I p.176,7 ff. = III 240,5 ff. K) that it is the Demiurge who is responsible for the beneficial effects of the sun for things on earth by making it move along the ecliptic at the right distance from the earth. We know how the story goes on from here. What Galen might find attractive about this account is that it involves a God who governs everything, including the sun, yet makes room for the central and divine role of the sun, that it emphasises the existence and the providence of God and the gods, and that it does not force him to decide on the nature of God or the soul and the intellect, respectively. If the Demiurge is the world-soul, Galen does not have to espouse the view, or to reject it, that the Demiurge is an immaterial intellect above the world of the kind Aristotle envisaged in the *Metaphysics*.

This, then, as far as I can make out, is Galen's theology. It is not surprising that it does not seem to have left an impact on later theological thought. It stays comfortably within the limits of what an educated person in Galen's time would have been ready to accept. Given his methodological principles, but also, I submit, his religious attitude, Galen does not allow himself to be drawn into developing a positive view on some of the issues which were of most concern to philosophers, like the nature of this world, of God, of the soul or the intellect, or of the stars. But to some extent one also is left with the feeling that Galen found it much easier to criticize the theological speculations of philosophers than to put his own mind positively to the resolution of some of the questions involved which crucially interested him, like the formation of the foetus or, more basically, the total mixture of elements. He, after all, did assume that the mixture does require a Divine power. On the positive side, the belief in God's providence clearly not just proved to be a fruitful heuristic principle for his study of the use of the parts of the body, but this study in turn helped to give a clear content to the ascription of such predicates as 'good', 'wise', 'just', 'provident', 'powerful', to God, which they often do not seem to have.

DISCUSSION

J. Barnes: It is puzzling how the discussion about what Galen knows and what he does not know about God is introduced in *Plac.Prop*. 2, 1 (p.56,14-17). Galen starts the chapter by saying that he does not know whether the world is generated or not, and whether there is anything outside the world or not. And he goes on to say that, since he does not know this, he also does not know the answer to certain questions about God, for instance whether he is incorporeal or corporeal, and where he is located. What is the connection between the two sets of questions?

M. Frede: I myself have been puzzled by the beginning of *Plac.Prop*. 2. There are two things I have been puzzled by, your question and, prior to that question, the question why Galen begins with issues concerning the world. The two questions may be related. As to the prior question, I believe that Galen is inclined to think, following in this Plato's *Timaeus*, that the sensible world is itself a god, or at least that he has to face this question, given the Platonist and, to some extent, the Stoic position. It seems to me that the issues Galen raises in chapter 2 to 4 all concern items which have been claimed to be in some way divine, claims Galen seems to have some sympathy with: the world, God, the soul, the stars. As to your question, one might be tempted to answer it in the following way, if one just looked at our text. Suppose the world were not generated even in the attenuated sense in which later Platonists take it to be created by a Demiurge, a view Galen himself seems to accept in *UP*. Then the world itself would be not just a god, but God. And in this case God would be corporeal at least in the sense of having a body. And he would have a location. But if the world is generated, even if only in this attenuated sense, then it seems that God must be something distinct from this world. And hence the question arises whether God in this case is not something incorporeal and without location. Along these lines one might be tempted to think that the second issue raised about the world, namely whether there is something outside and beyond it (cf. the Hebrew version), was not primarily the issue whether God was outside the world or not. But if one looks at the parallel sets of questions in *PHP* 9, 6, 21 and in 9, 7, 9 it becomes unclear as to whether this is what Galen can have in mind here. Hence I do not see a clear and satisfactory answer to your question.

J. Jouanna: Dans votre étude sur la théologie dans le *De usu partium*, j'ai été frappé par l'expression θεολογίας ἀκριβοῦς (II p.447,23 Helmreich = IV 360,13 K). Je me demande s'il convient d'établir un rapport entre cet adjectif ἀκριβοῦς et l'adverbe ἀκριβῶς, qui est employé quelques lignes plus haut à propos de l'examen de l'art de la nature. N'y aurait-il pas une relation entre un examen 'rigoureux' de l'art de la nature et une théologie 'rigoureuse'?

M. Frede: I completely agree with you that there is a question about the exact force of ἀκριβοῦς in *UP* 17, 1, II p.447,23, and I gladly accept your observation that we may be able to determine its force with the help of the ἀκριβῶς a few lines above in II p.447,14 (= IV 360,5 K). The theology can only be precise or rigorous, if it is based on facts which have been accurately, rigorously, precisely determined. Hence the need for an accurate or rigorous study, involving sophisticated anatomy, of how artfully the parts of the body are constructed. But I think more can and needs to be said about the exact force of 'rigorous' here. The study of the use of the parts is such that it allows us to determine the relevant facts rigorously, because it makes them manifest or evident. By contrast, Galen explains some lines further on (II p.448,5-9 = IV 361,3-6 K), if we go to the Eleusinian or Samothracian mysteries, what we are shown, when we are initiated, reveals nothing clearly and manifestly, so that we could base any reliable inferences on it. But another aspect of a precise theology, it seems to me, is exactly this, that we not only have clear, precise facts to rely on, but also that the inferences which we draw from them are rigorous and unassailable.

T. Tieleman: Somewhere near the beginning of your lecture you said that it has been questioned whether the reference to Gods power (*virtus*) in chapter 2 of *Prop.Plac.* as reconstructed by Vivian Nutton is an authentic feature of Galen's original exposition. I see no good reason to doubt this. In fact what we have in chapter 2 is the traditional threefold distinction between being (οὐσία), power (δύναμις), and activity (ἐνέργεια), reflected in the Latin version by the terms *substantia*, *virtus*, and *operatio*. Galen uses this distinction as an inferential chain, going from observable activities to powers and concluding from powers to the being (*i.e.* existence) of God, though remaining typically agnostic about His being in the sense of essence (2, 2, p.58,2-4). The distinction has old Platonic credentials. It goes back to Plato's own criterion of being as the power to act or be acted upon (*Soph.* 247 e 3-4). Both the distinction and the procedure (*i.e.* the inferences) connected with it are found in later Platonic literature dealing with God, or the soul: see, for instance, Tertullian, *Anim.* 14, 3, Iamblichus, *In Platonis Alcibiadem* Fr.4,12-16 Dillon (cf. also J.M. Dillon's commentary *ad loc.*). Galen applies the schema to the soul at *PHP* 9, 9, 42 ff. De Lacy (= V 803,10 ff. K).

M. Frede: I find your comments very helpful, and I agree that Galen here clearly is relying on a distinction between the existence of something, its power or powers, and the activity this power manifests itself in, and that hence a reference to God's power must be an integral part of Galen's original text in *Plac.Prop.* 2, rather than part of a translator's expansion of the text.

IV

Teun Tieleman

GALEN'S PSYCHOLOGY

1. *Introduction*

In the course of the 19th century psychology began to emancipate itself from philosophy, both conceptually and institutionally. In most western countries this process was completed around the middle of the last century. It was integral to the self-image of the young discipline that it saw itself as "the science of mental life".[1] As such, it favoured experimentation and quantitative methods. This approach was typical of Gustav Theodor Fechner (1801-87), Hermann von Helmholtz (1821-94), Wilhelm Wundt (1832-1920), who count as its founding fathers precisely for this reason. To be sure, it is possible to trace more distant ancestors but most histories of the discipline do not go further back than the 16th and 17th centuries, i.e. the period in which modern science arose. Descartes (1596-1650) and others were influential in propounding the view that the study of the mind should conform with, or at least not contradict, the discoveries made by the emerging science and indeed adopt its methods.[2]

[1] This definition constitutes the opening of William JAMES' (1842-1910) masterpiece *The Principles of Psychology* (New York 1890; several reprints).

[2] Over the past decades a great number of histories of psychology have appeared, see e.g. R. THOMSON, *The Pelican History of Psychology* (Harmondsworth 1968); W.S. SAHAKIAN, *History of Psychology. A Source Book in Systematic*

Strictly speaking, then, it is anachronistic to speak of psychology with reference to medieval or ancient philosophers, who lacked the very term.[3] Yet it may be pardonable to do so provided we keep a constant eye on the specific historical and philosophical context conditioning pre-modern theories on mental life. With this caveat in mind, we can also speak of Galen's psychology. As it is, his work in this area offers a striking anticipation of two features I have just marked out as distinctive of modern psychology. First, Galen too grafts his theories onto the most advanced scientific knowledge available in his day, in particular the anatomy and physiology as it had been developed by Hellenistic science and further enriched by himself and others. Of central importance here was the discovery of the nervous system.

Secondly, Galen was acutely sensitive to methodological issues and requirements. Here too scientists, most notably Herophilus, were his models both as to their effective use of experimental methods and as to their sense of the limitations on what could in any given case be scientifically established. However, Galen's methodology is not wholly derived from the scientific or medical tradition. He is also indebted to the later exegetical traditions connected with the Aristotelian *Organon* and the Platonic dialogues. In consequence, we have to take account of both the medical and the philosophical traditions when studying the way in which Galen addressed problems relating to the mind.

Earlier work in this area has, understandably, focused on two treatises in particular — *On the Doctrines of Hippocrates and*

Psychology (rev. ed. Itasca Ill. 1981); D. HOTHERSALL, *History of Psychology* (New York 1984).

[3] The term has been traced back to the Dalmatian humanist M. MARULUS (MARULIC), who is on record as having completed around 1520 a tract entitled *Psichiologia de ratione animae humanae liber I*. Its earliest extant occurrence is in J.TH. FREIGIUS' *Ciceronianus* (1579); cf. also the monograph by O. CASMANN entitled *Psychologia anthropologica sive animae humanae doctrina* (1594). See further E. SCHEERER, in *Historisches Wörterbuch der Philosophie*, hrsg. von J. RITTER — K. GRÜNDER, Bd. 7 (Darmstadt 1989), *s.v.* 'Psychologie', cols. 1599-1601, with further references.

Plato (*PHP*) Books I-VI and *The Capacities of the Soul Follow the Temperaments of the Body* (*QAM*). It is also marked by a heavy concentration on Galen's relation to past authorities such as Plato, Hippocrates and the Hellenistic scientists.[4] This *status quaestionis* calls for two things in particular. First, we should adduce more Galenic treatises. Some are not specifically devoted to the soul but contain a host of relevant observations and arguments illustrating Galen's attitude, or attitudes, toward this matter. Two texts of this kind have only recently been made accessible or better accessible, viz. Larrain's new edition of fragments of Galen's commentary on the Platonic *Timaeus*[5] and Nutton's edition of the *On My Own Opinions* (*Sent.Prop.*).[6] Secondly, it

[4] On psychological themes in the *PHP* see PH. DE LACY, "The Third Part of the Soul", in *Le opere psicologiche di Galeno*, a cura di P. MANULI e M. VEGETTI (Napoli 1988), 43-64; P. MANULI, "La passione nel *De placitis Hippocratis et Platonis*", in *Opere psichologiche*, 185-214; R.J. HANKINSON, "Galen's Anatomy of the Soul", in *Phronesis* 36 (1991), 197-233; ID., "Actions and passions: affection, emotion and moral self-management in Galen's philosophical psychology", in *Passions & Perceptions. Studies in Hellenistic Philosophy of Mind*, ed. by J. BRUNSCHWIG and M.C. NUSSBAUM (Cambridge/Paris 1993), 184-222; J. MANSFELD, "The Idea of the Will in Chrysippus, Posidonius, and Galen", in *Proceedings of the Boston Area Colloquium on Ancient Philosophy* VII (1991), 107-45; T. TIELEMAN, *Galen and Chrysippus On the Soul. Argument and Refutation in the* De Placitis *Books II and III* (Leiden 1996); ID., "Galen on the Seat of the Intellect. Anatomical Experiment and Philosophical Tradition", in *Science and Mathematics in Ancient Greek Culture*, ed. by T. RIHLL and C.J. TUPLIN (Oxford 2002), 256-73; ID., *Chrysippus On Affections. Reconstruction and Interpretation* (Leiden 2003). On *QAM* see L. GARCIA BALLESTER, "La 'Psique' en el somaticismo medico de la antiguedad. La actitud de Galeno", in *Episteme* 3 (1969), 195-209; ID., (1971) "La utilizacion de Platon y Aristoteles en los escritos tardios de Galeno", in *Episteme* 5 (1971), 112-20; P.L. DONINI, *Tre studi sull'aristotelismo nel secondo secolo d.C.* (Torino 1974), 132-57; G.E.R. LLOYD, "Scholarship, Authority and Argument in Galen's *Quod animi mores*", in *Opere psichologiche*, 11-42. A somewhat larger selection of relevant treatises underlies the brief overview in P. MORAUX, *Der Aristotelismus bei den Griechen von Andronikos bis Alexander von Aphrodisias* II (Berlin/New York 1984), 773-85; cf. also the observations made by DEUSE (see n.7). I have not been able to use the older monograph by E. CHAUVET, *La psychologie de Galien* I-II (Caen 1860-7).

[5] Carlos J. LARRAIN (Ed.), *Galens Kommentar zu Platons Timaios*, Beiträge zur Altertumskunde 29 (Stuttgart 1992).

[6] *Galen. On My Own Opinions.* Edition, Translation and Commentary by V. NUTTON, Corpus Medicorum Graecorum V 3, 2 (Berlin 1999).

may not be exaggerated to say that much current research has a blind spot where the contemporary philosophical backdrop is concerned.[7] In order to make up for this neglect I shall compare Galen's arguments with what is to be found in Platonist authors of the Imperial period such as Alcinous, Porphyry and Jamblichus whenever this seems appropriate and illuminating. By considering Galen against the backdrop of contemporary Platonism, we may also get a clearer picture of his own specific contributions.

By exploiting more material and comparing other philosophers we may gain a fuller understanding of Galen's project of bringing the Platonic tripartition of the soul scientifically up-to-date — a project that seems deeply problematical. I shall argue that Galen did obviate some of the most pressing problems. Further there is the issue of the substance of the soul. It is well known that Galen disclaims knowledge of this matter. Still he keeps returning to it and it seems worth taking a closer look at the options he considers and their philosophical presuppositions. This point of view will reveal how deeply Galen was immersed in the philosophical debates of his day.

2. *Galen On the Soul*

Did Galen mark off the soul as a separate object of study? He used the Old Academic but later more general division of philosophy into logic, physics and ethics, e.g. in his manifesto *The Best Physician Is Also a Philosopher*.[8] But more often he sets,

[7] Galen's position is considered against the Middle Platonist backdrop by W. DEUSE, *Untersuchungen zur mittelplatonischen und neuplatonischen Seelenlehre* (Wiesbaden 1983), 100-2, 49-51; cf. also H. DÖRRIE, *Porphyrios'* "Symmikta Zetemata" (München 1959), 169 f.

[8] Cf. A.C.J. HABETS, *Geschiedenis van de indeling van de filosofie in de Oudheid* (Diss. Utrecht 1983), 127 ff. On the marriage between medicine and (parts of) philosophy envisaged by Galen see M. ISNARDI, "Techne", in *La Parola del Passato* 16 (1961), 257-96; M. VEGETTI, "Modelli di medicina in Galeno", in *Galen: Problems and Prospects*, ed. by V. NUTTON (London 1981), 47-65; cf. ID.,

in Aristotelian fashion, theoretical and practical philosophy against each other, with logic as an instrument rather than a part of philosophy.[9] We need not doubt that he subscribes to the view shared by Aristotle, the Stoics and Platonists and reflected in the doxographic tradition[10] that the topics of the soul's nature, structure and bodily seat belong to physics, which is part of theoretical philosophy.[11] The soul's virtues and affections, by contrast, traditionally belong to ethics. This is not to say that the boundaries between ethics and physics are strict. Thus the theory of affection (or emotion) depends directly on the conception of the structure of soul, i.e. which, if any, parts or powers it comprises. The soul's substance, by contrast, is taken by Galen as a purely theoretical subject. This is particularly clear from the long-standing antagonism between Platonic and Aristotelian dualism on the one hand and Stoic monism on the other. Galen opted for the first alternative in its Platonic version, viz. the tripartition involving one rational and two non-rational parts, which he also ascribed to Hippocrates and to Aristotle (albeit with the important qualification that the latter spoke of powers rather than parts, see below, p. 142). The moral philosopher needs to know only this tripartition; he does not need to take a stand on the soul's substance (mortal/immortal, corporeal/incorporeal) or its location for that matter.[12] Galen took the distinction between the moral and physical approach to be illustrated by Book 4 of Plato's *Republic* and by the

"L'immagine del medico e lo statuto epistemologico della medicina in Galeno", in *ANRW* II 37.2 (1994), 1672-1717.

[9] *PHP* 9.7.9-17 (= V 779.16- 782.3 K); 9.9.9-10 (= 794.6-17 K); *Sent.Propr.* 15.5, p.120.9-13 Nutton.

[10] For Aristotle, see e.g. *De an.* 1.1, 402 a 6-7, 403 a 27-28; for the Stoics see DIOG.LAERT. 7.133. The later Platonist position is represented by ALCIN. *Didasc.* pp. 166 ff., 176 ff. Hermann. For the doxographic (*Placita*) tradition see esp. AËTIUS, chs. IV and V.

[11] On this and what follows cf. HABETS, *Geschiedenis van de indeling* (see n.8), 127 ff.

[12] See e.g. *Plat.Tim.* III: CMG Suppl. I, p.12.16-21 Schröder-Kahle; *On Traits of Character*, pp.192-3 Kraus; *Sent.Prop.* 14.5, p.114.19-23 N.

Timaeus respectively. In the former dialogue, Plato is supposed to have limited himself deliberately to the tripartition as such, whereas in the latter he also discussed the bodily seat of each of the three parts of the soul.[13] But insofar as the moral philosopher refers to the soul's structure, he is drawing on physics. Thus Galen on occasion refers to the soul's structure and related issues as belonging to the "physical (or: natural) part of moral philosophy".[14]

In his *On My Own Books* (*Lib.Prop.*) however he does avail himself of these distinctions. Here he lists several treatises concerned with the soul as "Treatises pertaining to Plato's philosophy".[15] Among them are the extant treatises *PHP*, *QAM* and *Sent.Prop.* *QAM* is wholly devoted to the mind-body problem and so in fact to the soul's substance. In *PHP* and *Sent.Prop.* too the soul is the main subject, though the question of its substance is avoided as much as possible. Another title that features among this group is *On the Parts and Powers of the Soul* in three books. It is no longer extant but looms behind the closing section of *PHP* Book 9 (9.9.42 & 46 = V 803.10-17 & 804.15-805.3 K), to which I shall return below. Later Platonists such as Porphyry and Iamblichus devoted tracts to the same issue.

When Galen assembles these treatises as pertaining to Platonic philosophy, this means of course that he discussed Platonic doctrines in all of them. But another aspect seems also involved in this heading, viz. the fact that Galen here discussed Platonist questions, that is to say questions concerning the soul that were topical or controversial among the Platonists of his day. This is confirmed by a comparison of their contents with the relevant sections from extant Platonist literature from the same period. I shall give some examples of this in due course.[16]

[13] Cf. *PHP* 5.7.1-2 (= V 479.14-480.4 K); *Sent.Prop.* 8.3, p.82.9-15 N.

[14] *PHP* 9.9.9 (= V 794.6-17 K); *Plat.Tim.* III 2, p.12.18-21 S.-K.; *Sent.Prop.* 13.7, p.108.18-25 N.

[15] *Lib.Prop.* 13, p.122.7-18 Müller.

[16] I may add that therapeutical concerns do not seem to have influenced the place assigned by Galen to psychological issues within his conception of medicine-

3. *Galen's Agenda*

So much for the place assigned by Galen to the issues concerning the soul in his enterprise of a medical philosophy as a whole. Let us now take a closer look at the issues themselves. A traditional agenda of topics had developed under the influence of Aristotle's *On the Soul* (Περὶ ψυχῆς, *De anima*) in particular. Aristotle's monograph stands at the beginning of a long line of treatises with the same title. The Stoic scholarch Chrysippus (c.280-204 BCE) wrote one and so did the Christian apologist Tertullian (c.160-240 CE) and the Platonist philosopher Iamblichus (c.250-330 CE) — to name but a few. Plato was incorporated in this tradition when his *Phaedo* received the alternative title *On the Soul* (Diog.Laert. 3.37). But of course the Platonic *Timaeus*, *Republic* Book 4, the *Phaedrus* and other dialogues were considered relevant as well.

The distinctive tenets of philosophers and physicians on each of the traditional issues could conveniently be looked up in doxographic literature by those who composed monographs dealing with the soul (see Aëtius, chs. IV and V). These traditional issues were: whether or not the soul exists, what its substance (οὐσία) is, how many powers it has, of which kind the powers are, where in the body they are located, etc. This agenda can be traced back to Aristotle's *On the Soul*,[17] but it became far more standarized than it had ever been in the work of the great master himself. It is also reflected in the arrangement of subject-matter over the first six books of *PHP*, in accordance with this programmatic statement from the opening of Book 2:

> Having proposed to inquire into the doctrines of Hippocrates and Plato I began with that which is first in importance, from which I showed that almost all particular details

cum-philosophy. He did not have our modern concept of psychiatry, see J. PIGEAUD, "La psychopathologie de Galien", in *Opere psichologiche* (see n.4), 153-83, esp. 182. This is not to say (as Vincent Barras reminds me) that he was lacking in interest in many afflictions that we today label psychiatric.

[17] See ARIST. *De an.* 1.1, 402 a 23 ff.

> follow. This is their teaching about the powers (δυνάμεις) that govern us, their number, the nature of each and the place that each occupies in the body (*PHP* 2.1.1 [V 211-212.3 K] = Book 1, Test. II, third text, De Lacy).[18]

Thus Books 1-3 and 6 are concerned with the question of location and Books 4-5 cover those of number and quality.[19] Conspicuously absent from Galen's check-list list are two standard issues, viz. those of existence and substance. He may have justified their omission in the lost beginning of Book 1. In other treatises Galen argues that the soul's existence is evident from the motion of the organism. This point can be paralleled from several Platonist (and other) authors.[20] It reflects the Platonic definition of the soul as the "source and principle of motion" (πηγὴ καὶ ἀρχὴ κινήσεως, *Phaedr.* 245 c 9). From the Platonist tradition Galen also takes the distinction between motion/power (δύναμις)/substance,[21] which goes back to Plato's definition of

[18] Similarly 3.1.1 (= V 285 K); cf. ARIST. *De an.* 1.1, 402 a 7 f., 402 a 23-b 2, 402 b 10-403 a 2; Ps.ALEX.APHR. *Mantissa*, p.101.1-2 Bruns; PORPH. Fr.253 Smith, *ap.* STOB. I p.353.2, 13-14 Wachsmuth. For the doxographic tradition see the Aëtian *Placita* IV 2-3 (the substance of the soul), 4 (its parts), 5 (location of the regent part), 6, 8-13 (various powers: sense-perception, imagination, thought, speech); cf. also STOB. I 49. pp. 318 ff. W. It is certain that Galen used doxographic schemas from the tradition represented by Aëtius, see J. MANSFELD, "Doxography and Dialectic. The *Sitz im Leben* of the Placita", in *ANRW* II 36.4 (1990), 3141 ff.; TIELEMAN, *Chrysippus On Affections* (see n.4), ch.2.

[19] For these items as determining the structure of Galen's discussion see also *PHP* 5.7.1-2, 7 (= V 479.14-480.4 & 481.4-8 K). From a methodological point of view the differentiation between the powers precedes their assignment to particular organs, see next p.

[20] *Sent.Prop.* 14.1, p.110.4-24; *Plat.Tim.* III 2, p.11.9-20 S.-K. For Platonists using this argument see CIC. *Nat.deor.* 2.32; ATTICUS fr.7, ll. 51-64 Des Places, *ap.* EUSEB. *PE* 15.9.10-11. Cf. also Ps.ALEX.APHR. *Mantissa*, p.101.3-4 Bruns; SEXT.EMP. *Math.* 8.155 (bodily motion an "indicative sign", ἐνδεικτικὸν σημεῖον, of soul). On the question whether or not the soul exists in doxographic literature see previous n. and J. MANSFELD, "Doxography and Dialectic" (see n.18), 3188.

[21] See TERT. *Anim.* 14.3, IAMBL. *In Alc.* 4.12-16 Dillon. Iamblichus arranges his subject-matter of his *On the Soul* on the basis of this distinction, see J.M. DILLON *ad loc.* (p.233), who points out that in later Platonist literature it has become a general metaphysical principle applicable to other spiritual forces also. Thus GAL. *Sent.Propr.* 2, p.56.16 ff. N. applies it to God, arguing that he does

the criterion of being as the power to act or be acted upon (*Soph.* 247 d 8-e 4).[22] In later authors such as Galen this definition is operative in philosophical method. Since motion, or activity, is obvious to perception, it permits us to infer the presence of a particular power, taken as the cause of the activity at issue. Power in turn is linked to substance as an active property of it. Philosophers who like Galen were saturated in the Platonist-cum-Peripatetic ontology took substance as ontologically prior to power and activity. From a methodological point of view, however, what comes first is the activity, i.e. the perceptible phenomenon.[23] That is to say, Galen starts from obvious activities to infer the presence of particular powers. Thus emotions and voluntary movements are *seen* to be different in kind and so point to two different causes or powers.[24]

In this context we should understand Galen's well-known if not notorious statement that whenever we are at a loss as to the being of something we use the term power (*Nat.Fac.* 1.4, II 9 K.; *Sent.Prop.* 14.1, p.110.15-21 Nutton). Thus, suspending judgement as to the soul's substance he prefers to speak of the powers that govern us (see e.g. *PHP* 2.1.1 [= V 211-212.3 K] quoted above).

not know His substance, just as he disclaims knowledge of the substance of the soul. See also the contribution of Michael Frede to this volume. On Galen's linking of activity and power as a Platonist motif see also M.R. Barnes, "The Background and Use of Eunomius' Causal Language", in *Arianism after Arius. Essays on the Development of the Fourth Century Trinitarian Conflicts*, ed. by M.R. Barnes & D.H. Williams (Edinburgh 1993), 217-36.

[22] Λέγω δὴ τὸ καὶ ὁποιανοῦν κεκτημένον δύναμιν εἴτ' εἰς τὸ ποιεῖν ἕτερον ὁτιοῦν πεφυκὸς εἴτ' εἰς τὸ παθεῖν [...] πᾶν τοῦτο ὄντως εἶναι· τίθεμαι γὰρ ὅρον τὰ ὄντα ὡς ἔστιν οὐκ ἄλλο τι πλὴν δύναμις.

[23] Obviously, this feature is more Aristotelian than Platonic in origin. The version Aristotelian methodology developed by Herophilus is also one of the influences to be reckoned with when it comes to explaining Galen's position, see H. von Staden (Ed.), *Herophilus. The Art of Medicine in Early Alexandria* (Cambridge 1989), 115-25, 130-4 (including T50a-b, T58, T59a). There can be no doubt that Galen's stress on empirical verifiability bears a Herophilean stamp.

[24] *PHP* 2.7.18 (= V 271.3-11 K); 5.7.9 (= V 481.13-17 K); 5.7.83-7 (= V 502.1-503.18 K); 6.3.5 (= V 520.13-521.1 K); cf. 5.4.2 (= V 454.11-15 K).

The existence of soul was almost universally accepted in ancient philosophy and science.[25] The persistence of the idea of soul may seem surprising in view of the thorough-going physicalism of Hellenistic science, in particular the physiological theories of Herophilus and Erasistratus. These scientists had limited the scope of soul to the two functions they had been able to ascribe to the nervous system, viz. perception and voluntary motions. Both designated the *pneuma* ("breath") in these vessels as the vehicle or even (Erasistratus) substance of the soul. They no longer attributed bodily processes such as digestion to the soul but demoted these to the status of natural operations. Galen too retained the concept of soul but again extended it to cover growth and digestion. He assigned these functions to the Platonic third or appetitive part of the soul as he understood it and which he situated in the liver.[26] I shall return to this (problematic) feature of his physiological system presently. Suffice it to note here that for all his dependence on Hellenistic science, Galen chose to stuck to the Platonist tradition on this particular point.

But his doubts as to the soul's substance also marks a departure from the position of at least Erasistratus. In *PHP* Book 7 we find an intriguing passage (too long to quote) where Galen does discuss the question of substance — although he reaches no positive conclusion. Both common experience and anatomical experiment show that the escape of the *pneuma* from the

[25] The Peripatetic philosopher Dicaearchus and the Herophilean physician Andreas stand out as exceptions, see H. VON STADEN, "Body, Soul and Nerves: Epicurus, Herophilus, Erasistratus, the Stoics, and Galen", in *Psyche and Soma. Physicians and metaphysicians on the mind-body problem from Antquity to Enlightenment*, ed. by John P. WRIGHT & Paul POTTER (Oxford 2000), 105.

[26] He was also willing to speak of 'nature' with reference to the functions in question: see e.g. *PHP* 6.3.7 (= V 520.5-18 K); cf. *Hipp.Epid.VI* 5.5, CMG V 10.2.2., p.272.27 ff. Wenkebach-Pfaff (= XVIIB 250.15 ff. K). 'Nature' was the Stoic term used, in line with the Stoic *scala naturae*, according to which 'nature' or 'natural pneuma' defines the mode of existence of plants (and embryos of animals), see A.A. LONG, "Soul and Body in Stoicism", in *Phronesis* 27 (1982), 34-57; T. TIELEMAN, "Diogenes of Babylon and Stoic Embryology. Ps. Plutarch, *Plac.* V 15.4 Reconsidered", in *Mnemosyne* 44 (1991), 106-125.

brain induces temporary loss of consciousness but not death. This, he argues, strongly suggests that the *pneuma* is the soul's "first instrument" (the Aristotelian term) rather than its substance (7.3.14-22 [= V 604.14-606.15 K]). In another part of the same book where he discusses sense-perception as involving optical pneuma, he returns to the question of the substance of the soul: this is either *pneuma* (a position he ascribes to both the Stoics and Aristotle) or incorporeal. The latter option — which represents the Platonist position — entails that the *pneuma* is the soul's "first vehicle (ὄχημα)" — the Platonic term.[27] Galen does not express a preference for either option. In the present context it is sufficient for him to argue that the psychic *pneuma* through its communion with the optical *pneuma* renders the latter luminous. It is intended to justify why Galen does not want to decide upon this question, i.e. whether the soul is incorporeal or corporeal, whether it is immortal or mortal — fundamental polarities in Platonism.[28]

4. *Options*

In *PHP* Galen operates with a division of the options open in the debate on the number of parts or powers of the soul.[29] As is clear from this division, this question is inextricably linked to that of their location. The fullest version of this schema is to be found at 6.2.5-6 (= V 515.12-516.6 K):

[27] See e.g. *Tim.* 44 e 2, 69 c 7; *Phaedr.* 247 b 2; cf. *Tim.* 41 e 2; *Phaedo* 113 d 5. For the Platonist tradition cf. ALCIN. *Didasc.* 23, p.176.14 Hermann.

[28] This passage should be compared with Galen's later reflections on the soul's substance at *Hipp.Epid.VI* 5.5, pp.270.21-274.11 W.-Pf. (= XVIIB 246.8-253.3 K). Referring to his discussion in *PHP* (*ibid.* p.271.8-9 = XVIIB 247.13-16 K), he sticks to his agnosticism in this matter and even argues that a Hippocratic passage which seems to state that the soul is innate heat cannot be authentic.

[29] For Galen's view that a complete "division of the problem" (διαίρεσις τοῦ προβλήματος) should constitute the basis for scientific or philosophical discussion see esp. *PHP* 4.1.15-17 (= V 365.4-366.5 K); cf. 5.6.40-41 (= V 477.9-18 K); 3.1.18. (= V 289.8-11 K).

> Plato, holding that they [i.e. the forms, εἴδη, of the soul] are separated by their location in the body and differ greatly in essence (ταῖς οὐσίαις πάμπολυ διαλ⟨λ⟩άττειν), has good reason to call them both forms and parts (εἴδη τε καὶ μέρη). But Aristotle and Posidonius do not speak of forms or parts of the soul but say that there are powers of a single essence which has its base at the heart (δυνάμεις ... μιᾶς οὐσίας ἐκ τῆς καρδίας ὁρμωμένης).[30] Chrysippus not only subsumes anger (θύμος) and desire (ἐπιθυμία) under one essence (οὐσία) but also one power (δύναμις) (*PHP* 6.2.5-6 ~ Posid. Fr.146 E.-K.).

The same division of options underlies the following passage from Book 5, where Galen offers a critique of the form of psychological monism represented by the Stoic scholarch Chrysippus:

> My purpose is to show that it is not in a single part (μόριον) of the soul nor by virtue of a single power (δύναμιν) of it that both judgements and affections (πάθη) occur, as Chrysippus claimed, but that the soul has both a plurality of powers of different kinds (ἑτερογενεῖς) and a plurality of parts. That the powers of the soul are three in number and that by them we desire, feel anger, and reason — this is granted by both Aristotle and Posidonius. But that they are also spatially separate from each other, and that our soul not only contains many powers but is composed of parts that differ in kind (ἑτερογενῶν) and in substance (οὐσίαις), this is the doctrine of Hippocrates and Plato (*PHP* 5.4.2-3 [= V 454.11-455.4 K]; transl. De Lacy's, slightly modified).

According to this division of options Plato is credited with three essentially different parts, situated in three different organs. By contrast, Aristotle and the Stoic Posidonius who opted for one central organ are credited with one form underlying three powers. Galen does not attempt to explain what it means for the soul or its parts to be in a certain place, having decided to skip

[30] For this phrasing see also *ibid.* 6.1.1 (= V 505 K); cf. PORPH. Fr.251, p.269,31 f. Smith, *ap.* STOB. I p.349.3-4 W.

the question of its substance, i.e. whether or not the soul is corporeal. On the other hand he links the aspects of part and bodily seat (but cf. Galen's later explication in his *QAM* that the parts of the soul are the forms immanent in the three vital organs, below p. 150). The term 'substance' or 'being' (οὐσία) here serves to bring out that in speaking of parts one refers to essentially different 'forms' or 'kinds'. The Greek term εἶδος had been used by Plato himself in a relevant sense, as when he said that plants "share in the third kind (εἴδους) of soul", viz. the appetitive part (*Tim.* 77 b 3-4).[31] As such, it feature prominently in the context of the above passage. Here Galen is not so much concerned to refute the Stoics or Peripatetics but takes part in a dispute among Platonists. Presumably under the influence of Peripatetic criticism certain Platonists had abandoned the idea of the soul having separate forms or parts as incompatible with its unity and hence immortality. Exactly which Platonists Galen has in mind here must remain uncertain. But a version of this view was advanced by the Platonist Severus, a contemporary of Galen's.[32] Versions of it are attested for Nicolaus Damascenus (c. 5 BCE- 64 CE)[33] as well as Porphyry's mentor Longinus (early 3rd c. CE, see below).[34] Against their view, Galen devotes the second chapter of Book 6 to showing that Plato himself had spoken about forms of the soul. As is clear from the above division, the postulate of parts (rather than powers) and their separate location presuppose one another. Of

[31] Michael Frede drew my attention to this passage as illustrating the relevance of the sense 'kind' born by the term εἶδος.

[32] See EUSEB. *PE* 13.17.1-6, II p.239.9 ff. Mras with DEUSE, *Untersuchungen* (see n.7), 102-108, esp. 104 ff. Cf. J. DILLON, *The Middle Platonists. A Study of Platonism 80 B.C. to A.D. 220* (London 1977), 262-64.

[33] See PORPH. *ibid.* (see n. 30) p.353.12-354.6 W.(= F 7 Roeper/T 9 Lulofs) with P. MORAUX, *Der Aristotelismus bei den Griechen* I (Berlin/New York 1973), 481-87.

[34] PORPH. Fr.253, p.272.32 ff. Smith, ap. STOB. I p.351.11-19 W. cited *infra*, p. 145; cf. also Fr.253, p.274.77 ff. Smith, ap. STOB. I p.353.1-11 W. Highly relevant is TERT. *Anim.* 14, insisting that the idea of powers (as opposed to parts) is fundamental to that of the soul's unity and immortality.

this Plato had not offered a *demonstration*, however. The mythic account of the *Timaeus* could hardly count as such. This then is what Galen has to provide himself. He sets out to do so in Books 1-3 and 6, where he demonstrates that each of the three organs is the seat of one of the Platonic parts (Books 4-5 establish the tripartition as such, irrespective of the status of the faculties as either parts or powers, in line with the schema at 6.2.5 [V 515.12-516.1 K]). This demonstration takes the form of an inquiry into the distinctive *function* of each of the three organs. Identifying function with essence (*PHP* 1.8.12-15 [V 202.17-203.14 K]), Galen successively establishes the 'being' or essence of each of these organs in order to determine whether this suits his definition of the Platonic parts of the soul. Thus the brain is shown through anatomical observation and experiment to be the functional centre of perception and voluntary motion and hence the seat of the Platonic rational part.

To be sure, this way of linking of essence and function with respect to particular organs is Aristotelian rather than Platonic in inspiration. Indeed Galen effectively operates with the notion of immanent form. But we should not forget that immanent form was cheerfully accepted and reconciled with that of transcendent form by many Platonists of Galen's day.[35] But what then is the relation between the essence of the brain and the soul? In *PHP* Galen does not go into this inevitable question. But in *QAM* he will take the obvious next step of identifying the three parts of the soul with the form of each of the main bodily organs (see below, p. 150).

The Platonist backdrop can be further illustrated by comparing *PHP* 6.2.5 (= V 515.12-516.1 K) with Porphyry Fr.253

[35] See e.g. DILLON, *Middle Platonists* (see n.31), 137, 274 (note that Galen's term εἶδος was used for immanent form, whereas ἰδέα was reserved for transcendent form); cf. J. WHITTAKER, "Platonic Philosophy in the Early Centuries of the Empire", in *ANRW* II 36.1 (1987), 110 ff., who notes that "a further prominent feature of the Middle Platonic scholastic tradition is the attempt to interpret Plato in the light of Aristotle and where possible to accomodate the one to the other" (p.110).

Smith, *ap*. Stob. I p.351.8-19 W. and Iamblichus, *De anima, ap*. Stob. I pp.367.10-369.4 W. (= Fr. 10-12 Finamore-Dillon). Porphyry writes:

> It should be said that power (δύναμις) differs from part (μέρους) because one part diverges from another in kind (κατὰ γένος) and character, but powers belong to one and the same kind (γένος). This is why Aristotle declined parts with regard to the soul, but accepted powers: for the differentiation between parts immediately introduces a difference of substrate, whereas the differentiation between powers also occurs in one substrate.[36] Longinus, too, held that the living being did not have a plurality of parts but was without parts, though not without a plurality of powers, saying that according to Plato the soul comes to have a plurality of parts in bodies, being without parts when on its own; but if it is without a plurality of parts, it does not thereby have but a single power; for it is possible for a single thing without parts to have more than one power.

The passage from Iamblichus (which is far too long to quote) distinguishes between the same options in the same terms. The pattern of similarities and differences that emerges indicates that none of these authors (Galen, Porphyry, Iamblichus) depends on one of the others but that all depend on a common tradition. The traditional schema featured three main options in terms of the part/power distinction we have just explained, viz. the Platonic, Aristotelian and Stoic conceptions of the soul's structure. These three passages provide a nice example of how a schema of this sort could be used for the particular purpose each of them was pursuing. Galen associates the allegedly deviant Stoic Posidonius with the Aristotelian position. This suits his project in *PHP* Books 4 and 5 of playing

[36] This sentence is translated from Wachsmuth's text. Smith inserts a sentence (l.34 τὸ δέ ἑτεροδύναμον … l.35-6 εἰσάγειν), which is grammatically incorrect (note the genitive ὑποκειμένου) and paleographically unaccountable.

off Posidonius against Chrysippus.[37] Similarly Porphyry links his teacher Longinus to Aristotle, while having little interest in the Stoic doctrine which he almost completely suppresses (but note the reference to the option of a single power near the end of our passage). Longinus strikes a compromise by opting for powers with respect to its disembodied state and parts when it has taken up residence in the body.[38] This saves both the Platonic reference to parts and the unity and immortality of the soul.

Iamblichus, like Porphyry, explains the concepts of part and power (pp.367.10-368.11 W.) before presenting the schema of options (pp.368.12-369.4 W.). He does not attach the name of a later philosopher to the traditional division, limiting himself to a *précis* of the three main options (Stoic, Aristotelian, Platonic). But in marked contrast to Porphyry and Galen, he expands on the Stoic view on the parts and powers of the pneumatic soul (cf. *SVF* II 826, 831). Common to all three authors is the way in which they regulate the relation between the concepts of being, part and power. This also holds good for Iamblichus, even if he is the only one to draw attention to the corporeal conception of the soul advocated by the Stoics.

The Platonist backdrop to Galen's argument in *PHP* becomes still clearer from its closing section, *viz.* 9.9.41-46 (= V 803.7-805 K). This passage lists a number of examples of how the logical method of diaeresis or division can be applied. The powers of the soul (like the powers of the physical elements) are given in illustration of the thesis that

[37] Opinions still differ as to the extent to which Galen's portrayal of Posidonius as an adherent of psychological dualism is historically accurate. See now Tieleman, *Chrysippus On Affections* (see n.4), ch.5, for a full discussion and further references. Galen's inclusion of Posidonius into the Platonist division of options under discussion here should exhort us to exercise a due amount of caution as to Posidonius' acceptance of the Platonic trifold division, albeit in terms of powers rather than parts.

[38] The key text here is *Tim.* 35 a (on the context of which see also *infra* p. 149), from which Platonists such as Longinus could derive some support, see esp. the phrase τῆς ... περὶ τὰ σώματα γιγνομένης μεριστῆς (scil. οὐσίας), 35 a 2-3.

> ... substances (οὐσίας) are not divided into the powers (δυνάμεις) in them but that each substance, being undivided, has some activity (ἐνεργεῖν τι) in accordance with the powers in it (45).

Thus they [i.e. anonymous philosophers referred to a little earlier, 44, p.608.21 De Lacy = V 804.11 K) do not say

> without qualification that the substance has a power but at one time they add of burning or cooling or drying or moistening,[39] at another time of receiving impressions and reasoning and moving itself, or some of the other activities of this kind that we do (ἐνεργοῦμεν) with the rational soul, which is itself one but has many powers... (46).

When we compare this passage with 6.2.5 (= V 515.12-516.1 K), we may infer, first, that the basic schema of options in Book 6 results from an application of the method of diaeresis or division, in keeping with Galen's insistence on this method elsewhere as an indispensable tool for stating the options that are open in any debate.[40] But in the account from Book 9 we receive some further information. The distinction between substance and powers is explained as one between "unqualified underlying substance and its properties" (τῆς ὑποκειμένης οὐσίας ἀποίου καὶ τῶν συμβεβηκότων αὐτῇ, 44, p.608.19-21). We may take it that substance here stands for corporeal substance, with the properties being taken as incorporeal.[41] On the other hand, the schema at 6.2.5 suggests the Aristotelian sense of secondary substance, i.e. essence or form. In that case the properties are accidental properties in the Aristotelian sense. But in regard to

[39] *Viz.*, in the case of the physical elements.

[40] See *supra*, n. 29.

[41] Cf. the argument directed by the author of the pseudo-Galenic tract *The Qualities Are Incorporeal* against the Stoic position on the properties (XIX 463-484 K); ALCIN. *Didasc.* ch. XI. Like these authors, Galen at *PHP* 9.9.45 (= V 804.12-14 K), argues that the Stoic view would entail an endlessly repeated division; cf. also IAMBL. *ap.* STOB. I p.367.17-22 W. (on the context of which see above in text).

PHP 6.2.5 too we have noted that the concept expressed by the term οὐσία presupposes underlying material substance. In sum, there seems to be an ambiguity involved in Galen's use of the term in *PHP*.

In addition, we find here another instance of the triad substance/power/activity in connection with the distinction between unqualified being or substance (οὐσία) and its properties we have just noted. I have already pointed to Plato's statement of the criterion of being (*Soph.* 247 d-e; above, p. 139). But one also hears an unmistakable echo of *Phaedrus* 270 c-d. Here Plato describes the Hippocratic method as applied to the nature of the soul: first one establishes through division simple substances and then the powers characteristic of these substances. Here too, then, division halts at substance and substance underlies the powers. The fact that Plato subscribes to what he takes as the method of Hippocrates suits Galen's central thesis in *PHP* of the basic agreement between the two great masters. We need not doubt that this well-known passage was among Galen's personal favourites.[42] Even so he does not cite it here or anywhere else in *PHP*. But then the particular mode of division applied to the soul in this passage was not designed by Galen directly on the basis of this Platonic passage. As De Lacy rightly notes in his apparatus of references, we have a very similar division of types of division in ch. 5 of Alcinous' Platonist handbook.[43] Right at the end of the book and following the passage we have just quoted there is a reference to a (lost) treatise (*PHP* 9.9.46). A little earlier in the same section Galen characterizes the same treatise as dealing with the forms of the soul in accordance with Plato's doctrine (*ibid.* 42).[44] In sum, there is no denying the Platonist scholasticism of the closing section of *PHP* Book 9.

[42] Cf. *MM* X 13-14 K; *Comp.Med.Gen.* XIII 594 K.

[43] De Lacy refers to Albinus but this once common mistake seems now at last to have been superseded, see e.g. WHITTAKER, "Platonic Philosophy" (see n.34), 83 ff.

[44] On this treatise see *supra*, p. 136.

Keeping the conceptual distinctions of *PHP* Book 9 in mind, we may turn now to a further piece of evidence, Galen's exegesis of a notoriously difficult passage from the Platonic *Timaeus*, 37 a-b, printed as nr. 11 by Larrain in his edition of additional fragments of Galen's commentary (see above, n.5). Here Plato describes how the Demiurg installs two kinds of motions in the human body, one analogous to the sphere of the fixed stars, the other to the sphere of the Zodiac. These circular motions (κινήσεις) or rotations (περίοδοι) represent the soul's cognitive activity. Clearly Plato wishes to make an epistemological point: human reason is capable of coming into contact with both unchangeable being and the world of becoming. The two circuits of the soul represent the two kinds of cognition, knowledge and opinion, corresponding to these two spheres of reality. What we have here, as Aristotle already saw,[45] is the common principle of knowing like by like.

For Galen, however, the problem arises how to explain these rotations from an ontological point of view. These rotations are clearly different. How then can they both belong to one entity, viz. human reason? His solution lies in the distinction between substance and properties we have encountered in *PHP* Book 9. Plato, he argues, speaks of the two circular motions in terms of substance (οὐσία), but what he really means to say is that they are *properties belonging to* the substance of the rational part of the soul. Galen goes on to explain these properties or motions in terms of mental functions such as opining and cognizing.

We may feel that Galen grossly distorts Plato's meaning. But the conventions of ancient exegesis allowed Galen ample scope to update Plato. Once again his use of the term makes οὐσία one wonder whether it indicates the transcendent being or corporeal substance. In the context he stresses, in typical fashion, the corporeal basis of psychic life. This may seem un-Platonic, but in

[45] ARIST. *De an.* 1.2, 404 b 16 ff. Cf. also ALCIN. *Didasc.* 6, p.158.18 ff. Hermann.

fact this kind of reading was not without parallel.[46] In fact Plato himself had drawn attention to the soul's dependence on bodily factors in *Timaeus* 86-88. Not surprisingly, this aspect features also prominently in other extant fragments of Galen's commentary (see Frs. 6-10 Larrain). Secondly, he employs the substance/power distinction in a way which he could take to be justified by the key passage from the Platonic *Phaedrus* I have just referred to (see above, p. 148). Galen, then, is applying the time-honoured exegetical principle of explaining *Homerum ex Homero* to Plato.

I proceed to another key passage, viz. *QAM* 4, pp.44.2-45.2 Müller (= IV 782.4-783.7 K). Galen's *QAM* has been excellently discussed by Lloyd and others (see above, n.4). I confine myself to a few observations on the points I have raised sofar. In *QAM*, as we have noticed (above, p. 143), Galen identifies the soul with the form (εἶδος) of each of the three main organs, form being explained in terms of the mixture of bodily elements. What we have here is the marriage of the Platonic tripartition-cum-trilocation with the Aristotelian definition of the soul as the form of the body. This clearly supports Galen's main thesis that corporeal factors influence our mental functioning including character in a morally relevant sense. From a historical point of view, the explanation of Aristotle's definition in term of the elemental qualities had been anticipated by Peripatetics such as Andronicus of Rhodes to whom Galen refers (*QAM* 4, pp.44.2-45.2 Müller). He caps the latter's view of the soul as the *power resulting from* the blend of elements, arguing that it is the mixture itself. This point may be related to the fact — we have repeatedly noted — that Galen sees power as an attribute of the underlying substance and hence ontologically derivative. But given the close connection between substance and power, the difference seems largely one of perspective. For Galen it held

[46] According to the account of Platonic philosophy transmitted by Diogenes Laertius, Plato considered the substance of the soul to be three-dimensional *pneuma*, 3.67.

the additional attraction of its affinity with Hippocratic ideas on powers as resulting from mixtures of the elements, or elementary qualities.[47] Further, we may note that Galen in this late treatise finally takes a stand as to the sense of οὐσία in relation to the soul, opting for immanent form according to Aristotle's distinction (see esp. *ibid.* pp.44.20-45.2).

G.E.R. Lloyd has demonstrated that Galen is not clear about exactly what is implied by the term "follow" in the title of the treatise: "The capacities of the soul follow the temperaments of the body".[48] At face value Galen seems to upheld a version of what is today called epiphenomenalism, denying any causal role to the soul. Still he upholds moral responsibility. And, more pertinently perhaps, he elsewhere does ascribe influence to the soul on bodily states: mental affections such as fear or distress can be lethal under certain circumstances. So it remains risky to apply modern labels in view of later connotations which do not fit Galen's original position.

5. *The Parts Of the Soul: Location and Interaction*

In *PHP* Books 4 and 5 Galen stresses the fact that the tripartition as such[49] can be based on obvious phenomena, i.e. the powers or motions that are "different in kind".[50] In other words,

[47] As Professor Jouanna has reminded me, Galen seeks support for the thesis of *QAM* from several passages from the Hippocratic *Airs Waters Places* illustrating the influence of the environment on the body and of the body on the soul. Other ideas from the Hippocratic writing may also help explain certain emphases in Galen's outlook, e.g. the prominence given to the concept of power (δύναμις). On its in Hippocratic physiology see J. SOUILHÉ, *Étude sur le terme* δύναμις (Paris 1919), 32-6; G. PLAMBÖCK, *Dynamis im Corpus Hippocraticum* (Wiesbaden 1964); M.R. BARNES, *The Power of God. Δύναμις in Gregory of Nyssa's Trinitarian Theology* (Washington 2001), 28 ff.

[48] See LLOYD, "Scholarship, Authority and Argument" (see n.4), 33 ff.

[49] That is to say, leaving aside the question of the status of the faculties distinguished as either powers or parts, see *supra*, p. 143.

[50] *PHP* 5.7.7-8 (= V 481.3-13 K); 5.7.83-85 (= V 502.1-16 K); 5.7.87-88 (= V 503.10-504 K); cf. *Sent.Prop.* 8.2, p.82.3-8 N.

these motions can be divided according to three powers, viz. the powers that had been distinguished by Plato and also, he holds, by Hippocrates, Aristotle and Posidonius (see *PHP* 6.2.5 [= V 515.12-516.1 K], quoted above, p. 142). He seems to be thinking of our experience of mental conflict whether through introspection or our observations of other people. He quotes Plato's story in *Republic* Book 4 about Leontinus wavering over whether to go and have a look at some corpses of executed criminals (*PHP* 5.7.45 ff. [= V 491.8 ff. K]). On a more technical level, Galen subscribes to Plato's use of the principle of non-contradiction in the same book as proving the necessity of differentiating between separate psychic faculties.[51]

When it comes to demonstrating the bodily seat of the three capacities and hence proving their status as parts or forms of the soul, Galen no longer appeals to obvious phenomena or common experience. This demonstration (which had not been undertaken by Plato) calls for technical experience, that is to say, anatomical observation and experiment. At first sight, Galen's project of providing Plato's psychology with a firm basis in anatomy and physiology seems a rather hazardous undertaking. (And his reading of Hippocrates as agreeing with Plato on this score seems downright frivolous.) In practice, he sets out to prove Plato correct in the light of later, mostly Hellenistic, science. Still, the task is somewhat less daunting than it might initially appear to be. In the *Timaeus* Plato draws extensively on the medical science of his own day. But he is often rather vague on anatomical details. The reason lies in the purpose in this dialogue. On the one hand Plato wanted to lend a degree of scientific respectability to his account of the cosmos. But on the other hand he selected those scientific insights which could be pressed into the service of an overriding philosophical aim — the determination of man's place in a providentially ordered cosmos. Thus his account of the human soul and its location in the body is governed by moral concerns rather than an interest

[51] *PHP* 5.7 (= V 479.14-504 K); 9.9.22 ff. (= V 797.10 ff. K).

in anatomical or physiological detail. This tendency of the Platonic *Timaeus* has been pointed out by several modern scholars beginning with Cornford and need not be dwelt upon.[52] What is less widely known is that there was even an ancient tradition which preferred to take the Platonic tripartition as having moral significance only.[53] Even so Galen could represent Plato as having had the correct insight about the function of the brain as the seat of reason and hence perception and voluntary movement. In his commentary on the *Timaeus* he acknowledges the fact that Plato and certain physicians in his day had no inkling of the nervous system and its workings (*Plat.Tim.* III 6, CMG Suppl. I, p.15.18-20 Schröder-Kahle). It was sufficient to show that Plato had at least been on the right track.

In regard to the spirited part residing in the heart the account at *Tim.* 69 d-70 d had only to be made more precise insofar as Plato does not distinguish between arteries and veins — which was a scientific insight of later date (entertained by e.g. Praxagoras, Erasistratus). Galen of course considers the heart as the centre of the arterial system only. The Platonic assumption that the heart was the seat of certain psychic functions (notably anger) and the centre of bodily heat continued to be widespread and respectable among philosophers and scientists well into Galen's day and beyond. In the schema of options employed by Galen, as we have seen, this assumption is common ground between the main contestants in the debate; that is to say, there was no difference from the Peripatetics and Stoics on this point.

More problematic was the third or appetitive part, which had been located by Plato in the belly (*Tim.* 70 d 7-e 2). Galen however assigns it to the liver as the structural and functional centre of the veins. He had to make this adjustment in view of the

[52] F.M. CORNFORD, *Plato's Cosmology: The* Timaeus *of Plato Translated with a Running Commentary* (London 1937), 20, 282; P. HADOT, "Physique et poésie dans le *Timée* de Platon", in *Revue de Théologie et Philosophie* 115 (1983), 113-33, esp. 118; C. STEEL, "The Moral Purpose of the Human Body. A Reading of Timaeus 69-72", in *Phronesis* 46 (2001), 105-128.

[53] Cf. PORPH. Fr.253, ll.14-15 Smith.

role assigned by post-Platonic science to the liver in the processes of digestion and growth.[54] Of course this made the liver exquisitely suited to house the appetitive part (though understandably Galen choses to ignore the fact that Plato in the *Republic* adds money as object of desire to food and drink and sex, *Rep.* 9, 580 e-581 a). Not only did Plato not assign any role to the liver with respect to nourishment, he gave this organ an altogether different role to play, viz. as a kind of television screen on which reason projects images that calm down unruly desire lurking in the belly (*Tim.* 71 a 3-d 4; cf. 80 d-81 e). Moreover, Galen ignores the role of the liver in divination accepted by Plato (*Tim.* 72 b-c). The attempt to bring Plato scientifically more up-to-date with respect to the liver (as well as other physiological points) can be paralleled from other Platonists.[55] This might help explain why he did not bother to acknowledge that there was a real difference between himself and Plato on this point.

Galen's anatomically based tripartition entails a rather strict separation between the parts, where Plato shows more interest in the coherence and interaction between the parts. We should not suppose that this strict separation is wholly due to Galen's anatomical reading and so peculiar to him. If we compare Alcinous' manual (which may or may not predate Galen), we find a very similar reading of Plato, including a reference to the brain as the centre of the nervous system (separation: chs. 23-24; nerves: 17, p.173.8 Hermann). Still, Galen's no doubt represents the most extensive and detailed attempt to reconcile the Platonic tripartition with the later advances in science. He offered a fairly coherent account of the three ἀρχαί of the organism — brain, heart and liver — as the centres of functions that corresponded

[54] This insight is first attested at ARIST. *PA* 3.7, 670 a 27; cf. N. MANI, *Die historischen Grundlagen der Leberforschung* I (Basel-Stuttgart ^{2}1965), 35 ff. (Plato), 41 ff. (Aristotle).

[55] Cf. PLUT. *Virt.Mor.* 11, 450 F; PS.TIM.LOCR. 46, p.218.10-1 Thesleff-Marg; PS.HERACLIT. *All.* 18, p.22 Buffière; APUL. (c. 155-? CE) *Plat.*; PORPH. Fr.253, ll.84-85 Smith. Cf. DILLON, *Middle Platonists* (see n.31), 326 f.; TIELEMAN, *Galen and Chrysippus* (see n.4), XXX f.

to the each of the three Platonic parts. But he fails to account for the anatomical and physiological basis for the necessary interaction between the three parts, or so it seems. This problem seems to subvert his whole enterprise.

It has been said that Galen omits to discuss the necessary interaction between the parts of the soul, to which Plato devotes ample attention.[56] His silence on this point is taken as an indication that he is in very serious trouble indeed. Galen's project of updating the Platonic tripartition entails a strict, anatomically based separation between the parts. But can he explain their interplay and conflict in physiological terms? How does desire in the liver and anger in the heart influence reason in the head and *vice versa*? A related problem is that Galen, having demonstrated the liver's role in digestion unwarrantably, it seems, infers that it is the seat of desire in the full-blown Platonic sense of a conscious, morally relevant mental phenomenon. Here too he fails to provide a justification, at least in his discussion in *PHP* Book 6.[57]

A few passages which have sofar been overlooked suggest that Galen did address the above problems. In a recently published fragment from his *Timaeus* commentary (Fr.14 Larrain) Galen repeats the point — which he had argued at length in *PHP* — that the heart is not the centre of the nervous system, but he adds something else: certain nerves reach the heart from the head *in view of the service the former needs to render the principle contained in the latter, i.e. reason.*[58] Contrast Galen's insistence in *PHP* on the mutual independence of the brain and the heart (esp. *ibid.* 2.6 [V 262.11-267.6 K]). In the same fragment

[56] Cf. MANSFELD, "The idea of the Will" (see n.4), 131 f.; HANKINSON, "Actions and passions" (see n.4), 208; cf. DE LACY, "Third Part" (see n.4), 61 f.

[57] See HANKINSON, "Anatomy of the Soul" (see n.4), 230; T. TIELEMAN, "Plotinus on the Seat of the Soul: Reverberations of Galen and Alexander in *Enn.* IV 3.23", in *Phronesis* 43 (1998), 321 f.

[58] On Galen's view on the heart, its automatism and connection with the nervous system see further R.E. SIEGEL, *Galen's System of Physiology and Medicine* (Basel/New York 1968), 44 ff.; C.R.S. HARRIS, *The Heart and the Vascular System in Ancient Greek Medicine. From Alcmaeon to Galen* (Oxford 1973), 267 ff.

from his commentary Galen says that the heart has "to take part in the higher principle", which must mean that it is capable of listening to it.[59] This point refers to Plato's well-known and graphic portrayal of anger arising in the heart, *Timaeus* 70 a 7-b 8.[60] Here the spirited part is said to respond to reason when this reports a certain wrong done to us and calling for revenge. This Platonic passage also inspired an intriguing passage from Galen's *On Preserving Health*:

> Anger is not simply an increase, but a kind of boiling, so to speak, of the heat in the heart; this is why the most distinguished philosophers say that its substance is of such a kind. For the craving for revenge is an inessential property rather than the substance of anger (2.9.5-6, p.61.24-28 Koch [= VI 138.7-12 K]).[61]

Galen argues that the definition of anger as a kind of seething or boiling pertains to its substance or being (οὐσία), whereas the definition of anger as a desire for retribution expresses an accidental feature (συμβεβηκός). Both definitions were widespread and not confined to one particular school.[62] But the distinction drawn by Galen clearly reflects Aristotle, *De an.* 1.1, 403 a 29-b 2, where Aristotle says that the first is typical of philosophers of nature and pertains to matter (ὕλην) and the second is used

[59] Fr.14, ll.1-14: ὅτι ἀπὸ ⟨τοῦ⟩ ἐγκεφάλου πάντα φαίνεται τὰ κατὰ τὸ ζῷον νεῦρα τὴν ἀρχὴν ἔχοντα, ἀφ' ὧν καὶ εἰς τὴν καρδίαν ἀποφύσεις μικραὶ παραγίνονται. καὶ γὰρ καὶ ταύτην ἔδει μετασχεῖν τῆς ἄνωθεν ἀρχῆς ὑπηρετήσειν ταύτῃ μέλλουσαν ....

[60] Cf. Galen's discussion of this passage, *PHP* 3.1.31 (= V 292.8-17 K).

[61] Ὁ μέν γε θυμὸς οὐδ' ἁπλῶς αὔξησις, ἀλλ' οἷον ζέσις τίς ἐστι τοῦ κατὰ τὴν καρδίαν θερμοῦ· διὸ καὶ τὴν οὐσίαν αὐτοῦ τῶν φιλοσόφων οἱ δοκιμώτατοι τοιαύτην εἶναί φασι· συμβεβηκὸς γάρ τι καὶ οὐκ οὐσία τοῦ θυμοῦ ἐστιν ἡ τῆς ἀντιτιμωρήσεως ὄρεξις.

[62] See Plat. *Tim.* 70 a-b (boiling: 70 b 3; revenge: 70 b 4); Arist. *De an.* 1.1, 403 a 29-32 (on which see in text); for Stoicism see Chrysipp. *SVF* II 886, *ap.* Gal. *PHP* 3.1.25 (= V 290.17-291.7 K), where Galen remarks on the similarity between Chrysippus' description and Plato's, *ibid.* 31; Stob. II p.91.10-11 W.; Diog.Laert. 7.113 (*SVF* III 395, 396); for Epicureanism see Philod. *De ira*, col. XLI 29 f. Indelli. Note also the very similar definitions from various schools collected by Seneca at *De ira* 1.2.3 with Cooper *ad loc.*

by dialecticians and refers to "the form and definition" (τὸ εἶδος καὶ τὸ λόγον), i.e. essence. Galen's reference to the most distinguished philosophers must refer to Aristotle and to Plato in view of passages such as *Timaeus* 70 a 7-b 8. But in fact Galen typifies the two definitions differently from Aristotle, taking the physical one as essential — quite in line with his general emphasis on corporeal factors. He retains the alternative definition in intentional terms, but, as we have noticed, demotes it to accidental status, presumably because it represents an evaluation of one's situation and hence reason. Galen, then, appears to have adapted Aristotle's well-known distinction so as to suit his understanding of the interaction between the two Platonic parts concerned. The physical effects shown by the heart and the judgement that revenge is called for are both involved in anger, as already Aristotle had taught. But Galen seems to take affections such as anger as blind, non-cognitive forces, though capable of interacting with reason.[63] A very similar picture of the respective roles allotted to the rational and spirited parts and of their communication is presented by Plato at *Tim.* 70 a 7-b 9.[64] In fact, Galen seems to read the Aristotelian distinction in the light of this Platonic passage in particular.

The passage from Galen's *Timaeus* commentary we have just mentioned indicates how their communication could be conceived on the anatomical and physiological level. Clearly this goes beyond anything to be found in the Platonic *Timaeus*. Indeed the original Platonic tripartition involves the ascription of both cognitive and motivational aspects to each of the three 'parts' of the soul. It seems that Galen for his part took the step to which his project of modernizing Plato scientifically had forced him to separate the two aspects.

[63] For a similar picture of the interaction between reason and non-rational functions as manifest from vehement emotions, see also *Loc.Aff.* VIII 227-228 K (a reference I owe to Jim Hankinson).

[64] Elsewhere Plato has no qualms about ascribing cognitive functions to the non-rational parts of the soul and even here describes the spritied part as obedient to the demands and threats of reason, *ibid.* b 7-9.

But is there any evidence for an analogous or similar solution in regard to the third or appetitive part? As De Lacy has already pointed out, Galen holds that hunger and thirst arise in the so-called mouth of the stomach, and they are transmitted by a nerve to the brain — not to the liver or to the brain by way of the liver.[65] But this seems to deprive the liver of its function as the centre of desire. The obvious next step to take is to locate desire as a mental phenomenon in the brain. But Galen sees no problem here, or so it seems. Is this a blind spot, caused by his Platonist bias? His attitude becomes more understandable and coherent once we realize that he equated the Platonic appetitive part with the level of soul possessed by plants, quite in line with Plato's ascription of this part to plants (*Tim.* 77 b). Thus in his *On the Use of Parts*, in explaining why there is only a small nerve to the liver, Galen argues:

> Insofar as this organ is the source of the nutritive soul, the kind that is also in plants, it appears to have no need for a nerve. I pass over the questions whether it should be called nature or nutritive soul (*UP* 4.13, I p.226.18-22 Helmreich [= III 308.17-309.3 K]).

Accordingly the activities of the liver are natural activities, and its powers are "natural powers" involved in nourishment and growth, *viz.* attraction, retention, alteration, expulsion.[66] So even if he is prepared to call these 'natural' functions psychic, he distinguishes between them on the one hand and others such as desire on the other.[67] This difference arises from the fact that

[65] *UP* 4.7, I p.201.19-202.2 Helmreich (= III 275.8-15 K); 16.5, II p.394.18-24 Helmreich (= IV 289.6-11 K); *Hipp.Epid.III* 3, 15, p.118.22-24 W.-Pf. (= XVIIA 664-665 K); cf. De Lacy, "Third Part" (see n. 4), 62.

[66] *Hipp.Epid. III* I 17, p.46.12-15 (= XVIIA 566 K), *ibid.* II A, p.71.6; *Hipp.Prorr.* CMG V 9, 2, p.56.4-8. See further De Lacy, "Third Part" (see n.4), 54 ff.

[67] This distinction also surfaces in the context of the issue of the soul's immortality. In one passage dealing with the soul's οὐσία Galen sides with those Platonists who ascribe mortality to the appetitive part (ἐπιθυμητικόν): *Hipp.Epid. V* 5, p.272.22-273.1 W.-Pf. (= XVIIB 250 K): τινὲς δὲ οὐ μίαν, ἀλλ' ἰδίαν ἑκατέρᾳ τὴν οὐσίαν εἶναί φασι καὶ οὐ σμικρῷ δέ τινι διαφερούσας, ἀλλ ' ὅλῳ τῷ γένει, ὅπου γε

desire and related emotions involve sensation and hence the nervous system. Thus desire, as we have noticed, includes the sensation of hunger and thirst. This dualism goes beyond the Platonic text. Presumably Galen adopted it under the influence Hellenistic predecessors such as Herophilus, who described as psychic those, and only those, functions that were operated by the nervous system they had just discovered. Herophilus too qualified other functions as 'natural'.[68] This involves a more restricted concept of soul, restricted, that is, to the orbit of consciousness and hence a purely mental phenomenon. This represents a striking anticipation of the modern concept of the mental as the subject-matter of psychology.

But where does this leave Galen and his defence of the Platonic tripartition? His explanation of the sensation of hunger and thirst is in fact more compatible with the Platonic text than his position in *PHP* Book 6. After all, as we have seen (above, p. 154), Plato installs desire in the stomach not the liver, saying that anger and desire are made obedient through "the narrow channels" (τῶν στενωπῶν, *Tim.* 70 b 5-7). This point could even be presented as anticipating the discovery of the nervous system.[69] Yet an appeal to Plato in this context would have revealed the discrepancy from *PHP* Book 6, where Galen assigns appetition to the liver without any qualifications (a move which, as we have noticed, entails a distortion of the Platonic account as well).

Another move which did involve an actual departure concerns the appetitive part as the locus of sexual desire. The liver qualified as the bodily seat of the Platonic ἐπιθυμητικόν because post-Platonic science had established its role in digestion and growth. But obviously it could not house the function of reproduction, which Plato also ascribes to his third part. In other

καὶ τὴν μὲν φύσεως φθαρτὴν εἶναι ἡγοῦνται, τὴν δὲ τῆς ψυχῆς ἄφθαρτον. Cf. DEUSE, *Untersuchungen* (see n.7), 101.

[68] See VON STADEN, "Body, Soul and Nerve" (see n.25), 89 ff.

[69] That Plato and his contemporaries did not know about the nervous system was acknowledged by Galen and was not at issue, see *supra*, p. 153.

works Galen elevates the testicles to the status of ἀρχή in addition to the three 'Platonic' ones of *PHP*.[70] It may seem surprising that this problem does not come up in the latter work (it can hardly be explained away by arguing that *PHP* Books 1-6 were written early in his career). In my view this feature bears witness to the fact that the discussion conducted here is to a large extent determined by the schema of fixed options set out at *PHP* 6.2.5 (as quoted above, p. 142). Another example (which we have already noted, above, p. 153) is Galen's omission to consider the possibility that the brain is the seat of the emotions as well as reason.[71]

We may conclude that Galen did address the problem of the interaction and coherence between the three Platonic parts by subsuming some of the relevant functions under the nervous system. He did so in works written some time after *PHP* Books 1-6 and in a way which meant an — unacknowledged — departure from some of the assumptions in these books.

6. *Conclusion*

In certain respects Galen behaves more like an empirical Platonist than a modern scientist engaged in an open-ended quest for knowledge. He remains caught in a traditional schema of options that are in principle open in the debate on the human soul. We have also seen that he follows a traditional agenda of topics. The ontological distinctions involved are Aristotelian in origin but had by Galen's day been fully absorbed by Platonism.

[70] *Ars Med.* 4, I 314 K; *MMG* 2.4, XI 97 K; *UP* 14.10, IV 186 ff. K. Véronique Boudon drew my attention to these passages and to the problem of their compatibility with the position taken by Galen in *PHP*.

[71] Doxographic schemas were used for what Galen calls 'dialectical' disputations on issues such as the seat of the soul, see *Loc.Aff.* VIII 157-159 K, esp. 157.17-18 with Mansfeld, "Doxography and Dialectic" (see n.18). Obviously these dialectical debates were not open-ended but aimed at reaching a verdict in favour of one of the competing options distinguished in such a schema.

Thus, as we have seen, certain Galenic key passages can be paralleled from more or less contemporary Platonist texts. Moreover we have found that he contributes to a contemporary debate among Platonists on the issue of whether the soul has parts or powers. This issue was connected with that of their location and that of the substance (οὐσία) of the soul. In *PHP* Books 1-6 Galen mounted an extensive vindication of the trilocation of the soul as presented by Plato in the *Timaeus*. The localization of reason, anger and appetite in three different organs committed him to the view that the soul consisted of three parts rather than powers. Put differently, there were three forms or kinds (εἴδη) of soul — the term already used by Plato. In *PHP* Galen suspends judgement as to its substance (corporeal/incorporeal, mortal/immortal) but in the work of his old age, *QAM*, he explicates his position in this matter by adapting a Peripatetic theorem: form is to be understood as the blend of corporeal elements of the main organs.

Galen's defence of the Platonic tripartition-cum-trilocation in the context of contemporary philosophical debate seems to sit uncomfortably with the ideal of a science free of partisanship and prejudice. Still it would be rash to conclude that philosophical schemas and debates were merely obstacles to scientific progress. Philosophical logic helped shape the sophisticated anatomical experiments designed by Galen to demonstrate the location of psychic functions.[72] Here the Platonic *Timaeus* left Galen ample room for his own innovations, most notably his exploration of the nervous system. Indeed, some new material suggests that he interpreted the Platonic tripartition-cum-trilocation of the soul in such a way that the brain as the functional centre of the nerves became the integrating factor in mental life.[73]

[72] Cf. TIELEMAN, "Galen on the Seat of the Intellect" (see n.4), 256-273.

[73] I want to record my gratitude to the other participants in the colloquium for their valuable comments and questions which are acknowledged at appropriate places in the text. Jonathan Barnes and Michael Frede also made a few suggestions of a more general kind which were equally helpful in preparing the final version. Of course, these scholars do not bear any responsibility for the resulting text.

DISCUSSION

J. Barnes: Your paper provides much food for thought, and is a model of the Utrecht school of ancient philosophy. I would like to raise one point which seems to me questionable. I agree that very many imperial authors used handbooks, epitomes, doxographies etc. as aids to writing their own works, if not as sources of information. But can it really be thought that Porphyry would go to a doxography to ascertain the views of Aristotle or of Longinus, or that Galen's central thesis about Plato and Hippocrates, authors whom he knew intimately, was taken from a manual?

T. Tieleman: To be sure, authors such as Galen and Porphyry were directly acquainted with the work of Plato, Aristotle and other philosophical classics and so did not *need* to rely on doxographies, manuals and the like to ascertain their views. But in practice, and contrary to present-day expectations and conventions, they also used literature of this sort. Thus Galen in *PHP* quotes extensively from Platonic and Chrysippean treatises but also uses a schema of options (e.g. 6.2.5 [= V 515.12-516.1 K], see above, p. 142), which can be paralleled from Porphyry and Jamblichus. That is to say, these authors avail themselves of the same division of three different options that are open in the debate on the parts of the soul, viz. associated with the names of Plato, Aristotle and the Stoics (Chrysippus) respectively. These options, as we have noticed, are based on same ontological distinction between the concepts of part and power. Galen and Porphyry embroider on the traditional schema by including Posidonius and Longinus respectively. The basic trifold division must be a product of the Platonist scholasticism of their age.

Similar use was made of the schemas of tenets provided by so-called doxographic literature. J. Mansfeld (Utrecht school) has demonstrated this for a wide range of philosophical authors including Galen ("Doxography and Dialectic" [see above, n.18]). Often they will have known such divisions of options (or at least a number of them) by heart, presumably as a result of their philosophical education. In sum, we should reckon with the possibility that Galen uses a pre-existing doxographic schemas. But if his use of doxography, manuals and the like can be established on the basis of parallels, the questions remains how and why he used this sort of literature. In his *On Affected Parts* he says that doxographic schemas were used for dialectical disputation (*Loc.aff.* VIII 157.17-18 K). Elsewhere he insists on the need to employ a division of the options that are open in a particular debate (*PHP* 4.1.14-17 [= V 364.12-366.5 K]; 3.1.10-20 [= V 287.16-290.4 K], where note the doxographic schema, *ibid.* 10-15; cf. Aët. 4.5). Particularly striking is his ascription to Zeno the Stoic and Epicurus (!) of the same view on the nature of emotion (*ibid.* 2.4-6) — an ascription which he clearly has not checked in any original texts (cf. *PHP* 5.6.40-42 [= V 477.9-478.9 K]). The view ascribed to Aristotle at *PHP* 6.2.5 (three powers — viz. the Platonic ones — located in the heart) does not appear to result from Galen's study of the relevant Aristotelian works either. In fact, he omits any mention of the standard Aristotelian distinction between five faculties as listed e.g. at *De an.* 2.3, 414 a 31-33). Nowhere does Galen corroborate his ascription by means of Aristotle's own words. As to Hippocrates and Plato, I think that we are agreed that Galen's admiration for them was genuine and based on his own readings of their works. It also inspired the main thesis of *PHP* that these two thinkers were in essential harmony on the most important issues (involving, as is only to be expected, a great deal of exegetical effort). In the case of the soul's structure Galen's thesis of their agreement can be paralleled from doxographic literature as well. I do not wish to argue that he simply took the idea from a specimen of this genre (Aët. 4.5.1, with Tieleman, *Galen and Chrysippus* [n.4], XXXIV-V). But I do believe that it makes sense to compare Galen's representation of the positions at issue with what is to be found in the kind of contemporary literature he is known to have used on a number of occasions. And why should we brush aside an indication that Galen was not the only one in his time to endorse this in our eyes odd thesis about the agreement between Plato and Hippocrates? To know something about the later *Rezeptionsgeschichte* of their work could help explain certain peculiarities of Galen's position and determine what was original and what traditional about it.

Your point about Porphyry's relation to Longinus fits in with I take to have been Galen's procedure. Porphyry had been a pupil of Longinus. There is no doubt that he was directly familiar with the latter's views. So I do not suggest that Porphyry turned to a traditional schema to 'ascertain' Longinus' view, as you seem to assume. Longinus did not feature in the traditional schema. But he happened to be of interest to his former student Porphyry. So he fitted Longinus into the pre-existing schema, presenting the latter's position as a compromise between two of the main options: Longinus is said to side with Plato as far as the incarnated soul is concerned and with Aristotle with respect to the disembodied soul. Similarly Galen links what he presents as Posidonius' position to that of Aristotle who, unlike Posidonius, featured in the original schema. Galen has a special interest in Posidonius because in books 4 and 5 of *PHP* he had played off this Stoic against Chrysippus.

V. Boudon: Je voudrais faire une remarque concernant le lien que vous avez très judicieusement établi entre psychologie et anatomie ou plus exactement entre psychologie et physiologie quand vous faites coïncider le siège des différentes parties de l'âme avec les trois ἀρχαί, les trois principes directeurs distingués par Galien, c'est-à-dire le cerveau, le coeur et le foie. Mais en face de cette tripartition que l'on rencontre, comme vous l'avez rappelé, notamment dans le *De placitis Hippocratis et Platonis*, on trouve ailleurs une quadripartition (cerveau, coeur, foie et testicules) dans l'*Ars medica* 5 (I 319.2-3 K), mais aussi le *Ad Glauconem De methodo medendi* 2, 4 (XI 97.2-4 K) et *De usu partium* 14, 10 (IV 186-187 K). Dans quelle mesure est-il possible, selon vous, de faire coïncider cette quadripartition galénique des ἀρχαί avec la tripartition platonicienne de l'âme?

T. Tieleman: Plato had situated the appetitive part in the belly. Galen transfers it to the liver in view of the central role played by the liver in digestion (a post-Platonic insight). However Plato had also ascribed sexual appetite to the soul's third part. Obviously this important function (connected with reproduction) could not be ascribed to the liver, so Galen in the works you mention added the testicles as the fourth ἀρχή. After all the reproductive organs were, if not indispensable for the individual organism, essential for the survival of the species. (Plato, *Resp.* 9, 581 a also attributes love of money to the appetitive part — a point understandably suppressed by Galen.) The difference between *PHP* and the three passages from other works reflects a feature of Galen's method in the former work, viz. his use of a fixed schema of pre-existing options, one of which is championed by Galen, viz. that the soul has three and only three parts, viz. those described by Plato and, he claims, Hippocrates. In the works where he assigns the status of ἀρχή to the testicles he is in a position to do more justice to the physiological facts.

M. Frede: Galen in the passage you quote (*PHP* 6.2.5-6 [= V 515.12-516.6 K]) says, quite rightly, that Plato speaks of both kinds (εἴδη) and parts (μέρη) of the soul, given that he believes that the parts of the soul separated from each other in place are very different in their οὐσία. One passage which he must have in mind is *Tim.* 77 a 6 ff., which he also discusses in *Sent.Prop.* 13. In the *Timaeus* Plato attributes to plants a soul. For, since they are alive, they are animals. They must have the third kind of soul (τὸ τρίτον ψυχῆς εἶδος, 77 b 3-4), the sort of the soul we have in the lower part of the body. This sort of soul in the case of a human being can be called, if one follows Plato, a part of the soul; in the case of plants, of course, it is not a part of the soul of the plant. Plato's way of speaking gives rise to a discussion as to whether we should speak of parts of the soul or kinds of soul; some thought we should speak of neither, and these spoke of powers (δυνάμεις) of the soul, that is *not* of parts of the soul or kinds of soul. One issue involved in this discussion was whether one οὐσία can have more than one δύναμις, especially an οὐσία which has no parts. This is affirmed by Longinus, obviously in opposition to authors who deny it. According to Galen (*loc.cit.*), it seems, it is denied by Chrysippus, who denies that the soul has parts and reduces all functions (i.e. θυμός and ἐπιθυμία) to one δύναμις (the rational ability to assent or not). According to Galen, Aristotle is wrong to assume that one οὐσία without parts (i.e. the soul) can have three δυνάμεις. Thus Galen seems to accept the view that an οὐσία without parts can have more than one δύναμις. As far as I can see, Galen does in fact think that there are three ἀρχαί in the human body, and thus three kinds of soul. Hence I think that the texts collected under "3. *Options*" have a complexity which is not captured by the scheme which you think is underlying them.

T. Tieleman: Thank you for reminding me of *Tim.* 77 a 6 ff. as relevant to the discussion conducted by Galen. I am inclined to assume that the preference of certain Platonists for the term 'power' was primarily motivated by their wish to save the soul's unity and hence immortality. Different powers could belong to a single underlying οὐσία, whereas different parts or kinds pre supposed different οὐσίαι for each of them. Hence Longinus' view that the soul has parts only when based in different bodily parts but powers *when separated from the body*.

In other words, I am not sure whether the term power was introduced as a way out of any exegetical problem arising from the fact that Plato had spoken both of kind (viz. with respect to plants) and of parts (with respect to humans). In fact, the terms εἶδος and μέρος were used interchangeably not only by Plato himself, but also by Aristotle and the late commentators in contexts concerned with division (diaeresis) in general or division of the soul in particular (for Plato see e.g. *Phaedr.* 253 c, 265 e-266 c; *Resp.* 6, 504 a; 9, 580 d-581 e; 9, 590 c; *Tim.* 73 b-d with M. Talamanca, "Lo schema 'genus-species' nelle sistematiche dei giuristi romani", in *La filosofia greca e il diritto romano* II, Accademia Nazionale dei Lincei 374, Quaderno 221 [Roma 1977], 3-319, 24 ff.). I have not come across any passage in Galen or elsewhere where the designation of the psychic faculties as parts as well as kinds/forms seems problematic or controversial (Alcin. *Didasc.* 5, p.156.29-32 Hermann; Gal. *PHP* 9.9.42-46 [= V 803.10-805 K]).

It does not follow from 6.2.6 (= V 516.1-6 K) that Galen thought that Aristotle was wrong to assume that one οὐσία can have more than one δύναμις. Rather Aristotle was wrong in assuming one οὐσία, i.e. a soul without parts located in one organ, viz. the heart. But having assumed one οὐσία, Aristotle rightly spoke of three *powers* rather than parts. This follows from Galen's conceptual apparatus, aligning the concept of part with that of οὐσία. One kind or part (i.e. of soul) may underlie a plurality of powers (see *PHP* 9.9.39-46 [= V 802.8-805] on which see above, p. 146 f.). As it was, Galen had demonstrated that there were three bodily seats and hence three parts and three οὐσίαι. Of course Galen's strict, anatomically based tripartition rendered the unity and coherence of the soul deeply problematic. However, he thought that this was what Plato had meant and what was indicated by the anatomical facts. I have pointed to some evidence that Galen sought to save the unity of the soul by assigning an integrative function to the nervous system (which of course entails a special status for the rational or regent part). But Galen did not provide a sustained treatment of this problem, leaving this to others such as Plotinus, who wanted to built on his anatomical work for their own theory of the soul (see my "Plotinus on the Seat of the Soul", referred to at n.57).

J. Jouanna: Dans votre étude si claire et si suggestive sur la psychologie de Galien, vous avez accordé sa juste place au *Quod animi mores*. Toutefois vous n'avez pas fait référence, me semble-t-il, aux nombreuses citations que Galien fait dans ce traité d'Hippocrate, *Airs, eaux, lieux* pour illustrer l'influence de l'environnement sur le corps et du corps sur l'âme. En quoi ce traité hippocratique apporte-t-il une illustration de ce que Galien voulait montrer?

T. Tieleman: In *PHP* Galen still clings to an agnostic position as to the substance of the soul. Nonetheless he already links psychic part and bodily part (*PHP* 6.2.5 [= V 515.12-516.1 K]). In the work of his late age, *QAM*, he takes the next step of actually identifying the substance of the soul with the form of the three main bodily organs, taking form in the sense of the blend of elementary qualities distinctive of each organ. In effect he comes out in favour of the Peripatetic view of the substance of the soul as the form of the body, combining this with the Platonic tripartition-cum-location. This view of the soul's substance suits Galen's thesis in *QAM* of the dependence of mental life on bodily states. Galen illustrates this in part by referring to the observations made in the Hippocratic *Airs Waters Places* on the influence of physical and environmental factors on mental life.

V. Barras: (1) Vous évoquez dans votre exposé le fait qu'il n'y a pas de 'psychiatrie' comme telle chez Galien (de même qu'on ne peut parler chez lui de 'psychologie' au sens strict et contemporain du terme). Il existe toutefois chez lui un très fort intérêt pour des situations cliniques 'psychopathologiques'. À votre avis, l'analyse de cette clinique galénique pourrait-elle malgré tout apporter quelques éléments à la compréhension de la 'psychologie' de Galien, de même que parfois l'examen de dysfonctionnements pathologiques permet de saisir le fonctionnement normal?

(2) À votre connaissance, Galien tente-t-il d'établir explicitement dans ses œuvres anatomiques une relation 'démontrable', évidente, entre le cerveau et d'autres organes sièges d'une part de l'âme, sous la forme d'une connexion nerveuse notamment?

T. Tieleman: (1) I take your point that Galen takes a keen interest in many afflictions that today are called psychiatric. A more comprehensive treatment of Galen's psychology would perhaps require a closer study of these phenomena. However, the relevance of psychiatric phenomena to the issues I have raised here seems on the whole limited. An exception is a passage from *On Affected Parts* (*Loc.aff.* 3.5, VIII 157 K). Here Galen points to the inconsistency of the Pneumatic physician Archigenes, who held that in the case of mental afflictions the heart is the affected part yet prescribed medication for the head. In this particular case, then, clinical experience is directly relevant to the question of the structure of the soul and its location in the body.

(2) In my paper I have pointed to two passages which strongly suggest that Galen assigned a role to the nervous system to account for the sensation of hunger and thirst and for the genesis of anger (see above, pp. 155, 158). This involves an anatomical connection (viz. through the relevant nerves) between the brain and the belly and between the brain and the heart respectively. I may add that Galen had earlier shown an interest in the anatomical connections between the main organs, when he conducted a vivisection experiment whereby he intercepted each of the three main kinds of vessel (arteries, veins, nerves) linking the brain and heart (*PHP* 2.6.1-17 [= V 262.11-267.6 K]). From the resulting observations he concluded that neither organ has any need of the other in operating its main functions; in other words, each is the source (ἀρχή) of its own set of functions. This experiment was directed against Chrysippus the Stoic who had suggested that even if the brain is the source of the nerves it does not follow that it is the set of the regent part of the soul since it may receive its orders from the heart. But if Galen succeeds in vindicating the status of the brain as the seat of reason, it is also clear that his theory, at least at this stage, stands in need of further refinement in view of the interactions between the parts of the soul. The two other passage reveal an increased awareness of the need to address this problem and to find a solution in the structure and workings of the nervous system.

V

Daniela Manetti

GALENO, LA LINGUA DI IPPOCRATE E IL TEMPO

Argomento di questa trattazione è l'insieme dei meccanismi usati da Galeno per analizzare il linguaggio ippocratico visto come esempio storico autorevole di linguaggio scientifico: si cercherà di coglierne i diversi nuclei e di capire come essi interagiscano a formare un quadro unitario. La scelta di questa prospettiva ha come conseguenza di tenere sullo sfondo l'elaborazione teorica che Galeno ha sviluppato sul linguaggio scientifico in generale e di considerare invece in primo piano la consapevolezza 'storica' di Galeno nei confronti di Ippocrate e dello sviluppo successivo del linguaggio della medicina di tradizione dogmatica, in cui Galeno si identifica. Ulteriore corollario di questa scelta è lasciare ai margini i numerosi elementi di polemica contro le manipolazioni del linguaggio operate dai suoi rivali. Il campo della ricerca è dunque costituito essenzialmente dai passi in cui Galeno riflette sullo sviluppo della medicina in generale o della tradizione dogmatica e soprattutto dalle sue opere esegetiche. Queste hanno ricevuto cure e attenzioni particolari negli studi dell'ultimo trentennio, specie per gli intrecci fra cultura filologico-grammaticale e esigenze ideologiche della dottrina medica propugnata da Galeno.[1] Si è focalizzata la costruzione dell'immagine di Ippocrate, forgiata da Galeno anche per mezzo di raffinati strumenti critico-letterari e filologici. Non si potrà

[1] Smith 1979; Manuli 1984, 1986; Manetti-Roselli 1994; Sluiter 1995a e 1995b.

prescindere però da una serie di approfondimenti recenti sulle opere logiche di Galeno e sulle sue riflessioni teoriche sul linguaggio.[2] Né si dovrà trascurare la sua relazione con la cultura contemporanea, che ha prodotto discussioni e posizioni anche radicali.[3] È risultato comunque chiaro che Galeno ha un posto autonomo, perché, pur influenzato dal clima generale atticistico e con un ruolo culturale analogo a quello di altri 'sofisti' del suo tempo, esercita tuttavia una critica consapevole contro gli eccessi del formalismo atticistico, grazie anche alla relativa libertà garantitagli dal 'genere' della medicina.

E proprio alla definizione dei 'generi' di scrittura della medicina Galeno ha contribuito con un'ampia riflessione, che ha alcuni momenti decisivi nei commenti a Ippocrate. Egli ha compiuto una classificazione per generi dei testi di Ippocrate come opere di scienza e parallelamente ha ridisegnato compiti e confini del commento scientifico nei confronti di quello letterario.[4]

Galeno riconosce in Ippocrate non solo un grande medico ma anche un grande scrittore, già nel primo commento ai trattati chirurgici: *Hipp.Fract.* XVIIIB 324,4 K: ἔδοξεν ἐν αὐτοῖς Ἕλλησιν ἄριστος ἰατρός τε καὶ συγγραφεύς. E per quanto teorizzi che il commento medico deve avere come fine preminente la trasmissione dell'utile per la *techne* (degradando spesso l'esegesi puramente grammaticale ad esercizio sofistico), ricche, frequenti e preziose sono le osservazioni di carattere linguistico-grammaticale che Galeno profonde nei suoi commenti.

[2] BARNES 1991, 1993a e 1993b, 1997; FREDE 1981; HANKINSON 1994d; VON STADEN 1995. Poco conosciuto, ma molto dettagliato lo studio di KOTZIA PANTELE 1995. DEICHGRÄBER 1957, 8 ss., fa una presentazione sintetica degli studi linguistici perduti di Galeno, occupandosi specialmente di *Sui nomi medici*; VON MÜLLER 1897 ricostruisce il *De demonstratione*. Per il *De captionibus* (o *De sophismatibus*, d'ora in poi *Soph.*) cf. EDLOW 1977; SCHIAPARELLI 1999a e 1999b, 2002.

[3] Dopo i classici studi di BOWERSOCK 1969 e REARDON 1971, vedi KOLLESCH 1981; BRUNT 1994; DEBRU 1995; KOTZIA PANTELE 1995, 81 ss.; SWAIN 1996; VON STADEN 1997.

[4] MANETTI-ROSELLI 1994.

Ma qui interessa mettere a fuoco e commentare non la vasta erudizione di Galeno, ma la sua visione di insieme del linguaggio ippocratico, che si ricostruisce dai commenti e da altre opere. Lo scopo è capire se e quali elementi di carattere generale e/o teorico sono presupposti o fatti operare nell'analisi di un modello storico di linguaggio medico e se la consapevolezza della tradizione del linguaggio medico precedente può a sua volta chiarire meglio alcuni punti dell'elaborazione teorica di Galeno.

In effetti, dall'esame dei molti passi che Galeno dedica alla discussione della lingua di Ippocrate risulta un disegno abbastanza definito di uno scrittore fornito di uno stile preciso che si sostanzia di tre qualità o virtù: la chiarezza,[5] σαφήνεια, in primo luogo; la correttezza o ἑλληνισμός; e infine la brevità, βραχυλογία (o meno spesso συντομία). La chiarezza è ottenuta con l'uso di un linguaggio semplice e corrente, cf. p. es. *Hipp.Epid. III*, CMG V 10, 2, 1, p.126,10 ss. dove si attribuisce all'Ippocrate di *Aforismi* e *Prognostico* la chiarezza che viene dall'uso delle parole comuni, chiamate dai retori πολιτικά.[6]

La chiarezza di Ippocrate è presupposta a tal punto che, in quei passi dove il testo non corrisponda a questo standard, si può sospettare una interpolazione o una corruzione. Essa può tuttavia non essere riconosciuta a causa del passare del tempo, perché Ippocrate è scrittore antico: Ippocrate segue infatti la *synetheia* del suo tempo, ma la *chresis* è cambiata e per questo può apparire oscuro in certi casi, cf. *Hipp.Art.* XVIIIA 537,4 ss.:

> χρησαμένου τοῦ Ἱπποκράτους τῇ "ῥοιβοειδέα" φωνῇ σαφηνείας μὲν ἕνεκεν, ἥτις παράδειγμα λέλεκται πρὸς αὐτοῦ, μείζονα δ' ἀσάφειαν ἐργαζομένη αὐτοῦ τοῦ γιγνωσκομένου πράγματος ἢ τῆς σαφηνείας ἕνεκα παράδειγμά τι ὤφθη. τότε μὲν οὖν ἴσως ἦν ἡ φωνὴ

[5] Cf. *MM* X 424,15; *Hipp.Art.* XVIIIA 303,16; 375,4 ss. K ecc.

[6] Il testo è: ὁ γάρ τοι τοῦ Ἡρακλείδου υἱὸς Ἱπποκράτης ... φαίνεται συνηθεστάτοις τε καὶ διὰ τοῦτο σαφεστάτοις ὀνόμασι κεχρημένος, ἃ καλεῖν ἔθος ἐστὶ τοῖς ῥητορικοῖς "πολιτικά". Sull'uso di πολιτικὰ ὀνόματα vedi anche *Hipp.Art.* XVIIIA 414,15 ss. K: questa prima parte dà per scontati alcuni risultati delle ricerche di MANETTI-ROSELLI 1994 e SLUITER 1995a e 1995b.

συνήθης ἢ οὐκ ἂν εἴρηκε "ῥοιβοειδέα τρόπον". ἐν δὲ τῷ μετὰ ταῦτα χρήσεως αὐτῆς ἐκβληθείσης εἰς ἀσάφειαν ἧκε.[7]

La chiarezza del testo ippocratico deve dunque talvolta essere ricostruita attraverso il confronto con altri scrittori antichi. Questo basilare ragionamento di critica storico-filologica si era già imposto negli studi ippocratici da tempo: esso è esplicitato nel proemio del *Lessico Ippocratico* di Erotiano e Galeno ne mette in pratica costantemente le conseguenze. Contro i detrattori che lo accusano di oscurità voluta, Erotiano e Galeno non hanno mai messo in dubbio che il linguaggio di Ippocrate ricerchi la chiarezza.[8] Alla chiarezza è strettamente connessa la correttezza o ἑλληνισμός, che pone però gli stessi problemi di 'ricostruzione storica', poiché Galeno deve affrontare molti punti difficili: tuttavia essa è normalmente presupposta, tanto che alcuni casi di solecismo sono considerati indizi di non autenticità (interpolazione nel caso citato di *Hipp.Epid. III*).[9]

Come è noto, la teoria delle qualità della λέξις comincia con Aristotele, che per primo identifica la virtù del discorso nella chiarezza, che include lo ἑλληνίζειν, cioè la correttezza linguistica. Nel privilegiare la chiarezza dunque Galeno si inserisce nella tradizione che discende da Aristotele, anche se la sua insistenza sulla prevalenza del contenuto dottrinale rispetto alla forma linguistica potrebbe far pensare che egli svaluta la correttezza.[10]

[7] Si tratta dell'applicazione del principio, stabilito nel proemio del commento a Fratture (*Hipp.Fract.* XVIIIB 318 ss. K), della distinzione fra oscurità assoluta e oscurità relativa: quest'ultima segnala un disturbo nella comunicazione fra destinatore e destinatario, che in questo caso è appunto costituito dal passare del tempo e dal cambiamento nell'uso. Sul concetto di oscurità cf. MANSFELD 1994, 148 ss.

[8] Cf. *Hipp.Fract.* XVIIIB 326, 327, 335 ecc. Sulle accuse ricorrenti all'oscurità di Ippocrate e sul tema polemico della chiarezza di Ippocrate in Erotiano, cf. MANSFELD 1994, 148 ss.; MANETTI 1999, 363 ss.

[9] Cf. p. es. *Hipp.Prorr.* 13,27. Sul tema cf. SLUITER 1995a, 522 ss. e KOTZIA PANTELE 1995, 73 e n.65 (la quale rimanda la coppia *sapheneia-hellenismos* alle due virtù necessarie in CIC. *De orat.* 3, 38).

[10] SLUITER 1995a, 529. La tolleranza (teoricamente affermata, ma non spesso applicata nei fatti) di imprecisioni o solecismi in Galeno è complementare al rifiuto del purismo eccessivo degli atticisti (cf. p. es. *Alim.Fac.* VI 579,10 ss. K) ed è la faccia speculare del suo privilegiare la ricerca sui *pragmata*, tuttavia non

La sistemazione più influente della teoria si deve a Teofrasto, che definisce quattro virtù: chiarezza, purezza, ornato, convenienza. L'aggiunta della brevità è attribuita agli Stoici ma diventa ben presto parte del patrimonio comune.

È ovvio vedere nel quadro che Galeno costruisce il riflesso della cultura retorica del suo tempo, tuttavia vale la pena di approfondire le consonanze con alcuni testi. In effetti le tre virtù dello stile ippocratico risultano da una selezione nella quale si può scorgere una certa affinità con la ripartizione fra virtù 'necessarie' e virtù 'accessorie' dello stile in Dionigi di Alicarnasso,[11] come è esplicitata nell'opera *Su Tucidide* 22,2.

Le qualità necessarie sono attribuite in blocco all'insieme degli storici anteriori a Tucidide e alla guerra del Peloponneso, quelli almeno di cui Dionigi conosce le opere (*Thuc.* 23,4-6).[12] La definizione finale della loro lingua è καὶ γὰρ καθαρὰ καὶ σαφὴς καὶ σύντομός ἐστιν. Le tre virtù 'necessarie', correttezza, chiarezza e brevità, di Dionigi sono in effetti le stesse attribuite da Galeno a Ippocrate. È importante tenere presente che in *Thuc.* 5,3-4 Dionigi attribuisce agli storici più antichi, autori di storie locali di Greci o di barbari, anche *un unico scopo di comunicazione*, quello di portare a conoscenza comune, senza togliere né aggiungere niente, le memorie salvate dei popoli, dei luoghi sacri e delle città:

basta ad avvicinarlo all'affermazione attribuita a Crisippo, che in nome della supremazia della brevità e dell'attenzione ai contenuti più che alla forma (un tema caro anche a Galeno) ammette oscurità, ellissi e solecismi (PLUT. *Stoic.rep.* 28, 1047B). La chiarezza resta sempre l'elemento imprescindibile, come è chiaro dalla discussione sulla virtù della buona significazione in *Soph.*, cf. SCHIAPARELLI 1999a e 1999b (l'immagine del sistema linguistico in *Soph.* si avvicina ad un linguaggio artificiale o di tipo scientifico): raccolta di passi su σαφήνεια in LÓPEZ-FÉREZ 1994.

[11] La divisione è anteriore a Dionigi, probabilmente formatasi fra III e II sec. a.C.; cf. BONNER 1939, 19; anche lo stile di Tucidide viene considerato buono, quando egli non si discosta troppo dalle virtù 'necessarie', cattivo quando se ne discosta troppo a lungo, cf. D.H. *Thuc.* 49,1.

[12] Dionigi, *Thuc.* 23.2, dice che, per i nomi dei più antichi di cui non si conservano le opere, come Cadmo di Melto e Aristea di Proconneso, non si può sapere se erano semplici e disadorni, mirando all'utile e al necessario, oppure se preferivano uno stile solenne e pieno di ornamenti.

> ἕνα καὶ τὸν αὐτὸν φυλάττοντες σκοπόν, ὅσαι διεσῴζοντο παρὰ τοῖς ἐπιχωρίοις μνῆμαι κατὰ ἔθνη τε καὶ κατὰ πόλεις, εἴ τ' ἐν ἱεροῖς εἴ τ' ἐν βεβήλοις ἀποκείμεναι γραφαί, ταύτας εἰς τὴν κοινὴν ἁπάντων γνῶσιν ἐξενεγκεῖν, οἵας παρέλαβον, μήτε προστιθέντες αὐταῖς τι μήτε ἀφαιροῦντες ... λέξιν τε ὡς ἐπὶ τὸ πολὺ τὴν αὐτὴν ἅπαντες ἐπιτηδεύσαντες, ὅσοι τοὺς αὐτοὺς προείλοντο τῶν διαλέκτων χαρακτῆρας, τὴν σαφῆ καὶ κοινὴν καὶ καθαρὰν καὶ σύντομον καὶ τοῖς πράγμασι προσφυῆ καὶ μηδεμίαν σκευωρίαν ἐπιφαίνουσαν τεχνικήν.

Di questa unicità di scopo è immediato riflesso un'unità stilistica (all'interno della scelta del dialetto letterario). Allo scopo comune dunque corrisponde un linguaggio corrente (κοινὴ λέξις), che è adeguato ai fatti e non mostra alcun artificio tecnico. Se poi si considerano in dettaglio gli scritti che Dionigi dedica agli oratori antichi, ci si accorge che il modello di oratore più vicino alla caratterizzazione di Ippocrate in Galeno è Lisia.[13] Lisia infatti possiede le stesse qualità: 1) è corretto (*Lys.* 2,1 καθαρός ἐστι τὴν ἑρμηνείαν); 2) usa parole comuni, rifugge da figure poetiche (3,1-2) e ottiene la chiarezza (4,2); 3) è conciso e denso (4,4; 5,1).

Le caratteristiche attribuite a Ippocrate sono in sostanza quelle considerate necessarie ed essenziali per chiunque voglia scrivere una buona prosa,[14] ma sono in particolare le virtù riconducibili allo stato più antico della storiografia. Sono inoltre le virtù specifiche di uno degli autori modello della corrente atticistica che appartiene alla generazione più antica (D.H. *Orat.vett.* 4,5). La particolare vicinanza di Ippocrate ad un autore come Lisia[15] (di cui Dionigi dà una datazione più alta rispetto alla critica moderna) è consonante anche con la sua 'cronologia' tradizionale come

[13] Gli accosta la descrizione della lingua greca in *Diff.Puls.* VIII 585,16 s.; DEICHGRÄBER 1957, 32 n.1.

[14] Da considerarsi parallela la tradizione epicurea, che vede in chiarezza, sintesi e *hellenismos* (p. es. SEXT.EMP. *Math.* II 56) i tratti essenziali dello scrivere filosofico, cf. MILANESE 1989, 67-106 e *infra* n.19.

[15] In Galeno Lisia forma coppia con Demostene come riferimento al genere oratorio, cf. *Diff.Puls.* VIII 717,16 ss. K, dove egli li indica come modelli, dopo aver descritto lo ἄριστος διδάσκαλος che si esprime con chiarezza, brevità e precisione; "Lisia, Demostene e gli altri oratori" anche in *MM* X 12,1 K.

autore antico, così come coerente con questo è anche il fatto che la lingua di Ippocrate, a cui Galeno dice di aver dedicato un trattato, era definita 'attico antico', come quella degli storici anteriori alla guerra del Peloponneso (che è comunque affine allo ionico, cf. *Thuc.* 23,4), secondo Dionigi, e come la lingua di Omero.[16]

La serie delle tre virtù della lingua ippocratica trova ulteriori consonanze nella teoria dei *genera dicendi* (elevato, tenue e medio) che si è sviluppata nel tempo e sovrapposta alla teoria delle virtù del discorso. Da questo punto di vista la lingua ippocratica si avvicina alle caratteristiche del *genus tenue*, che persegue chiarezza, correttezza, concisione ma niente ornamento.[17] La coincidenza è tutt'altro che casuale perché uno degli scopi per cui è appropriato il genere 'sottile' o 'tenue' è appunto l'istruire (Quint. *Inst.* 12,10,59; Cic. *Orat.* 69) e uno dei *leit-motivs* di Galeno nei commenti e in tutta la sua opera è definire la scrittura di Ippocrate come rivolta all'insegnamento;[18] inoltre spesso

[16] Per la lingua di Ippocrate, cf. *Hipp.Fract.* XVIIIB 322,11 ss. K: Galeno sembra essere in parte dissenziente, ma rimanda al suo trattato *Sulla lingua di Ippocrate*, di cui purtroppo non sappiamo niente. Comunque, in un altro passo (*Hipp.Art.* XVIIIA 414,15 ss. K), Galeno paragona lo stile ippocratico a quello di Senofonte, per il fatto di usare per lo più parole correnti (πολιτικά) e anche τροπικά καὶ γλωσσηματικά come lui, ma in misura maggiore. Il termine γλωσσηματικά indica voci regionali o di singole città (*schol.ad* DION.THR., in *Gramm.Gr.* I 3, p.14,17, 739,27) e l'osservazione di Galeno si coordina bene con l'attenzione che egli dedica di volta in volta a spiegare nei commenti espressioni ioniche, cf. p. es. *Hipp.Prog.*, CMG V 9, 2, p.225, e anche derivate 'dal dialetto di Cos', cf. *Hipp.Epid. VI*, CMG V 10, 2, 2, p.79,15. D'altra parte, nel corso dei commenti, Galeno osserva dettagliatamente le figure (τροπικά), soprattutto metafora (p. es. *Hipp.Art.* XVIIIA 617,8 K) e *katachresis* (*Hipp.Art.* XVIIIA 482,1 K), ma anche l'ironia (*Hipp.Art.* XVIIIA 465,5 K). Se l'aggettivo πολιτικός, come sostiene HERBST 1911, 5 ss., equivale di fatto a 'attico', ne risulterebbe che la lingua di Ippocrate consta di un fondo antico-attico in cui sono però relativamente frequenti parole ioniche o 'regionali' e espressioni figurate (cf. *infra*). Per la lingua di Omero cf. Ps.PLUT. *De Homero* 8-12 (lingua mista di tutti i dialetti, ma *soprattutto* attica); CHOEROBOSCUS, Georgius, in *Gramm.Gr.* IV 2, p.86,17 ss. (dialetto attico antico). Sulla tradizione biografica antica su Ippocrate, cf. JOUANNA 1992, 13-40.

[17] Cf. per esempio la presentazione di Cicerone, *Orat.* 20.

[18] Cf. SLUITER 1995a.

questo genere è presentato come tipico della filosofia.[19] La scelta di queste particolari virtù dello stile è perciò un passo essenziale per disegnare la figura di scienziato di Ippocrate, che ha un suo specifico scopo di istruzione e che si distingue dai poeti, perché non contiene niente di ridondante e di superfluo come Omero, ma si differenzia anche da storici come Erodoto che scrivono per dilettare o come Tucidide.[20]

La brachilogia fra dialettica e retorica

Non credo sia un caso che le virtù essenziali siano attribuite da Dionigi agli storici più antichi: ciò naturalmente risponde ad uno schema evolutivo che va dal semplice al complesso.[21] Dionigi non attribuisce un carattere negativo alla semplicità stilistica degli esordi. Egli disegna un quadro fortemente unitario, attribuendo agli storici antichi anche una strategia comunicativa univoca e diretta, semplicemente il trasmettere la tradizione. Anche Ippocrate è inserito da Galeno in una fase arcaica: è scrittore παλαιός[22] e con gli scrittori suoi contemporanei condivide principalmente due caratteristiche: 1) un corretto uso del linguaggio, cioè non sofistico, che esprime un corretto rapporto con il destinatario della comunicazione; 2) la brevità, che è strettamente connessa alla prima caratteristica. Solo la brevità, fra le sue virtù, è esplicitamente e ripetutamente collegata ad una arcaicità di Ippocrate.

[19] MILANESE 1989 mostra (in generale e spec. 57 e nn., cf. 86 ss.) che una parallela e autonoma tradizione epicurea cerca di definire lo stile filosofico in opposizione alla tradizione retorica, esaltando la *sapheneia* basata sulla retta conoscenza.

[20] Temi già trattati in MANETTI-ROSELLI 1994; SLUITER 1995b.

[21] Analoga, ma di segno negativo (*subobscuri*), perché in un contesto antiprimitivistico, la situazione dell'oratoria antica (esemplata da Tucidide) in CIC. *Brut.* 29. Per la convivenza di schemi che vedono negli antichi un'età dell'oro e schemi che li vedono come imperfetti e su elementi comuni di diverse teorie, vedi GATZ 1967, 150 s.; sull'idea di progresso in Cicerone, cf. NOVARA 1982, I 199-270.

[22] Talvolta detto ὁ παλαιός per antonomasia, cf. p. es. *Di.Dec.* IX 885,17 K; *MM* X 772,16 K.

Ma prima di tutto gli antichi si ponevano uno scopo comunicativo molto semplice e diretto, farsi capire dal pubblico senza troppe sottigliezze. Per esempio a *Hipp.Art.* XVIIIA 646,14 ss. K[23] Galeno dice che Ippocrate come tutti gli antichi non conosceva ancora la *leptologia* diventata di moda fra i moderni, ma voleva solo farsi capire dal pubblico; a *Hipp.Art.* XVIIIA 685,12 ss. K[24] dice che Ippocrate si preoccupa solo di significare l'oggetto del suo discorso e che tutti gli antichi avevano lo stesso scopo. Non si può fare a meno di notare l'analogia con lo schema dionisiano che attribuiva agli storici antichi una unicità di intenti. Questi (e altri) passi mettono in contrasto esplicito il passato (un po' idealizzato) con un presente di segno negativo. Il presente è simbolizzato dalla *leptologia* o *mikrologia*, cioè da una preoccupazione eccessiva di distinzione fra le parole, il cui campione è per antonomasia Prodico.[25] La polemica di Galeno contro le sofisticherie linguistiche di certi suoi rivali è uno dei suoi ritornelli più noti ed è costruita in modo quasi esclusivo su una contrapposizione fra antichi (Ippocrate, Platone, Aristotele) e moderni.[26]. L'uso costante del riferimento ai sofisti del V secolo a.C. è uno dei segni più evidenti di quanto il problema del linguaggio e della terminologia medica sia affrontato da Galeno in termini platonici e rivestito di 'citazioni' e allusioni platoniche.[27]

[23] XVIIIA 646,14 ss. K δῆλον ὅτι μὲν ἰσχίον εἴρηκεν ἐκπίπτειν ἀντὶ τοῦ κατ' ἰσχίον ἄρθρου. εἴρηται γὰρ ἡμῖν πολλάκις, ὡς οἱ παλαιοὶ πάντες, οὔπω τὴν ὕστερον ἀσκηθεῖσαν εἴδεσαν ἀκριβολογίαν τε καὶ λεπτολογίαν ἐν τοῖς ὀνόμασιν, ἀλλ' ἱκανὸν ἦν αὐτοῖς ἑρμηνεύειν, ἑνὸς μόνου στοχαζομένοις τοῦ (τὸ Kühn) παρακολουθεῖν τοῖς λεγομένοις τοὺς ἀκούοντας.

[24] XVIIIA 685,12 ss. K ῥητέον οὖν πρὸς τὰ τοιαῦτα ζητοῦντας ὃ καὶ ἔμπροσθεν ἤδη μοι λέλεκται, τοῦ σημᾶναι τὸ λεγόμενον πρᾶγμα μόνον φροντίζειν τὸν Ἱπποκράτην, καθάπερ καὶ ὁ Πλάτων ἡμᾶς τε ποιεῖν ἀξιοῖ τοῦτο καὶ πρῶτον αὐτὸς πράττει. δέδεικται δ' ἡμῖν ἑτέρωθι, ὅτι οἱ παλαιοὶ πάντες οὐκ ἄλλον ἢ τοῦτον εἶχον τὸν σκοπόν. μόνος γὰρ φαίνεται Πρόδικος ἐζηλωκέναι αὐτὴν ἐν τοῖς ὀνόμασι μικρολογίαν, ὡς εἰώθασι προσαγορεύειν οἱ τὰ Προδίκου ζηλώσαντες.

[25] Cf. *Hipp.Art.* XVIIIA 535,13 ss.; 544,12 ss. K; *HVA*, CMG V 9, 1, p.261,3: è meschino opporre all'imprecisione degli antichi la *leptologia* dei moderni.

[26] Hankinson 1994b, 1779; Vegetti 2001.

[27] Si ricordi p. es. in *Resp.* III 405 d 3-4 la polemica di Platone contro le invenzioni terminologiche degli 'Asclepiadi raffinati'. Ma uno dei punti più influenti è la specificazione che i nomi sono uno strumento didascalico in *Crat.* 388 b-c ὄνομα

Il motivo che si debba disprezzare lo zelo sui nomi e occuparsi della conoscenza dei fatti, è basato da Galeno esplicitamente sul richiamo a Platone (*Polit.* 261 e) che ricorre più volte.[28] In questi casi ci è presentata spesso la coppia Ippocrate-Platone come guidata da un identico criterio: tale sorta di endiadi fa sì che per una proprietà transitiva sia attribuita a Ippocrate non solo l'assenza di *mikrologia*, ma anche un ruolo di consapevole opposizione ai sofisti, al pari di Socrate.[29] Infatti a *Hipp.Fract.* XVIIIB 513,5 ss.

ἄρα διδασκαλικόν τί ἐστιν ὄργανον καὶ διακριτικὸν τῆς οὐσίας e 428 e διδασκαλίας ἄρα ἕνεκα τὰ ὀνόματα λέγεται. Galeno ripete spesso che l'uso della denominazione è ἕνεκα συντόμου διδασκαλίας: cf. p. es. *Sui termini medici* = Meyerhoff-Schacht 1931 (d'ora in poi *Med.Nam.*), 8; *Temp.* I 546,4 K; *MM* X 461,2; 603,14 K ecc., ma in particolare *Hipp.Epid. I*, CMG V 10, 1, p.117,3 ss. ἄμεινον οὖν ἐστι τῶν μὲν ὀνομάτων, ὡς εἴρηται, καταφρονεῖν, ἀσκοῦντα διαγνώσεις τε καὶ προγνώσεις καὶ θεραπείας ἑκάστου τῶν πυρετῶν. ἐπεὶ δὲ σαφεστέρα τε καὶ συντομωτέρα διὰ τῶν ὀνομάτων ἡ διδασκαλία γίνεται ... ἀκριβῆ τριταῖον ὀνομάσομεν ἕνεκα συντόμου διδασκαλίας. Insomma è l'insegnamento, la necessità di comunicazione del sapere, a rendere necessario l'uso dei nomi (*Diff.Puls.* VIII 493,3 ss. K) e a giustificare l'esigenza di un linguaggio scientifico adeguato. Quanto all'uso frequente di νομοθετεῖν, νομοθεσία ecc. in Galeno, esso deriva naturalmente da Platone (p. es. *Crat.* 389 d-e), ma il termine era stato assunto anche dagli Stoici (cf. p. es. Varro *Ling.* 8,7). Forse non a caso Galeno caratterizza di solito il νομοθετεῖν come l'azione arbitraria dei *neoteroi* e lo riferisce esplicitamente a Crisippo (*Diff.Puls.* VIII 631,1 ss. K), 'antenato' di Archigene, uno dei suoi obbiettivi polemici.

[28] Per la ricerca sui *pragmata* piuttosto che sui nomi, cf. *Crat.* 439 b ὅντινα μὲν τοίνυν τρόπον δεῖ μανθάνειν ἢ εὑρίσκειν τὰ ὄντα, μεῖζον ἴσως ἐστὶν ἐγνωκέναι ἢ κατ' ἐμὲ καὶ σέ· ἀγαπητὸν δὲ καὶ τοῦτο ὁμολογήσασθαι, ὅτι οὐκ ἐξ ὀνομάτων ἀλλὰ πολὺ μᾶλλον αὐτὰ ἐξ αὑτῶν καὶ μαθητέον καὶ ζητητέον ἢ ἐκ τῶν ὀνομάτων. Per i passi galenici cf. p. es. *AA* 6, 13, II 580-81 K; 10, 9, 79-81 Simon (= Garofalo 1991, in part. 898); 12, 2, 144 Simon (= Garofalo 1991, 958) e molti altri citati da Kotzia Pantele 1995, 61 s.

[29] Cf. *AA* 12, 2 *cit.* L'accoppiamento con Platone può aver riverberato almeno in parte su Ippocrate, autore usualmente ignorato dalla critica retorico-letteraria (unica citazione in Demetr. *Eloc.* 238; cf. Sluiter 1995a), anche l'immagine che il suo stile godeva nella tradizione retorica. Lo stile platonico è secondo Dionigi una mescolanza dello elevato e del tenue, è cioè un genere medio, ma il giudizio sui passi in cui egli segue il genere tenue ricorda la caratterizzazione galenica di Ippocrate: *Dem.* 5,3 ὅταν μὲν οὖν τὴν ἰσχνὴν καὶ ἀφελῆ καὶ ἀποίητον ἐπιτηδεύῃ φράσιν, ἐκτόπως ἡδεῖά ἐστι καὶ φιλάνθρωπος. καθαρὰ γὰρ ἀποχρώντως γίνεται καὶ διαυγής, ὥσπερ τὰ διαφανέστατα τῶν ναμάτων, ἀκριβής τε καὶ λεπτὴ παρ' ἡντινοῦν ἑτέραν τῶν [εἰς] τὴν αὐτὴν διάλεκτον εἰργασμένων. τήν τε κοινότητα διώκει τῶν ὀνομάτων καὶ τὴν σαφήνειαν ἀσκεῖ, πάσης ὑπεριδοῦσα κατασκευῆς ἐπιθέτου (cf. Gal. *Hipp.Elem.* I 501,6 K = CMG V 1, 2, p.148,12).

si dice che Ippocrate, come tutti gli antichi, disprezza la *mikrologia*, quella che in seguito viene chiamata *akribeia*, precisione.

Accanto alla *mikrologia*, anche la *makrologia* così tipica dei sofisti è assente dal linguaggio degli antichi.[30] La lingua di Ippocrate si presenta dunque in primo luogo sul versante negativo, cioè come assenza di disquisizioni sui nomi: in particolare, il 'socratismo' dell'Ippocrate galenico comporta anche la sua scelta di brevità in contrapposizione alla *leptologia* di sofisti come Prodico da una parte, ma anche alla *makrologia* di sofisti come Protagora e Gorgia dall'altra,[31] e in seguito di Stoici come Crisippo. E tuttavia questa brevità ha subito una considerevole manipolazione rispetto al modello platonico, perché non corrisponde più alla forma dialogica difesa da Socrate.

La scelta linguistica dell'Ippocrate galenico è costruita con una impostazione retorica evidente, come capacità di dire l'essenziale senza alcun artificio, cioè ornamento (κατασκευή è il termine tecnico), secondo i precetti scolastici più noti, ma va al di là del livello retorico nella misura in cui è anche originata da un rapporto fiduciario con il suo pubblico, come è chiaro da *Hipp.Elem.*, CMG V 1, 2, p.148,10 ss. (= I 501,6 ss. K) e da *Diff.Puls.* VIII 494, 8 ss. K:

> "Per questo penso che il mio discorso sarà più lungo a causa della confutazione di questi sfrontati, mentre il discorso di Ippocrate che scrive proprio ciò che appare chiaramente senza nessun artificio è breve e sintetico, perché non sospetta neanche che qualcuno ignori cose del genere o le rifiuti (ὁ λόγος ... Ἱπποκράτει δὲ βραχὺς καὶ σύντομος αὐτὸ τὸ φαινόμενον ἐναργῶς γράφοντι χωρὶς ἁπάσης κατασκευῆς τῷ μηδ' ὑπονοῆσαι μηδένα μήτ' ἀγνοῆσαί ποτε τὰ τοιαῦτα μήτ' ἀρνήσασθαι)".
>
> "È facile scoprire che gli antichi usavano i nomi semplicemente, preoccupandosi solo di rivelare il contenuto di pensiero. I moderni invece argomentano quasi su ciascuna sillaba e amano la contesa e

[30] MANETTI 1998.

[31] Sull'indifferenza dei mezzi formali della trattazione in relazione agli argomenti trattati *Prot.* 329 b, 335 b-c; *Grg.* 449 b-c: Socrate invece si dichiara incapace di fare lunghi discorsi.

non fanno che litigare sui nomi (τοὺς μὲν οὖν παλαιοὺς ἁπλῶς ἔστιν εὑρεῖν χρωμένους τοῖς ὀνόμασιν, ἑνὸς μόνου φροντίζοντας ἀεὶ τοῦ δηλῶσαι τὸ νοούμενον. οἱ δὲ νεώτεροι μόνον οὐ (οὐ add. Barnes) καθ' ἑκάστην συλλαβὴν σοφίζονταί τε καὶ φιλονεικοῦσι, καὶ οὐδὲ παύονται περὶ τῶν ὀνομάτων ἐρίζοντες.)".[32]

La lingua di Ippocrate dunque discende naturalmente da quell'atteggiamento di comunicazione diretta e senza 'malizia' che è proprio degli antichi e si rivela come disposizione psicologica ed etica prima che come abilità retorica.

Tuttavia il parlare sinteticamente ma in modo chiaro è un difficile equilibrio, che comporta dei rischi, come insegnano i manuali di retorica: l'eccessiva brevità è a scapito della chiarezza, genera oscurità e diventa un vizio, si possono infatti omettere elementi necessari.[33] Galeno è ben consapevole di questo rischio e si preoccupa di chiarire bene la differenza fra brevità e omissione.

De sanitate tuenda II 4,4 (VI 105-106 K = CMG V 4, 2, p.48,4-8): "Il tipo di espressione antica è così breve che egli spesso sembra omettere nel discorso molte delle cose che conseguono necessariamente a ciò che viene detto (τὸ δὲ τῆς παλαιᾶς ἑρμηνείας εἶδος οὕτως ἐστὶ βραχυλόγον, ὡς πολλὰ πολλάκις ὑπερβαίνειν δοκεῖν τῇ λέξει τῶν ἐξ ἀνάγκης ἑπομένων τοῖς λεγομένοις). E per questa ragione, penso, scriviamo commenti ai suoi testi, guidando coloro che per mancanza di esercizio non sono in grado di seguire la sintesi della dizione antica, così come facciamo in questo discorso".[34]

Lo stile breve degli antichi può dare l'impressione di omettere elementi utili,[35] di lasciare implicite le conseguenze di ciò che

[32] Cf. anche *Cris.* IX 570,7 ss. K.

[33] Cf. p. es. DION.HAL. *Thuc.* 55,2: quella di Tucidide è una brevità αἰνιγματώδης. Osservazioni sul carattere negativo della brevità anche negli scoli omerici, cf. p. es. *Schol.ad Il.* 11, 300 b1.

[34] Si noti in primo luogo, a proposito dell'apparenza di omissione, l'affinità con il giudizio di Dionigi su Lisia, *Lys.* 5,1 (συνέστραπται δὲ εἴ τις καὶ ἄλλος καὶ πεπύκνωται τοῖς νοήμασι, καὶ τοσούτου δεῖ τῶν οὐκ ἀναγκαίων τι λέγειν, ὥστε καὶ πολλὰ καὶ τῶν χρησίμων ἂν δόξειε παραλιπεῖν). Per passi simili in Galeno, cf. p. es. *Cris.* IX 760,14 K: coloro, la maggior parte, che non sono allenati a seguire la brevità degli antichi, pensano che manchi qualcosa.

[35] Sul rischio di oscurità e di omissione di elementi utili, cf. *Cur.Rat.Ven.Sect.* XI 267,1 K; *HVA*, CMG V 9, 1, p.140,1-141,14.

viene detto, ma essa è solo dovuta ad una carente preparazione del pubblico comune e dei commentatori precedenti. La caratterizzazione del testo ippocratico come ellittico è infatti una soluzione esegetica praticata già prima di Galeno, ma egli talvolta la critica:

> *Hipp.Off.Med.* XVIIIB 730,5 ss. K: "... i manoscritti antichi e i commentatori conoscono il testo scritto in maniera incompleta (καί τά γε παλαιὰ τῶν ἀντιγράφων καὶ οἱ ἐξηγησάμενοι τὸ βιβλίον ἐλλιπῶς ἴσασι γεγραμμένην τὴν λέξιν), perché non c'è scritto ἀνίσως καὶ ἀνομοίως, e poiché c'è solo ἄνισα καὶ ἀνόμοια dicono di sottintendere ἀνίσως καὶ ἀνομοίως, da lui tralasciato per la ragione che esso apparirebbe chiaramente dalla conseguenza di ciò che è detto. In realtà la forma dell'espressione non è propria della brachilogia ma è un chiaro errore. Era meglio, se questo era stato trovato scritto, considerare che, come molti altri primi manoscritti, essi erano sbagliati e che questo è successo perché il primo copista li ha tralasciati e l'errore si è conservato fino ad oggi".

In questo caso Galeno contesta ai commentatori di aver considerato l'omissione di ἀνίσως καὶ ἀνομοίως nei manoscritti una semplice ellissi, che lascerebbe non esplicitata la conseguenza, τὸ ἀκόλουθον, ricavabile facilmente dai lettori. Galeno non accetta questa soluzione e, da buon filologo, afferma che essi avrebbero dovuto in primo luogo chiedersi se non si trattava di un semplice errore di tradizione. A maggior ragione dunque, secondo Galeno, è necessaria la mediazione del commento per chi non sia abituato alla dizione antica.

La matrice apologetica[36] dell'operazione con cui Galeno definisce la brachilogia una delle qualità dello stile di Ippocrate è del tutto evidente. In effetti, che la brevità del testo ippocratico ponesse talvolta forti problemi di comprensione era innegabile. Fra gli scritti commentati da Galeno la concisione è rappresentata specialmente in *Officina del medico* e *Aforismi* e nel commento a queste opere spesso Galeno ammette le difficoltà.[37] Ma

[36] Sulle accuse di oscurità rivolte ad Ippocrate, cf. *supra* n.8.

[37] Il *Prorretico*, ugualmente sintetico, è però considerato non autentico da Galeno e distinto dagli altri, perché non solo brachilogico ma anche pieno di solecismi (cf. *Hipp.Prorr.* CMG V 9, 2, p.13,27).

Galeno riconduce i problemi esegetici particolari di queste opere — quando, come si è visto, siano da escludersi errori di tradizione — a situazioni stilistiche specifiche, come il genere letterario degli aforismi o delle *gnomai* e delle epitomi o sommari.[38] Servendosi della classificazione dei 'generi' degli scritti ippocratici, egli può affermare che di fronte a forme diverse di espressione (μακρολογία o βραχυλογία) bisogna prima di tutto indagare lo scopo dell'esposizione didattica (τοὺς σκοποὺς τῆς διδασκαλίας), cf. *Hipp.Fract.* XVIIIB 324 ss. K. Talvolta egli difende esplicitamente la dizione ippocratica brachilogica perché *non tralascia* niente. Nel commento a *Officina del medico*, un'opera estremamente sintetica, sostiene che Ippocrate ἐν ὅλῳ γὰρ τῷ βιβλίῳ φυλάττει τὴν βραχυλογίαν, ἀλλὰ (*lege* ἅμα) τῷ βουληθῆναι μηδὲν παραλιπεῖν τῶν χρησίμων (*Hipp.Off.Med.* XVIIIB 668,4 ss. K). La brevità ippocratica si accompagna dunque alla chiarezza e proprio per questo è lodevole.[39] Ma Galeno è costretto ad ammettere che il testo 'breve' è talvolta carente e oscuro in modo irrimediabile, anche se trova quasi sempre giustificazioni specifiche, richiamando il fatto che Ippocrate è il primo ad aver ricercato certe cose o che il passo fa parte di un'opera non destinata alla pubblicazione.[40] Tuttavia mi preme insistere che, al di là dell'insieme di strategie giustificative del testo ippocratico, la brachilogia ippocratica spicca come un tratto caratteristico di Ippocrate e degli antichi, che definisce soprattutto una connotazione morale e un atteggiamento corretto nei confronti dei

[38] *Hipp.Aph.* XVIIB 462,10; 518,10; 876,15 K ecc.

[39] *Hipp.Fract.* XVIIIB 540,5 ss. K ἴδιόν ἐστι τῆς Ἱπποκράτους βραχυλογίας ἅμα σαφηνείας διὰ τῶν ἐπιφερομένων ἐπιδείκνυσθαι τὸ παραλελειμμένον ἐν τῷ προειρημένῳ λόγῳ, τοῦτ' οὖν ἐποίησε νῦν; *Hipp.Off.Med.* XVIIIB 761,9 K τὴν τοιαύτην βραχυλογίαν ἐπαινεῖν προσῆκεν, εἰ δι' ἑνὸς ὀνόματος δηλοῦται σαφῶς ὁ λόγος, ὥσπερ καὶ νῦν.

[40] *Cris.* IX 669,14; 670,6; 760,13 K. In *MM* 9, 8 (X 632,5 ss. K) Galeno riconosce che il discorso terapeutico da lui fatto è stato iniziato da Ippocrate, il quale però, in quanto πρῶτος εὑρετής non ha dato il giusto ordine a tutto, non ha definito in modo completo, ha tralasciato delle qualificazioni e ἀσαφῶς τε τὰ πλεῖστα διὰ παλαιὰν βραχυλογίαν ἑρμήνευσεν. Sul motivo delle opere non finite cf. *Hipp. Off.Med.* XVIIIB 790,10 K. Sul tema cf. SLUITER 1995a e MANETTI-ROSELLI 1994.

destinatari della comunicazione. Come gli storici antichi in Dionigi, anche Ippocrate vuole offrire al suo pubblico una comunicazione più efficace e diretta.

> *De difficultate respirationis* (VII 908-909 K): "Bisogna che d'ora in poi noi non ci comportiamo come la maggior parte dei contestatori di Ippocrate, nello scoprire facilmente le difficoltà e rimanere incapaci di trovare soluzioni, ma che in primo luogo scopriamo una via di soluzione e in seguito proviamo con la dimostrazione ciò che si è trovato attraverso quella. Qual è la via di soluzione? Bisogna cominciare da qui: una prima via è la comune consueta brevità di tutti gli antichi, una seconda la grandezza d'animo di Ippocrate stesso (χρὴ γὰρ ἐντεῦθεν ἄρξασθαι· μία μὲν ἡ κοινὴ πάντων τῶν παλαιῶν συνήθης βραχυλογία· δευτέρα δὲ Ἱπποκράτους αὐτοῦ μεγαλοφροσύνη). Ho dimostrato che spesso egli è abilissimo nel passar via gli argomenti che sono noti agli altri medici, nella convinzione che essi non possono essere ignorati da chi esercita l'arte, e al contrario nello spiegare con chiarezza e accuratamente tutto ciò che è ignorato da costoro".

La scelta di una scrittura breve si rivela dunque un atteggiamento consapevole di Ippocrate, teso verso un massimo grado di comunicazione didattica, e ha forti connotazioni etiche, ciò che potrebbe suggerire, al di là della comune cultura di scuola, un influsso dell'esaltazione della brevità specifica della retorica stoica,[41] perfettamente consonante inoltre con l'insistenza di Galeno sulla prevalenza del contenuto sulla forma del discorso. In effetti la definizione di brevità che Galeno formula nel commento a *Sulla dieta nelle malattie acute* (*HVA*, CMG V 9, 1, p.286,20 s. ἐν ὀλίγῃ γὰρ τῇ λέξει δύναμίς ἐστι πολλή, καθάπερ ἐν τοῖς Ἀφορισμοῖς) richiama da vicino le caratteristiche di brevità degli Stoici, specialmente attribuite al capostipite Zenone, p. es. in Plut. *Vita di Focione* 5,3 s.[42]

[41] Cfr. *MM* 2, 7 (X 150,17 K) in cui si attribuisce agli uomini una naturale inclinazione alla *syntomia* (e HANKINSON 1991, 226). In particolare sulla brevità della retorica stoica e i miti del laconismo spartano, cf. MORETTI 1995, 52 ss. Sull'influenza (in genere da lui non riconosciuta) della retorica stoica in Galeno, cf. PEARCY 1983.

[42] ...ἔχων βραχυλογίαν. ὡς γὰρ ὁ Ζήνων ἔλεγεν, ὅτι δεῖ τὸν φιλόσοφον εἰς νοῦν ἀποβάπτοντα προφέρεσθαι τὴν λέξιν, οὕτως ὁ Φωκίωνος λόγος πλεῖστον ἐν ἐλαχίστῃ

Se fino a qui è venuta in evidenza la sostanza retorica della caratterizzazione dello stile ippocratico, nell'analisi dei casi specifici, in cui Galeno rileva esempi della βραχυλογία ippocratica, si scopre un aspetto un po' diverso, che non sembra far riferimento ad una matrice retorica scolastica. La συντομία dei manuali è infatti soprattutto la ricerca di un linguaggio semplice e piano, senza orpelli, che non deve aggiungere elementi superflui ma non omettere tuttavia niente di necessario.[43] Invece l'aspetto principale che risulta dall'analisi dettagliata dei casi specifici è proprio il carattere *ellittico* dello stile di Ippocrate e degli antichi in generale. Eppure Galeno sembrava aver rifiutato una tale soluzione nel brano citato sopra del commento *Hipp.Off.Med.* XVIIIB 730,3 ss. K. Una tale caratterizzazione esce dall'ambito della retorica, per la quale la *brevitas* deve soprattutto evitare di aggiungere orpelli al grado della denotazione.[44] Un brano ci fornisce un esempio di come Galeno riporta difficoltà testuali di carattere grammaticale alla comune dizione 'breve' degli antichi.

> *Hipp.Fract.* XVIIIB 343, 12 ss. K (lemma *Fract.* 2: "il braccio dunque, l'argomento di cui stiamo parlando, τὴν οὖν χεῖρα περὶ οὗ ὁ λόγος"): qualcuno dei medici che passano per sapienti, correggendo come credeva la frase presente, ritenendola scorretta, la ha scritta così "il braccio dunque del quale stiamo parlando

λέξει νοῦν εἶχε. ... ὡς γὰρ ἡ τοῦ νομίσματος ἀξία πλείστην ἐν ὄγκῳ βραχυτάτῳ δύναμιν ἔχει, οὕτω λόγου δεινότης [ἐ]δοκεῖ πολλὰ σημαίνειν ἀπ' ὀλίγων: cf. *Praec.ger.reipubl.* 7, 803E e VAN DER STOCKT 1990; su Zenone, cf. anche DIOG.LAERT. 7, 16 ss. La connotazione fortemente ideologica della brevità ippocratica è sottolineata inoltre, per contrario, dal fatto che i casi in cui Ippocrate dice qualcosa di *perittos* sono sì rilevati, ma non sottolineati o caratterizzati (cf. p. es. *HVA*, CMG V 9, 1, p.280,4-10; *Hipp.Epid. III*, CMG V 10, 2, 1, p.84,10; p.113,22 ss.), fatta forse eccezione per l'uso dell'esempio della Libia e degli Sciti alla fine di *Prognostico* (cap. 25), che Galeno considera uno scarto dallo stile brachilogico del trattato (*Hipp.Prog.*, CMG V 9, 2, p.376,25 ss.).

[43] Cf. la definizione di συντομία, tradizionalmente parte della *narratio*, in Teone, *Progymn.* p.83,14 ss. Spengel ὁμοίως δὲ ἔσται καὶ σύντομος ἡ διήγησις ἐκ τῶν πραγμάτων καὶ τῆς λέξεως. ἔστι γὰρ ἡ συντομία λόγος τὰ καιριώτατα τῶν πραγμάτων σημαίνων, μήτε προστιθεὶς τὸ μὴ ἀναγκαῖον μήτε ἀφαιρῶν τὸ ἀναγκαῖον κατὰ τὰ πράγματα καὶ τὴν λέξιν.

[44] Cf. ancora Teone, *Progymn.* p.84 (evitare sinonimi, usare nomi piuttosto che perifrasi o parole semplici invece di composte ecc.).

(τὴν οὖν χεῖρα, περὶ ἧς ὁ λόγος)", indicandoci chiaramente l'educazione ricevuta dai grammatici e dai retori, tale da ignorare la forma più comune della dizione di tutti gli antichi, che si realizza chiaramente per mezzo di ellissi: la frase completa, che noi dobbiamo sottintendere è di questo genere... (ὡς ἀγνοεῖν τὸ συνηθέστατον εἶδος τῆς ἑρμηνείας, ἅπασι τοῖς παλαιοῖς ἐλλειπτικῶς δηλονότι γιγνόμενόν· ἔστι τὸ πλῆρες, ὃ δεῖ προσυπακούειν ἡμᾶς τοιόνδε).

Alcuni commentatori avevano ravvisato nella *concordantia ad sensum* del passo ippocratico (con l'uso di un neutro generalizzante in riferimento ad un termine femminile) un errore e l'avevano corretto: nell'opinione di Galeno essi dimostrano di aver ricevuto un'educazione grammaticale e retorica, ma di ignorare il carattere della dizione antica. Si tratta in realtà, per Galeno, di una costruzione ellittica e il bravo commentatore deve fornire la versione 'completa' del discorso, recuperando ciò che è sottinteso. Le ragioni per cui un problema sintattico venga ricondotto alla categoria dell'ellissi non ci interessano in questo momento[45] quanto piuttosto la definizione della dizione antica come *generalmente* ellittica.

Questo carattere ellittico non è però negativo né casuale e non corrisponde certo a carenze espressive di Ippocrate e degli antichi, non è, in altre parole, espressione di 'primitività', ma segue certe regole che devono essere individuate: nel passo sopra citato del commento a *Off. Med.* Galeno osservava che τὸ τῆς ἑρμηνείας εἶδος, "la forma dell'espressione", non era propria della brachilogia e per questa ragione egli rifiutava un'interpretazione simile in quel caso. Per essere definita brachilogia in senso positivo, la dizione antica deve perciò rispondere a certe esigenze formali. Una serie di passi nei commenti e in *De methodo medendi* ci indica la via verso l'identificazione di criteri di riferimento.

[45] L'ellissi è considerata fenomeno legato alla *brevitas* come figura *per detractionem* (LAUSBERG 1973, §688 ss.) e i casi di ellissi considerati nella manualistica concernono lo stile nominale, l'uso di infinito storico, varie forme di zeugma, fra cui però non rientra un esempio come questo, anche se si può seguire facilmente il ragionamento galenico.

Hipp.Prog., CMG V 9, 2, p.271,15: "abbiamo dimostrato che è in lui abituale indicare gli opposti per mezzo degli opposti, tralasciando di nominarli (σύνηθες γὰρ αὐτῷ τοῦτο πολλάκις ἐδείξαμεν ὃν ἐκ τῶν ἐναντίων ἐνδείκνυσθαι τἀναντία, παραλείποντι τὰς προσηγορίας αὐτῶν)";
Hipp.Prog., CMG V 9, 2, p.274,10-14: "(lemma *Prog.* 11: bisogna che l'evacuazione si condensi quando la malattia si avvia alla crisi) si condensa chiaramente ciò che è acquoso e leggero, non ciò che è denso e duro, così da riguardare il discorso coloro che hanno evacuazioni liquide fin dall'inizio. Ma questo è caratteristico della brachilogia antica e soprattutto abituale in Ippocrate, l'indicare qualcosa simultaneamente per mezzo degli opposti, tralasciando di menzionarli per nome (ἴδιον δὲ τοῦτο βραχυλογίας παλαιᾶς καὶ μάλιστα σύνηθες Ἱπποκράτει τὸ διὰ τῶν ἀντικειμένων ἐνίοτε συνενδείκνυσθαί τινα παραλείποντι μνημονεύειν αὐτῶν ὀνομαστί)";
HVA, CMG V 9, 1, p.229,30-230,12: "si potrebbe discutere opportunamente per quale ragione Ippocrate ha omesso di parlare in particolare di questa specie di vini... neppure questo infatti è possibile dire, che egli ignorava un vino del genere... dicendo perciò con precisione e chiarezza gli elementi di riconoscimento del vino 'vinoso' e spiegando come influisca sulla testa e la mente, ha ritenuto sufficiente l'insegnamento anche per la specie opposta a questa (*scil.* il vino 'acquoso'), dal momento che noi possiamo comprendere col ragionamento che ha le caratteristiche contrarie (ἱκανὴν ἐνόμισεν εἶναι καὶ περὶ τοῦ ἐναντίου αὐτῷ τοῦ ὑδατώδους τὴν διδασκαλίαν, ἡμῶν δυναμένων λογίσασθαι τἀναντία ὑπάρχειν αὐτῷ)";
Hipp.Off.Med. XVIIIB 845 K: "e tuttavia ho dimostrato[46] che non solo in questo libro, ma anche in molte altre opere Ippocrate, insegnando per mezzo di uno o due fatti, mostri con evidenza per loro tramite dottrine di carattere universale quando naturalmente ciò che è insegnato si differenzi in cose che pertengono allo stesso genere (τὸν Ἱπποκράτην δι' ἑνὸς ἢ δυοῖν πραγμάτοιν διδάσκοντα λόγους καθολικούς, ὅταν πραγμάτων ὁμογενῶν διαφέρει τὸ διδασκόμενον, ἐναργῶς ἐπ' αὐτῶν φαίνεσθαι), come qui...";[47]

[46] δείκνυσιν Kühn: propongo e traduco δέδεικται.
[47] Sarebbe da indagare l'utilizzazione che Galeno fa dei *paradeigmata* nell'esegesi ippocratica: all'uso degli esempi aveva dedicato un trattato (come all'induzione), cf. VON MÜLLER 1897, 428 s. Anche in questo caso la *Retorica* di Aristotele fornisce qualche riscontro p.es. a proposito della diversa quantità di esempi necessari se portati a dimostrazione o a conclusione, a 2, 20, 1394 a 15.

Hipp.Aph. XVIIB 425,13 ss. K: "negli aforismi precedenti ha dato insegnamenti sulla quantità nella dieta, ora tratta della qualità, insegnando molti e utili elementi dell'arte in un discorso brevissimo.... (427,13) se qualcosa non è stato menzionato esplicitamente in questo aforisma, che faccia parte dello stesso giudizio detto, anche questo bisogna considerarlo detto in potenza, infatti ha ricordato l'età e l'abitudine: tu potresti ragionevolmente ricordare anche la costituzione naturale e la stagione e il luogo, che talvolta anche lo stesso Ippocrate aggiunge, talvolta invece, menzionando una o due cose, omette le altre che appartengono alla stessa serie (καὶ εἴ τι μὴ ῥητῶς ὠνόμασται κατὰ τὸν ἀφορισμὸν ἐκ τῆς αὐτῆς ὑπάρχον τῆς εἰρημένης κρίσεως, καὶ τοῦθ' ἡγητέον εἰρῆσθαι δυνάμει, ἡλικίας μὲν γὰρ ἐμνημόνευσε καὶ ἔθους· σὺ δ' ἂν καὶ τῆς φυσικῆς κράσεως καὶ ὥρας καὶ χώρας εὐλόγως μνημονεύσεις, ἅπερ ἐνίοτε καὶ αὐτὸς μὲν Ἱπποκράτης προστίθησιν, ἐνίοτε δ' ἑνὸς ἢ δυοῖν μνημονεύσας τὰ λοιπὰ τῶν ἐκ τῆς αὐτῆς συστοιχίας παραλείπει)"; *MM* 4, 4 (X 274-275 K): "Forse sarebbe meglio, per quanto non avessi programmato di parlare qui della intenzione di Ippocrate, dire qualcosa su di essa anche se sommariamente: questo discorso potrebbe essere nondimeno una spiegazione dell'intenzione degli antichi. Infatti dal momento che quegli uomini non erano ancora schiavi per scelta delle dottrine, ma con intelletto semplice e puro si occupavano di scoprire qualcosa di utile per le terapie (ἐκεῖνοι γὰρ οἱ ἄνδρες, ἅτε μήπω δουλεύοντες αἱρέσει δογμάτων, ἀλλὰ καθαρᾷ καὶ ἁπλῇ τῇ διανοίᾳ σπουδάζοντες ἐξευρίσκειν τι χρηστὸν εἰς τὰς ἰάσεις), erano intenzionati a scoprire qualcosa per mezzo dell'esperienza, qualcos'altro per mezzo della ragione. E avrebbero scritto ciò che avevano scoperto molto spesso senza aggiungere il modo della scoperta, talvolta invece insieme a questo. E questo lo avrebbero deciso a vantaggio dei lettori: se infatti avessero sperato che conoscere il modo della scoperta avrebbe facilitato i posteri in un'abile utilizzazione delle scoperte, allora lo avrebbero scritto accuratamente. Se invece avessero ritenuto superfluo dirlo, lo avrebbero tralasciato. Che la brevità era in modo straordinario onorata dagli antichi, lo sanno tutti, anche se non lo dico io. Ed è certo per questo motivo che non solo Ippocrate ma tutti gli altri antichi talvolta sorvolando il termine medio congiungono il terzo al primo (καὶ ἡ βραχυλογία τοῖς παλαιοῖς ἐτετίμητο, πάντες ἤδη τοῦτο γινώσκουσι κἂν ἐγὼ μὴ λέγω· καὶ διά γε ταύτην τὴν αἰτίαν οὐχ Ἱπποκράτης μόνον, ἀλλὰ καὶ οἱ ἄλλοι παλαιοὶ τὸ μέσον ὑπερβαίνοντες ἐνίοτε τῷ πρώτῳ τὸ τρίτον συνάπτουσιν). Dunque se il primo termine è segno del secondo e a questo necessariamente segue il terzo, così essi riferiscono il terzo al primo saltando il secondo. Ho mostrato spesso che, fra tutti gli altri antichi, Ippocrate in particolare scrive in questo modo e che colui che vuole divenire familiare con il modo di esprimersi degli antichi deve esercitarsi in quegli (autori)".

In tutti questi passi l'analisi operata da Galeno tende ad identificare nel testo alcuni nuclei argomentativi, secondo la tradizione dialettica che deriva dai trattati aristotelici. C'è anche una spia lessicale precisa: nel passo di *Hipp.Aph.* XVIIB 427 si usa la parola συστοιχία che è rivelatrice e riconduce direttamente a Aristotele, *Top.* 2, 9, 114 a 39:

> "è chiaro che una volta mostrato come buono e lodevole un solo qualsivoglia termine tra quelli costituenti la stessa serie linguistica, risulteranno provati anche tutti i rimanenti".

Il passo di *De methodo medendi*, con la sua allusione ai segni, richiama la discussione aristotelica sui segni in *An.Pr.* 2, 27 (70 a 3 ss.), ma può in particolare essere avvicinato a *Retorica* 1, 2, 1357 a 18-21, dove si accenna a una relazione transitiva analoga:

> "perché se una di queste (premesse) è nota, non è necessario esprimerla in quanto è l'ascoltatore stesso ad aggiungerla: ad esempio, per dimostrare che Dorieo ha vinto una gara che comporta una corona come premio è sufficiente dire che ha vinto i giochi di Olimpia, e non c'è bisogno di aggiungere che il premio a Olimpia è una corona, in quanto tutti lo sanno".[48]

È perché si identificano nel testo ippocratico argomenti di transitività e di implicazione, in altre parole perché si individuano in essi strutture logico-dialettiche, che l'ellissi originata dalla brevità degli antichi non può essere accusata di essere omissione negativa.[49]

[48] Cf. BURNYEAT 1994, in part. 22.

[49] Nella tradizione posteriore retorica e dialettica sono intrecciate, anche per influsso della logica stoica (cf. MORETTI 1995, 152 ss.) e nella manualistica l' 'entimema', specialmente a proposito di opposti, è definito una forma 'breve'; a differenza del sillogismo dialettico, l'entimema lascia inespressi alcuni nodi dell'argomentazione, che devono essere integrati dagli ascoltatori, come troviamo teorizzato nel περὶ ἐπιχειρημάτων 3 di Minucianus rhetor (*Rhetores Graeci* I

Modelli concorrenti?

Il quadro del linguaggio antico tracciato da Galeno sembra alludere a un rapporto più 'naturale' fra chi usa il linguaggio e i suoi destinatari. Tale schema 'storiografico' si rivela abbastanza diffuso, soprattutto nelle teorie sullo sviluppo dell'eloquenza. Si può per esempio comparare un passo delle *Epistole* di Seneca (59,6), che allude ad una simile concezione dello stato antico del linguaggio, nel commentare alcune caratteristiche di stile (l'uso di figure) nel suo corrispondente Lucilio. Seneca afferma che gli antichi si esprimevano *simpliciter et demonstrandae rei causa*, usando solo metafore necessarie e non come quelle dei poeti.

Caratteri analoghi presenta la teoria contro cui polemizza Quintiliano in *Inst.* 12, 10, 40-42: i suoi sostenitori affermavano che le parole avevano solo lo scopo di mostrare il significato (*quibus solum natura sit officium attributum, servire sensibus*), le cose avevano un nome proprio (*cum sua cuique sint adsignata nomina*) e gli antichi oratori parlavano *secundum naturam*, ma in seguito si comportarono come i poeti introducendo figure e altri tropi (*mox poetis similiores extitisse* etc.). La teoria combattuta da Quintiliano è stata avvicinata ad alcuni passi della *Retorica* di Filodemo, con la sua insistenza su uno stile φυσικός che deve essere subordinato ad esprimere i contenuti sensoriali e di pensiero e perciò utilizzare i κύρια ὀνόματα ed evitare un linguaggio poetico.[50]

Sia Quintiliano sia Seneca si riferiscono ad un ideale stilistico di una *lexis* subordinata alle pure esigenze di comunicazione, in opposizione ad un certo sviluppo successivo della retorica che viene rifiutato. Galeno in realtà, a parte la difesa della tradizione

p. 419,12 ss. Spengel). Sull'interpretazione posteriore dell'entimema come sillogismo incompleto, cf. BURNYEAT 1994.

[50] Cf. MILANESE 1989, 93 ss., che, sulla scia di Radermacher, ravvisa una identità di vedute ma non di linguaggio fra Dionigi di Alicarnasso, Filodemo, Epicuro stesso e i *quidam* cui si riferisce Quintiliano (97 e nn.). Si potrebbe qui aggiungere che anche Galeno partecipa di questo quadro generale.

ippocratico-platonica e la creazione del conseguente idolo polemico dei 'sofisti' contemporanei, è tutt'altro che propenso a vedere nel presente un'epoca di decadenza della medicina (almeno per quel che riguarda la 'sua' tradizione dogmatica), anzi, in particolare, è profondamente consapevole dello sviluppo storico del linguaggio scientifico e lo collega esplicitamente ad un progresso delle conoscenze, cf. p. es.:

> *PHP* 8, 4, 8-9 (CMG V 4, 1, 2, p.500,3-12, in part. 10 ss. = V 673,11 ss. K): "che cosa chiamo 'corpi primi', lo chiarirò subito, affinché non ci sia niente di oscuro nel mio discorso. Ippocrate per parte sua non nominò 'corpo primo' o 'secondo', come Aristotele. Platone invece parla di una composizione 'seconda' dei corpi, ma non nomina la 'prima' neppure lui: ma dal fatto di parlare di una seconda è chiaro che prima di questa poneva una composizione che Aristotele denominò con il termine di 'omeomeri', quando esamina diffusamente le parti degli animali e la loro generazione. Infatti con quanta maggiore precisione e sottigliezza si tratta della natura degli oggetti, tanto maggiore diventa il bisogno di designazioni (ὅσον γὰρ ἄν τις ἀκριβέστερόν τε καὶ λεπτομερέστερον ἥντινοῦν φύσιν πραγμάτων ἐξεργάζηται, τοσούτῳ πλεόνων ὀνομάτων αὐτῷ γίγνεται χρεία)".

Dunque c'è sempre più bisogno di nomi, quanto più le conoscenze si affinano. Galeno in effetti non può negare gli enormi progressi compiuti dalla medicina posteriore a Ippocrate, specie nel campo dell'anatomia, che hanno comportato una evoluzione ed un arricchimento terminologico. Questa coscienza dell'evoluzione del linguaggio si inserisce in uno schema cronologico generale, che è dominato dall'opposizione fra antichi e moderni.[51] I confini fra i due campi non sono precisi e inoltre si spostano a seconda del tema che Galeno sta affrontando:[52] il punto di discrimine può essere prima e dopo Alessandro Magno (*Hipp.Epid. VI*, CMG V 10, 2, 2, p.399,8 ss.), oppure prima e dopo Erasistrato (*Nat.Fac.* II 141,17; 166,11 K), o il passaggio fra Academia antica e Academia scettica (*Opt.Doct.* I 40,4 K,

[51] Cf. Vegetti 2001.
[52] Manetti-Roselli 1994, 1633 ss.

cf. *PHP* 9, 7,3, CMG V 4, 1, 2, p.586,16). Due autori contemporanei come Erasistrato e Erofilo si collocano in campi diversi. Erofilo è l'ultimo degli antichi, mentre Erasistrato si trova in un punto di cerniera, è il primo dei *neoteroi* per la rottura dottrinale che lo contraddistingue (*Diff.Resp.* VII 853,5 K)[53] e anche, di conseguenza, per ragioni linguistiche, perché segna un punto di passaggio decisivo del linguaggio medico (cf. *Hipp.Aph.* XVIIIA 6-7 K = Garofalo 1988, frr. 261a; 13), in particolare per i casi di πυρετός e φλεγμονή.[54] Solo ragioni ideologiche spingono Galeno a separare Erofilo da Erasistrato e a porre quest'ultimo all'origine della degenerazione successiva. Tuttavia, nel campo dell'anatomia, si riconosce che un grande progresso è avvenuto, anche per le conquiste di conoscenza dovute a entrambi i grandi medici ellenistici. Il campo anatomico è quello in cui più si manifesta l'arricchimento e la variazione di nomi e Galeno in *De anatomicis administrationibus*, anche se continua a rifiutare la disputa sui nomi con il solito richiamo a Platone,[55] distingue la diafonia sui fatti da quella sui nomi, valutando quest'ultima come solo apparente, se il referente anatomico resta lo stesso (*AA* II 235-236 K, dove allude alla sua opera *Sulle divergenze anatomiche*). Galeno afferma la continuità con la tradizione soprattutto per esigenze didattiche: bisogna cominciare comunque dai testi degli *endoxoi*, per non turbare i giovani, poi inserire le precisazioni necessarie (II 239-242 K). Perciò nei *Procedimenti anatomici* Galeno, al seguito di una lunga tradizione di 'genere' (di cui è esempio per noi l'opera *Sui nomi delle parti del corpo* di Rufo di Efeso[56]), si fa raccoglitore e catalogatore di una

[53] Cf. Vegetti 2001, 88 ss.

[54] Su 'cronologia' recente di Erasistrato, cf. anche Ps.Gal. *Int.* XIV 729,7 K; *Hipp.Vict.Morb.Ac.*, CMG V 9, 1, p.370,17; *Nat.Fac.* II 117,12, 140,18 K. Per la discussione di πυρετός e φλεγμονή, cf. *Sui termini medici* 26,28 ss.; 35,4 ss. ecc.; su φλεγμονή *Hipp.Fract.* XVIIIB 548,1 ss. K.

[55] Cf. *AA* 6, 13, II 580-81 K; 10, 9, 79-81 Simon (= Garofalo 1991, 897-98); 12, 2, 144 Simon (= Garofalo 1991, 959).

[56] Su Rufo di Efeso, cf. Kotzia Pantele 1995, 104 ss. Rufo, a differenza di Galeno, afferma che bisogna proprio cominciare dalla conoscenza dei nomi, ma la distanza è più apparente che reale.

ricca messe di sinonimi, senza che il suo insegnamento ne sia turbato minimamente.[57]

Da questo punto di vista, il linguaggio dei medici antichi in sé si presenta, è ovvio, come carente, spesso per una ragione dichiarata (in particolare per Platone), il non avere pratica di dissezione.[58] L'assenza di nomi o l'errata designazione sono causate da difetto di conoscenza o da errate opinioni sulle cause.[59]

Lungi da vedere nel passato un'epoca idealizzata, dove tutto era regolato e in ordine, per Galeno l'irregolarità dei nomi è fenomeno che pertiene al linguaggio fin dall'antichità, ai *nomothetai* della tradizione medica:

> *MM* 2, 2, X 81 ss. K:[60] "Avendo posto queste definizioni, bisogna esaminare attentamente l'irregolarità dei nomi che hanno prodotto coloro che per primi hanno imposto nomi alle malattie: spesso hanno posto i nomi a partire dal nome della parte danneggiata. ... spesso dai loro sintomi... spesso da tutti e due insieme... spesso dalla causa supposta... talvolta dalla somiglianza con oggetti esterni ecc.".

Insomma, la storia dei nomi di malattia rivela che non esisteva in antico un criterio coerente di denominazione: inoltre i nomi dei singoli tipi di una classe generale, per esempio ἕλκος, non

[57] Un campo analogo è la farmacologia, perché il mondo botanico o minerale è naturalmente ricco di omonimi e sinonimi anche solo regionali: cf. BARNES 1997. Sulle serie sinonimiche cf. anche MANULI 1986. Bisogna aggiungere che neanche l'omonimia di differenti parti anatomiche risulta problematica per Galeno nei *Procedimenti anatomici*, se si basa su una evidente analogia funzionale (cfr. p.es. *AA* 12, 8, 164 Simon = GAROFALO 1991, 976).

[58] Cf. *Plat. Tim.*, CMG Suppl. I, 14,10 ss. (Platone, al pari di Omero, ignora l'anatomia, a proposito di μυελός); 15,9 ss. (ignora la funzione dei nervi); per gli anatomisti in generale, cf. *AA* 1, 9, II 266 K ecc. Anche errori sostanziali come sulla sede dello ἡγημονικόν derivano da incomplete osservazioni anatomiche, p. es. nel caso di Aristotele, cf. VEGETTI 1999, 344.

[59] Anche se Galeno dichiara che gli antichi apprendevano l'anatomia nella pratica e non avevano bisogno di scriverla, questa difesa non basta a compensare le numerose volte in cui Galeno afferma la distanza fra antichi e moderni in fatto di pratica anatomica, cf. nota prec. (diversamente VEGETTI 2001, 89). Per il famoso caso dell'inadeguatezza del nome greco tradizionale per cervello (ἐγκέφαλος), vedi *infra*.

[60] HANKINSON 1991, 164 s.

sono dati secondo le *differentiae* specifiche — se non sporadicamente — ma seguono la stessa varietà di modi appena descritta, in cui le metafore o altri tropi sono molto presenti (cf. 2, 2, X 83,6-84,10 K: οὕτως οὖν ἀνωμάλου τῶν ὀνομάτων τῆς θέσεως τοῖς ἀρχαίοις γεγενημένης).

La stessa imprecisione viene di volta in volta segnalata nei commenti ippocratici e imputata agli antichi, cf. p. es.: *Hipp.Fract.* XVIIIB 512,7 K:

> "Bisogna dunque ricordarsi di questo, non potresti trovare curata la precisione dei nomi propri riguardo a molti fatti in nessuno degli antichi, ma essi parlano, in parte abusando, in parte trasferendo (τὴν ἀκρίβειαν τῶν κυρίων ὀνομάτων οὐδὲ παρ' ἑνὶ τῶν παλαιῶν Ἑλλήνων εὕροις ἂν φυλαττομένην, ἀλλὰ τὰ μὲν καταχρώμενοι[61] τὰ δὲ μεταφέροντες λέγουσι)...(513,9) è evidente che egli usa i nomi in modo un po' vario, come ho detto fanno anche gli altri antichi" (cf. sopra).

Metafora e *katachresis* sono fenomeni connaturati al linguaggio comune,[62] come già diceva Aristotele (*Rhet.* 3, 2, 1404 b, cf. Demetr. *Eloc.* 86), ma l'attribuzione di questi strumenti agli antichi rientra anche nella coscienza di una particolare condizione storica. L'uso di figure nella designazione da parte degli antichi è dovuto alla mancanza di *kyria onomata* per classificare gli oggetti, ad una sproporzione fra parole e oggetti: così anche Ippocrate ricorre a questi mezzi per la cosiddetta *inopia verborum*, cf. *Hipp.Art.* XVIIIA 482,1 ss. K:

> "(lemma *Art.* 40:"se l'orecchio si frattura ecc.") l'interruzione di continuità nelle parti carnose è detta 'ferita', nelle ossa è detta 'frattura': poiché quella che avviene nelle cartilagini non ha un nome proprio, Ippocrate la ha chiamata, abusando, con il nome di 'frattura' (τὸ δὲ ἐν χόνδρῳ γενόμενον οὐκ ἔχον ἰδίαν προσηγορίαν καταχρησάμενος ὁ Ἱπποκράτης τοῦ κατάγματος ὀνόματι προσηγόρευσεν)".[63]

[61] Correggo il χρώμενοι di Kühn.

[62] Cf. anche PHLD. *Rhet.* 2, coll. XLI 27-XLII 11, p.74-75 Sudhaus = 129 Longo Auricchio; GAL. *Hipp.Aph.* XVIIB 406; XVIIIA 16,6 ss. K.

[63] Talvolta l'utilizzazione di *katachresis* corrisponde alla difficoltà di descrivere le fasi di un processo degenerativo continuo (come quello della cancrena) e rientra

Si delinea dietro tutti questi passi una visione storica del linguaggio che muove dall'imprecisione alla precisione, dalla povertà alla ricchezza (fino a diventare vittima delle sofisticherie dei moderni), con una concezione di progresso cumulativo — fatto di arricchimenti successivi e di precisazioni e specificazioni.[64] Si presuppone una *inopia verborum* degli antichi e il fatto che molte cose senza nome con il tempo sono state nominate attraverso criteri simili a quelli che Galeno dà ai suoi contemporanei per la formazione dei neologismi.[65] Dunque il linguaggio si evolve per eliminare omonimie,[66] che sono anch'esse connaturate al linguaggio comune (*MM* X 130-131 K); la metafora e la *katachresis* sono due strumenti essenziali per assegnare nomi, già fino dall'antico,[67] il fattore di ogni evolu-

nei limiti che Galeno riconosce al linguaggio medico: cf. *Hipp.Art.* XVIIIA 688,1-3 K "in effetti talvolta ci serviamo per abuso dei nomi delle affezioni vicine per quelle che arrivano ad esse, ma non hanno ancora la loro forma e natura". Un esempio analogo di *katachresis* osservata nella descrizione di processi in divenire, in *PFlor.* 115, un frammento papiraceo contenente resti di un commento a Ippocrate *De alimento* (cf. MANETTI 1995, 40 per il testo, 48 per il commento), in cui ci si rifa ad esempi noti come 'tessere una veste' o 'scavare un pozzo'.

[64] Per esempi di specificazione dell'uso di οἴδημα e φλεγμονή, *Hipp.Fract.* XVIIIB 547 K: si noti che la specializzazione del significato avviene con Erasistrato, cf. *supra.* Un classico esempio di specializzazione è πάθος, che passa da 'alterazione' qualsiasi per gli antichi a 'affezione morbosa' per i moderni, cf. *Symp.Diff.* VII 44-45 K; per μήνιγξ (da 'membrana' in generale a 'membrana che circonda il cervello') cf. *AA* 9, 2, II 716 K; 14, 2, GAROFALO 1991, 233-34, ecc. In generale sulla concezione di progresso in Galeno, cf. HANKINSON 1994b.

[65] Sulle cose senza nome in antico per carenze cognitive, cf. p.es. *Syn.Puls.* IX 431-435 K. In *Morb.Temp.* VII 417,13 ss. K si danno i criteri per i neologismi: se mancano i nomi della *synetheia*, bisogna usare metafora o *creare* nuovi nomi per analogia (ἀναλογία) con qualcuno degli oggetti già nominati o usare *katachresis*; cf. *AA* II 615,12 ss. K (sulla derivazione di nomi da altri esistenti). Sui neologismi, KOTZIA PANTELE 1995, 94 ss.

[66] Cf. p. es. *Comp.Med.Loc.* 1, XIII 2,6 ss. K.

[67] Cf. *AA* II 615,13 K. Su *katachresis* come fenomeno corrente del linguaggio comune (κατὰ τὸν βίον), come di quello medico, cf. *Hipp.Aph.* XVIIB 406,10 ss. K. Quanto afferma VON STADEN 1995, 504-505 (vd. anche KOTZIA PANTELE, 95 ss.), a proposito dell'opposizione di linguaggio κύριος e linguaggio figurato, con una sostanziale identificazione di metafora e *katachresis*, va precisato: nella valutazione di questi fenomeni è decisivo il punto di vista (normativo, polemico o analitico) di volta in volta assunto da Galeno.

zione è l'ἔθος, cioè la consuetudine, che mantiene o risolve omonimie.[68]

Nel caso di Ippocrate, non si negano affatto le sue incoerenze terminologiche, anche se all'interno del quadro giustificativo delineato sopra: per esempio si discute al lungo dell'incoerenza dell'uso di γνάθος e γένυς (*Hipp.Art.* XVIIIA 444,3 ss. K). In realtà la situazione degli antichi è certo migliore dal punto di vista morale,[69] ma non sul piano del linguaggio. Analizziamo solo un esempio di carenza del linguaggio degli antichi: in *Symp.Diff.* si dice che i difetti di digestione non hanno tutti nome e perciò bisogna partire dall'esame della natura dei fatti, cf. *Symp.Diff.* 4, VII 65,11 K:

> "Di nuovo si divide in due uno dei due (difetti), il (digerire) male, se anche non puoi indicarlo con dei nomi chiaramente, perché non è in uso nel loro caso nessun nome: perciò tentando di esprimerti con una definizione, per quanto è possibile, (dico) che il digerire male, preso a sé, da una parte sarà digerire in modo insufficiente, dall'altra digerire in modo sbagliato".

Ma dei due tipi di difetti individuati, il digerire insufficientemente e il digerire male, solo il primo ha un nome proprio (βραδυπεψία). Inoltre la designazione dei difetti non corrisponde bene alla loro descrizione, come è spiegato a VII 66,7 ss. K. Alla facoltà di digestione pertengono due difetti diversi: l'uno, il digerire lentamente, ha un nome appropriato βραδυπεψία, ma l'altro, il digerire male, viene detto ἀπεψία, con un nome che si riferisce anche alla privazione della facoltà e dunque abbiamo a

[68] Cf. *ethos* e omonimia in *Alim.Fac.* VI 579,14; 606,14 K, ma anche *HVA*, CMG V 9, 1, p.344,28: il campo dei nomi di piante è specialmente interessato dall'omonimia, cf. *supra* n.57.

[69] Galeno condivide il pessimismo moralistico generale del suo tempo, quando osserva che, all'epoca di Ippocrate, *ethos* coincideva con *physis* ed era bene, mentre al suo tempo, con la decadenza dei costumi, un *ethos*, ovviamente corrotto, prevale sul naturale, il che è negativo per la salute: si osservi che questo incide sul grado di verità del testo ippocratico quando fa riferimento all'*ethos* (*Hipp.Prog.*, CMG V 9, 2, p.270,1-12); cf. anche HANKINSON 1994b. La decadenza dei costumi è un *topos* comune nelle teorie sullo sviluppo dell'eloquenza, cf. p. es. HELDMANN 1982, 84 ss.

che fare con un caso di omonimia. Ecco perché bisogna affidarsi all'osservazione diretta delle cose e non lasciarsi ingannare dai nomi. Galeno attribuisce una denominazione così carente a lacune di conoscenza o errori di giudizio degli antichi, richiamando allusivamente il discorso di Socrate in *Cratilo* 436 a ss.:[70] ancora una volta il *Cratilo* forma la trama sulla quale Galeno costruisce le proprie considerazioni sulla storia del linguaggio. Una designazione coerente e chiara degli elementi del sistema avrebbe dovuto chiamare solo la privazione della facoltà ἀπεψία, mentre avrebbe dovuto designare la digestione lenta con βραδυπεψία, la digestione sbagliata con δυσπεψία. In realtà sarebbe stato agevole farlo, perché tale nome si poteva ricavare facilmente per analogia da tante altre parole formate allo stesso modo indicanti fenomeni simili,[71] secondo un meccanismo ben noto a Galeno.

Ippocrate non è collocato nel polo dell'antichità solo in maniera statica, perché anch'egli si inserisce nel corso di un processo evolutivo e vi partecipa creativamente: Galeno talvolta osserva che Ippocrate forgia designazioni nuove, spesso per mezzo di metafora o *katachresis*.[72] Così p. es. in *Hipp.Fract.* XVIIIB 459,15 K spiega come ha creato il termine ναυσιώσεις: ναυσιώσεις ὠνόμασεν ἰδίως ἀπὸ τῶν ναυτιώντων καὶ διὰ τοῦτ' ἐμούντων ποιήσας τοὔνομα, cf. anche *Hipp.Art.* XVIIIA 661,2 K.[73]

Sulla stessa scia, anche Galeno crea parole nuove e, in coerenza con i precetti dati in *Sui termini medici* (*Med.Nam.* 16,31 ss.) e altrove (cf. n.65), lo fa ispirandosi alla tradizione ippocratica (la *synetheia* dei medici antichi): p. es. in *Morb.Temp.* VII

[70] GAL. *loc.cit.*: ἀλλὰ γὰρ, ὅπερ ὁ Πλάτων ἔλεγεν, ἀγνοοῦντες οἱ παλαιοὶ τὰ πλεῖστα τῶν πραγμάτων τὰ μὲν οὐδ' ὅλως, τὰ δὲ οὐκ ὀρθῶς ὠνόμασαν. οὔκουν ἐξαπατᾶσθαι χρὴ τοῖς ὀνόμασιν, ἀλλ' εἰς αὐτὴν ἀποβλέπειν τῶν πραγμάτων τὴν οὐσίαν.

[71] Il ruolo dell'analogia grammaticale nelle opere esegetiche di Galeno meriterebbe un'indagine a parte; per un ragionamento analogico sui composti con *dys-* cf. *Diff.Resp.* VII 753,3 ss. K (vd. *infra*).

[72] Cf. *Hipp.Prog.*, CMG V 9, 2, p.225,12: da ὑποφαίνεσθαι Ippocrate ha fatto la parola ὑπόφασις che è declinata al modo ionico ὑποφάσιες.

[73] Οὐδὲν ὄνομα σύνηθές ἐστι τῷ τοιούτῳ σχήματι. διόπερ ὁ Ἱπποκράτης, ὡς ἔφην, αὐτὸ καμπύλεσθαι προσηγόρευσεν, οἰκείαν τῷ δηλουμένῳ πράγματι φωνὴν ἐξευρών.

414,1 ss. K afferma di aver dato il nome διάλειμμα alle fasi di assenza di febbre, sulla base dell'uso di Ippocrate: διότι καὶ ὁ Ἱπποκράτης οὕτως ὠνόμασεν. In realtà la parola non è attestata nel *Corpus Hippocraticum*, ma è caratteristico l'uso che Ippocrate fa del verbo διαλείπω riguardo alle febbri intermittenti (p. es. *Epid.* 1, 1; 5, 1; 6, 8; 6, 21 ecc.): quindi Galeno si è ispirato ad un termine tecnico ippocratico e ne ha ricavato una nuova parola servendosi dell'ἀναλογία e della παραγωγή.

Designare 'correttamente' le cose è dunque frutto di una conoscenza delle cose stesse, che si acquisisce con il tempo, della memoria della tradizione medica e della *synetheia*. Non è affatto necessario che ad ogni nome corrisponda un solo oggetto e viceversa, se si utilizza un punto di vista storico: la corrispondenza 1:1 fra nomi e cose è sentita come un'esigenza importante da seguire per i neologismi,[74] ma non è affatto considerata un tratto originario né 'naturale' del linguaggio, anzi al contrario, cf. *Sui termini medici* (*Med.Nam.* 16, 7 ss.); *Syn.Puls.* IX 434,11 ss. K. Dunque si deve sottolineare che l'auspicata univocità del significato dei termini si inserisce nello sforzo di Galeno di 'costruire' nel presente un linguaggio scientifico adeguato e non in un nostalgico atteggiamento rivolto al passato: la corrispondenza uno a uno davvero necessaria è solo quella fra *pragmata* e definizioni (cf. *Diff.Puls.* VIII 569 ss. K), le quali sono il termine di mediazione fra l'irregolarità dei nomi e le esigenze di classificazione dei concetti.[75]

Questo schema storiografico è certamente coerente con la formazione peripatetica di Galeno, ma è interessante notare un'analogia generale nel modo di affrontare lo sviluppo del linguaggio in Epicuro, *Ep. ad Her.* 75-76 (e Diog.Oen. fr. 12 Smith[76]). La cosa

[74] Cf. in particolare *Symp.Diff.* VII 45,8 ss., 51,17 ss. K. Sul tema 'univocità', cf. HANKINSON 1994a; VON STADEN 1995, 506 ss.

[75] Le definizioni permettono anche di ovviare alla mancanza di nomi propri, cf. *Diff.Puls.* VIII 507,6 ss. K; *Dig.Puls.* VIII 912,15 K. Sulle definizioni cf. BARNES 1991, 72 ss.; HANKINSON 1991b; 1994a.

[76] Diogene di Enoanda, nella polemica contro la teoria platonico-stoica del *nomothetein*, parla inoltre di dare i nomi ἕνεκα ῥαδίας δηλώσεως, che ricorda

non deve stupire troppo — al di là del fatto che l'epicureismo è fra gli avversari dottrinali di Galeno — se si ricorda l'attenzione che anche Epicuro ha dedicato alle necessità del discorso scientifico-filosofico.[77] In Epicuro si spiega che, dopo una fase originaria, riconducibile ai meccanismi istintuali di reazione alle sensazioni,[78] si sviluppa una seconda fase, in cui le parole sono formate razionalmente e in base ad un accordo sociale, per migliorare le condizioni della comunicazione interpersonale e infine si ha una terza fase, che introduce nuove parole in seguito al progresso delle conoscenze.

> *Ep. ad Her.* 76: "Infine di comune accordo a seconda di ciascun popolo furono stabilite le espressioni proprie perché le comunicazioni reciproche fossero meno ambigue e si comunicasse con maggiore brevità. E chi essendone esperto introduceva cose non note dava loro determinati nomi, alcuni costretti a emettere certi suoni, altri scegliendo con il ragionamento, secondo la causa più forte, di esprimersi così (ὕστερον δὲ κοινῶς καθ' ἕκαστα ἔθνη τὰ ἴδια τεθῆναι πρὸς τὸ τὰς δηλώσεις ἧττον ἀμφιβόλους γενέσθαι ἀλλήλοις καὶ συντομωτέρως δηλουμένας. τινὰ δὲ καὶ οὐ συνορώμενα πράγματα εἰσφέροντας τοὺς συνειδότας παρεγγυῆσαί τινας φθόγγους τοὺς ⟨μὲν⟩ ἀναγκασθέντας ἀναφωνῆσαι, τοὺς δὲ τῷ λογισμῷ ἑλομένους κατὰ τὴν πλείστην αἰτίαν οὕτως ἑρμηνεῦσαι)".

È evidente una visione razionalistica analoga, che disegna un processo di raffinamento del linguaggio, attraverso l'eliminazione di ambiguità e la sintesi. Il progresso conoscitivo porta alla creazione di nuove parole; sono i 'competenti' (συνειδότες)

l'espressione usata da Galeno per giustificare l'uso dei nomi, cioè ἕνεκα συντόμου διδασκαλίας (cf. *supra* n. 27).

[77] Affinità in un contesto generale con gli epicurei su alcune tematiche relative alla comunicazione linguistica sono state rilevate sopra, cf. nn. 14,19. Che una connessione fra l'impostazione di Epicuro e quella aristotelica fosse riconoscibile è già stato fatto osservare da più parti, cf. ARRIGHETTI 1973², 518-522; sul tema vedi MILANESE 1989; sulla teoria epicurea cf. il vecchio studio di DAHLMANN 1928, 5 ss. Altri brani rilevanti per la storia del linguaggio umano all'interno della civilizzazione, come Diodoro 1, 8, o Cicerone *Rep.* 3, 3, sono meno caratterizzati o insistono più genericamente sul motivo dell'utilità.

[78] Sul fatto che la naturalità del linguaggio in Epicuro non si riferisca affatto ad una connessione naturale fra *onomata* e significati, come per gli Stoici, ma solo al problema storico delle origini cf. SCHRIJVERS 1974: il rapporto fra parola e significato resta convenzionale anche per Epicuro.

che danno i nomi, come atto che risulta da una conoscenza, attraverso una indicazione naturale (onomatopea?) oppure con un ragionamento (λογισμός) di tipo causale. Esiste un processo analogo ma diverso all'interno di ogni comunità linguistica. In Galeno ovviamente la fase originaria di Epicuro è omessa, perché estranea e incompatibile con i suoi interessi, ma le modalità di sviluppo del linguaggio della tradizione medica, da lui descritte in passi diversi, mostrano una parziale analogia con quelle abbozzate da Epicuro per la seconda e la terza fase.

Galeno, si sa, è sostenitore del carattere convenzionale del linguaggio, a tal punto da attribuire questa consapevolezza anche ad Ippocrate, quando in *Sui termini medici* (*Med.Nam.* 22,13 ss.) analizza espressioni ippocratiche come "nella febbre cosiddetta semiterzana" ἐν δὲ τῷ ἡμιτριταίῳ καλεομένῳ in *Epid.* 1, 11 (II 674,4 L) e simili.[79] L'uso di questo tipo di formule dimostra, secondo Galeno, che Ippocrate è perfettamente conscio sia dei diversi livelli linguistici sia del fatto che il designare è operazione convenzionale, così come l'attacco di Ippocrate, in *Sulle malattie acute*, contro i nomi delle malattie forniti dagli autori delle *Sentenze Cnidie* fa di lui un rappresentante della lotta contro chi si occupa di nomi invece che di fatti.[80]

In *Sui termini medici* la polemica è rivolta esplicitamente contro coloro che vedono un legame inscindibile fra nomi e πράγματα (*Med.Nam.* 22,25: *dass sie sich einbilden, die Namen und Bezeichnungen wären mit den benannten und bezeichneten Dingen unlösbar verbunden*) e sembra diretta contro medici di formazione stoica (come Archigene, citato a 14,5 ss.) che confondono livello ontologico e semantico, perché non sono capaci di riconoscere

[79] Del valore di simili espressioni Galeno parla anche in *HVA*, CMG V 9, 1, p.243,6 ss. dove ne dà una triplice spiegazione: 1) sono termini *non ancora* in uso; 2) o termini impropri; 3) o termini tecnici. Con ciò egli presuppone un linguaggio che fa uso consapevole o di una specializzazione d'uso (3) o di una innovazione personale (1) o delle parole comuni non tecniche (2). Sulla dubbia interpretazione di simili espressioni cf. *Hipp.Art.* XVIIIA 429,6 K (su muscoli *krotafitai* e *masseteres*, cf. *AA* II 422,2 ss. K).

[80] E' notevole che nel commento allo stesso passo di *Sulla dieta nelle malattie acute* non compaia affatto un'osservazione di questo genere.

verità e falsità del discorso, ignorando la distinzione fra discorso e designazione (24,42 ss.: *dabei wissen sie nicht einmal, was "richtig reden" und "falsch reden" bedeutet, da sie nicht wissen was der Unterschied zwischen Rede und Benennung ist*). Per Galeno, sulla scia del *De interpretatione* di Aristotele,[81] questo è inaccettabile, perché per lui il livello di verità è quello del discorso e non del nome.

Del buon uso dell'etimologia: storie di nomi

Poco dopo, in *Sui termini medici* (*Med.Nam.* 26,17 ss. e 31,15 ss.), Galeno riprende il discorso dei criteri di indagine sul significato dei nomi e fissa tre criteri di riferimento: 1) indicazione della parola (*den Hinweis der Worte, aus dem Hinweis des Wortes selbst*), 2) uso degli antichi (*die Gewohnheit der Alten, auf Grund des Gebrauches dieses Namens durch die Alten*), 3) uso dei moderni (*die Gewohnheit der Wunderlichen unter unseren Zeitgenossen, auf Grund des Gebrauches dieses Namens durch die Menschen*). In questo contesto egli menziona a 26,17 ss. l'esempio di Prodico e la sua analisi del significato di flegma in modo abbastanza neutrale: *Was den Hinweis der Worte anlangt, so liegt er im Falle des Prodikos vor, der, als er das meinte, was alle Welt Galle nennt, es Schleim* (φλέγμα) *benannte. Er tat das, weil sich der Name* φλέγμα *auf griechisch, wenn man sich seine Etymologie überlegt als von "Entzündung" und "Brennen" abgeleitet ergibt, und weil dieses Temperament, nämlich das gallige, auf diesem Weg entsteht.* Non seguono le solite osservazioni sarcastiche sulla stoltezza del comportamento di Prodico. Può stupire, perché il sofista è il *mikrologos* per antonomasia,[82] ma bisogna osservare che

[81] *Int.* 1, 16 a 12 ss.

[82] Cf. *Nat.Fac.* II 130,3 ss. K; *PHP* 8, 6, 50, CMG V 4, 1, 2, p.522 (De Lacy); *Diff.Feb.* VII 348,1 ss. K; *Hipp.Art.* XVIIIA 685,18 ss. K; *Hipp.Prog.*, CMG V 9, 2, p.204,26 ss. Galeno cita sempre e solo l'esempio di 'flegma' e pare dunque non avere a disposizione un testo di Prodico, il quale tuttavia doveva essere ancora letto nel II sec. d.C, a giudicare dal commento a Tucidide del gram-

in questo contesto (che è di carattere storico e non prescrittivo) anche Galeno usa positivamente l'etimologia accanto agli altri criteri di indagine del significato della parola πυρετός (cioè le testimonianze dell'uso comune e di autorità come Aristotele, Teofrasto, Cleante, Crisippo, Zenone e infine Aristofane). A 31,25 egli dice "*wir erschliessen die Bedeutung dieses Namens in der Sprache der Griechen aus dem Hinweis des Wortes selbst, nämlich dass es etymologisch von dem Namen"Feuer"abgeleitet ist*".

In questa occasione l'etimologia ha dunque un suo valore, eppure l'impostazione antistoica di tutto il passo non può non richiamare la fortissima polemica di Galeno contro l'uso che gli Stoici fanno dell'etimologia. Sembra una contraddizione che egli qui sia così 'neutrale', pur contestando solitamente Prodico o attaccando Crisippo e la sua etimologia di ἐγώ in *De placitis* 2, 2, 5 ss. (*PHP*, CMG V 4, 1, 2, p.104,6 ss.: τὴν βελτίστην ἐτυμολογίαν).[83] Bisogna in effetti constatare che Galeno utilizza abbastanza spesso un'analisi delle parole di tipo etimologico, sia nei commenti sia nelle altre opere. È vero che tende a escludere dal commento i problemi di analisi grammaticale in genere e in particolare l'etimologia.[84] Tuttavia, pur se egli prende le distanze, le etimologie ritornano di volta in volta senza alcuna connotazione negativa. Non mi sembra soddisfacente ricondurre l'apparente sfasatura al semplice condizionamento della tradizione filologica alessandrina, da cui pure Galeno è fortemente influenzato,[85] anche se bisogna ricordare che la pratica etimologica faceva ormai parte della γραμματικὴ τέχνη (cf. *infra*) e Galeno aveva a disposizione molti strumenti, che offrivano un ricco

matico Antillo, che fece un confronto sistematico fra le espressioni tucididee e le *lexeis* di Prodico (cf. LUZZATTO 1993, 187 ss.).

[83] Cf. DE LACY 1966, 264 s.

[84] Per es. *Hipp.Art.* XVIIIA 395,3 ss. K; *Hipp.Fract.* XVIIIB 364,3 K τὰ ἐξέχοντα τῶν χειρῶν ὀνομάζουσι θέναρα παρὰ τὸ θείνειν, ὡς ἔνιοι βούλονται τῶν χαιρόντων ἐτυμολογίαις; cf. KOTZIA PANTELE 1995, 91 n.144.

[85] Un esempio potrebbe essere la spiegazione etimologica del poetico μελεδόνας con τὰ μέλη ἐδούσας a *Hipp.Art.* XVIIIA 362,16 ss. K, perché la parola è assente dal lemma ippocratico e la trattazione ha l'aria di un *excursus* dotto fine a se stesso.

materiale di questo genere. Vale però la pena di riflettere sul modo in cui Galeno utilizza l'etimologia, per capire se vi è una reale contraddizione o se la situazione è più complessa. Nei *Procedimenti anatomici* egli si inserisce, come dicevo, in una tradizione ricca di nomenclatura tecnica e ad essa normalmente si richiama.[86] Egli è solito spiegare l'origine dei nomi di parti anatomiche (p. es. κέκληταί γε μὴν περιτόναιον ἀπὸ τοῦ περιτετᾶσθαι πᾶσι κτλ. a *AA* 6, 4, II 550,7 K = Garofalo 1991, 357,28 ss., cf. II 554 K = Garofalo 1991, 363,14 ss.), collegandola a determinate caratteristiche fisiche dell'oggetto e fornendo talvolta una sorta di 'dossografia' delle denominazioni di una stessa parte anatomica: cf. 6, 6, II 563,8 K (= Garofalo 1991, 373,28 ss.):

> "Il 'mesenterion', che chiamano anche 'mesaraion', avendo posto ambedue i nomi sulla base degli accidenti: 'mesenterion' [che sta in mezzo agli intestini] è detto dalla posizione, 'mesaraion' [a struttura lassa] dall'essenza propria".

I due nomi μεσεντέριον e μεσάραιον indicano lo stesso oggetto ma hanno un'etimologia differente: a Galeno interessa chiarire le ragioni che hanno portato alla diversa designazione, e collocare entrambe, con un grado maggiore o minore di correttezza, nell'ambito della tradizione accettata. Non è certamente un caso che il termine usato da Galeno sia μεσάραιον,[87] ma μεσεντέριον sia termine aristotelico (p.es. *HA* 574 b 32), cioè parte della tradizione a cui Galeno fondamentalmente si ispira nel campo anatomo-fisiologico e che quindi il suo atteggiamento sia pregiudizialmente favorevole. La posizione favorevole di Galeno nei confronti della tradizione di cui sta parlando è certamente rilevante, ma egli ama comunque dare spiegazione etimologica individuale di ogni termine tecnico.[88] In una certa misura

[86] Vedi il frequente uso delle locuzioni ὁ καλούμενος, ὀνομάζεται ὑπὸ τῶν ἰατρῶν, ὀνομάζειν δ' ἔθος ἐστίν ecc.

[87] Gal. *UP* III 339,1 K; 343,3 e 13 K; *Loc.Aff.* VIII 369,13 K ecc.; cf. anche Ruf. *Part.corp.nom.* 167 e 171; *Corp.hum.anat.* 51.

[88] Cf. p. es. *AA* 7, 2, II 591 K ὑπεζωκώς; 9, 3, II 719-720 K τὰ καλούμενα χοριοειδῆ; 10, 1, Garofalo 1991, 35-36, i nomi della membrana che avvolge i muscoli dell'occhio; 14, 2, Garofalo 1991, 233, su τόνος e νεῦρον.

l'etimologia contribuisce a tracciare un quadro 'storico' articolato della medicina attraverso il punto di vista linguistico: e questa è senz'altro un'utilizzazione che va al di là di come viene normalmente concepito lo scopo dell'etimologia in ambito grammaticale.[89] Il rispetto che Galeno nutre per la tradizione dogmatica della medicina è profondo e leale, anche quando si tratta di una nomenclatura che nella sua motivazione rivela gli errori delle generazioni passate.[90]

> *Hipp.Aph.* XVIIIA 1,4 ss. K: "La 'lienteria' è una veloce fuoruscita attraverso ventre e intestini dei cibi e delle bevande, le quali escono nello stato in cui sono state ingerite. Si potrebbe definire l'affezione più brevemente una assenza di cozione, dal momento che non avviene nello stomaco alcuna alterazione del colore, della composizione o dell'odore o di qualunque altra qualità. L'affezione fu chiamata così perché coloro che posero il nome ritenevano che avvenisse a causa dello stato liscio delle pareti interne degli intestini, per la quale non trattenevano più ciò che era al loro interno, come se, allo stato naturale, essi lo trattenessero per la loro ruvidità. E' certo giusto lodare per molti altri motivi coloro che per primi dettero nome alle cose (ὠνομάσθη δὲ τὸ πάθος οὕτως ὑπονοησάντων τῶν πρώτως θεμένων τὴν προσηγορίαν αὐτῷ διὰ λειότητα γεγονέναι τῆς ἔνδον ἐπιφανείας τῶν ἐντέρων, δι' ἣν οὐκέτι ἀντιλαμβάνεται τῶν ἐμπεριεχομένων ἐν αὐτοῖς, ὡς ἂν ὅτε κατὰ φύσιν εἶχε τῇ τραχύτητι κατεχόντων αὐτά. πολλὰ μὲν οὖν καὶ ἄλλα τῶν πρώτως ὀνομασάντων τὰ πράγματα δίκαιον ἐπαινεῖν), ma non posso accettare, almeno nel caso delle lienteria, uomini che ignorano che è compito specifico dello stomaco avvolgere i cibi per un certo tempo, perché li serra e li trattiene e poi li spinge in basso ecc.".

Le posizioni teoriche di Galeno gli impediscono di vedere qualsiasi legame naturale fra parola come sequenza di suoni e

[89] Cf. SLUITER 1997, 160 s.; sulla funzione dell'etimologia come criterio, cf. SIEBENBORN 1976, 140 ss. La mancanza di senso storico è vista generalmente come il principale ostacolo ad uno sviluppo scientifico dell'etimologia antica: cito, per tutti, CAVAZZA 1981, 18 s.

[90] Cf. anche il caso delle vene carotidi: *AA* 14, 7, GAROFALO 1991, 264, cf. 266 l'etimologia rivela che la designazione è sbagliata, perché riflette un'opinione errata dei medici antichi, ma ciò non elimina il nome.

significato. Egli insiste, sia nelle sue opere teoriche come *De captionibus* o *Sui termini medici* sia in frequenti passi sparsi in varie opere, che il linguaggio è convenzionale, il significato è frutto di un contratto, tanto è vero che viene da lui paragonato alla moneta.[91] È allora illuminante un passo di *Thrasybulus* 32 (*Scripta minora* III p.76,25 ss. Helmreich), in cui si ribadisce l'assoluta convenzionalità del legame fra parola e significato. Galeno afferma che non si può dire niente di sapiente sulle parole di una lingua, p. es. Assira, o Persiana ecc. se non chiederne il significato agli Assiri, ai Persiani ecc.: infatti la parola pronunciata di per sé non indica niente. Ma ci sono persone che affermano che la parola è per loro sempre indicativa: allora Galeno vuole metterli alla prova interrogandoli, ma può farlo solo su parole di lingua greca. Propone allora la parola λιμήν che ha un significato diverso in greco comune (porto) e in tessalico (ἀγορά): la sua conclusione è che non si può imparare niente sul significato dei nomi se non da coloro che li hanno posti.[92]

Galeno fa dunque riferimento a coloro che credono che le parole abbiano un loro valore referenziale autonomo e ribadisce che l'analisi del significato rientra nelle competenze esclusive di un determinato gruppo linguistico, riporta dunque il legame fra parola e significato all'*ethos* di un gruppo sociale, ad un consenso. È da considerazioni teoriche come queste che scaturisce il ruolo

[91] Il passo è notissimo: *Diff. Puls.* VIII 567,17 K; per il paragone cf. p. es. QUINT. *Inst.* 1, 6, 3: *consuetudo vero certissima loquendi magistra, utendumque plane sermone ut nummo, cui publica forma est.* Anche Plutarco utilizza il paragone linguaggio-moneta ma in modo diverso, con riferimento alla sinteticità del linguaggio, cf. VAN DER STOCKT 1990.

[92] *Thras.* 32 (*Scr.min.* III p.76,25-77,18)... τὸ γὰρ ὄνομα ῥηθὲν αὐτὸ καθ' αὑτὸ μόνον οὐδὲν ἐνδείκνυται. ... εἰσὶ δ' οἳ λέγουσιν ἐνδείκνυσθαι σφίσι τοὔνομα καὶ τούτους ἐγὼ πάμπολλα συναθροίσας ὀνόματα Κελτῶν καὶ Θρᾳκῶν καὶ Μυσῶν καὶ Φρυγῶν ἐκέλευον ἐφ' ἑκάστου λέγειν τὸ δηλούμενον πρᾶγμα· τῶν δ' ἐν τῇ τῶν Ἑλλήνων φωνῇ μόνῃ δύνασθαι τοῦτο ποιεῖν εἰπόντων, ἑξῆς προὔτεινα λιμένα· τῶν δ' εἰπόντων, ἵναπερ αἱ νῆες ὁρμοῦσιν, ἀλλὰ Θετταλούς γ' ἔφην τὴν ὑφ' ἡμῶν προσαγορευομένην ἀγορὰν οὕτως ὀνομάζειν. οἱ δ' ἠρνοῦντο τὴν τῶν Θετταλῶν ἐπίστασθαι διάλεκτον, ὥσπερ οὐκ αὐτὸ δὴ τοῦθ' ὁμολογοῦντες, ὅπερ ἐξ ἀρχῆς ἐλέγετο, μηδὲν τῶν ὀνομάτων, ἐφ' οὗ κεῖται πράγματος, ἄλλως δύνασθαι μαθεῖν ἢ παρ' αὐτῶν τῶν θεμένων διδαχθέντα.

privilegiato che egli assegna alla *synetheia*, sia degli antichi che dei moderni, come afferma in *Sui termini medici*. Non ha alcuna importanza che il legame originario fra significante e significato sia convenzionale: dal momento in cui esso si è costituito all'interno del gruppo (in un'epoca che va al di là dell'interesse di Galeno), l'uso di quel gruppo resta l'unico criterio 'storico-naturale' di indagine. Si può aggiungere che l'analisi del significato delle parole ci riporta esclusivamente a quelle competenze specifiche o, per dirla in termini platonici, ci rivela solo le intenzioni, le opinioni di coloro che hanno imposto i nomi.[93] In questo senso, il ruolo di riferimento del *Cratilo* platonico, che fornisce una visione certo critica delle etimologie ma non distruttiva,[94] non va assolutamente sottovalutato per comprendere come Galeno consideri le parole prodotto della *doxa*, giusta o fallace che sia, di uomini del passato e per queste ragioni comunque meritevoli di indagine. Infatti essere consapevoli delle opinioni che sono alla base delle parole in uso aiuta il compito del medico-scienziato, che deve distinguere il piano delle parole da quello dei fatti.

Anche se sul piano teorico, Galeno non può che rifiutare il valore gnoseologico dell'etimologia di tipo stoico, tuttavia non può evitare di dare importanza al contenuto semantico delle parole: si pensi solo al passo famoso del *De usu partium* in cui egli considera il nome latino *cerebrum* di cervello più appropriato del termine greco ἐγκέφαλος (*UP* 8, 4, III 628,13 ss. K = I p.455,21 ss. Helmreich). Per quanto ossequiente nei confronti della tradizione platonico-aristotelica, Galeno ha una nozione del ruolo del cervello più complessa, per cui il nome tradizionale di 'encefalo', etimologicamente 'ciò che sta dentro la testa', è assolutamente inadeguato a designare un organo con funzioni direttive, perché basato su un fattore accidentale (la

[93] Cf. p. es. *Loc.aff.* VIII 191,17 ss. K ἅπαντες γοῦν ὀνομάζουσιν τὸ πάθος τοῦτο μελαγχολίαν, ἐνδεικνύμενοι διὰ τῆς προσηγορίας τὸν αἴτιον αὐτοῦ χυμόν.

[94] D'altra parte Platone stesso fa uso autonomo e pregnante di analisi etimologiche 'non cratilee'; cf. CLASSEN 1959, 85 ss.

localizzazione nella testa nell'uomo, mentre altri animali non dotati di testa ce l'hanno nel torace), mentre il latino *cerebrum* sarebbe per lui un termine più chiaro ed efficace:

> "... perché tu apprenda più chiaramente e con più evidenza — dico — se lo chiamerai con il nome romano, non derivato dalla posizione né da qualche altro accidente, ma comunicante l'essenza stessa, saprai chiaramente che niente ti impedisce di dire che il *cerebrum* è nella testa degli uomini (infatti lo chiamano così) ma nei granchi è nel petto".

Va sottolineato però che l'efficacia che Galeno attribuisce al termine latino non gli deriva affatto da una sua trasparenza di significato, ma al contrario, rispetto al trasparente 'encefalo', da una sua maggiore 'opacità',[95] che non svierebbe gli utenti in modo ingannevole, una volta accettata per convenzione la nuova nomenclatura: l'opacità serve qui ad esaltare la funzione denotativa, la funzionalità del linguaggio medico. In questo caso infatti il contenuto semantico di 'encefalo' non solo è sorpassato dalla maggiore consapevolezza della medicina postellenistica, ma può creare imbarazzo.[96] Ciò significa ribadire il rifiuto di ogni valore descrittivo delle parole: Galeno è consapevole del rischio di farsi fuorviare dalle opinioni o credenze che si accompagnano, come una sorta di superfetazione, ai nomi, come è detto esplicitamente in *MM* X 84,16 ss. K:

> "Bisogna dunque tentare in tutti i modi, se si punta alla verità stessa, di tenersi lontani dalle opinioni aggiuntive che si basano sui nomi (ἀποχωρεῖν μὲν τοῦ προσδοξαζομένου τοῖς ὀνόμασιν), ma andare all'essenza stessa delle cose e questa osservare e indagare".[97]

[95] Nonostante il fatto che anche il termine latino sia ugualmente connesso con la nozione di testa, cf. ERNOUT-MEILLET, *s.v.*

[96] Cf. LONGO 1994-95.

[97] La frase è a conclusione di una analisi di nomi di malattie, come ἐπινυκτίς, ἀκροχορδών, νυκτάλωψ, che rimandano a opinioni non sempre corrette sulle malattie stesse. BARNES 1991, 75 e n.86, osserva come il passo utilizzi una nozione fondamentale (τὸ προσδοξαζόμενον) nell'epistemologia epicurea, cf. HANKINSON 1994a: cf. EPIC. *Ep. ad Her.* 62. Sarebbe un ulteriore elemento in comune fra Galeno e alcune riflessioni epicuree. Il verbo è comunque usato anche con connotazioni scettiche in SEXT.EMP. *PH* 1, 30; 3, 236 ecc. Galeno lo usa un'altra volta

Forse allora il ruolo che ha l'etimologia nel discorso scientifico, ma soprattutto nell'esegesi scientifica di Galeno, è proprio quello di evitare il rischio di 'opinioni aggiuntive' attraverso una consapevolezza del modo in cui i nomi sono stati assegnati. Un passo di *Diff.Resp.* (VII 753,2 ss. K) ci fornisce un altro indizio sulla funzione dell'analisi etimologica:

> "Che *dyspnoia* sia un danno della respirazione, come *dysaisthesia* lo è della sensazione e *dyskynesia* lo è del movimento, lo indica sufficientemente il nome: quante invece siano le differenze del danno e per quali cause si verifichino e in che modo bisogna fare la diagnosi, non è possibile che sia insegnato dalla sua denominazione ma la natura stessa della respirazione lo indicherà (τι μὲν ἡ δύσπνοια βλάβη τις τῆς ἀναπνοῆς ἐστιν, ὥσπερ ἡ δυσαισθησία τῆς αἰσθήσεως, καὶ ἡ δυσκινησία τῆς κινήσεως, ἱκανὸν ἐνδείξασθαι τοὔνομα· πόσαι δὲ τῆς βλάβης διαφοραί, καὶ διὰ τίνας αἰτίας γιγνόμεναι, καὶ πῶς ἑκάστην αὐτῶν χρὴ διαγινώσκειν, οὐκ ἐκ τῆς προσηγορίας διδαχθῆναι νῦν ἔστιν, ἀλλ' ἡ φύσις αὐτὴ τῆς ἀναπνοῆς ἐνδείξεται)".

Il passo ci mostra il parallelismo che Galeno instaura fra il piano dell'osservazione dei sintomi e quello della significazione, tanto è vero che usa lo stesso verbo, ἐνδείκνυσθαι. L'espressione è usata altre volte in riferimento alla capacità del nome di 'indicare' più o meno chiaramente il proprio contenuto semantico, anche se non ha un uso specializzato tale da farne un termine tecnico.[98] Il verbo ha però connotazioni importanti nella teoria diagnostica di Galeno. La ἔνδειξις dei nomi sembra qui avere un ruolo parallelo a quello della ἔνδειξις sul piano della diagnosi,[99] ma infinitamente più debole e incerto, perché il linguaggio è governato dalla convenzione e dall'uso.[100] Tuttavia le parole, pur non

in *Di.Dec.* IX 795,7 K riferendosi a medici di impostazione empirica (che evitano di προσδοξάζειν sull'evidenza fenomenica).

[98] Credo che sia da escludere ogni relazione con la teoria dei segni, distinti in rammemorativo e indicativo.

[99] Sul tema, cf. BARNES 1991, 98 ss.; HANKINSON 1991a, 202 (*ad* 2, 7); KUDLIEN 1991, 103 ss.

[100] Cf. *Hipp.Prog.*, CMG V 9, 2, p.291,19-292,12: l'analisi grammaticale (della *paragogé*) del termine πρασοειδής usato in un contesto di termini di colore dovrebbe portarci a identificare il termine πρωτότυπον (πράσον), ma tali analisi sono quanto mai incerte, dunque bisogna occuparsi dei nomi solo nella misura

avendo un valore 'descrittivo' assoluto dell'oggetto, hanno valore 'indicativo' all'interno della storia linguistica di una comunità.

Con tutti i suoi limiti, l'indicazione delle parole è la loro capacità di avere una maggiore o minore 'trasparenza' o 'evidenza' del significato, o un'utile opacità (come ὀφθαλμός, οὖς, che indicano solo la funzione dell'organo, in *UP* 8, 4, il seguito del passo citato sopra) o, peggio, un'evidenza ingannevole, fuorviante, che è bene identificare per evitarne i rischi. Essa è importante nella terminologia medica, a tal punto che, come si è visto, Galeno propone di sostituire il termine corrente ἐγκέφαλος con il latino *cerebrum*: e tuttavia una tale argomentazione non elimina affatto il nome tradizionale. Per contrastare le opinioni ingannevoli suscitate dalle parole è sufficiente una consapevolezza 'storica' del valore e delle ragioni delle designazioni. È a queste condizioni che si manifesta il valore relativo dell'etimologia, come mostrano molto bene i *Procedimenti anatomici*, ma anche la sua effettiva utilizzazione da parte di Galeno all'interno dei commenti. Si trovano spesso conferme di questo valore più o meno 'indicativo' dei termini medici, che costituiscono momenti della riflessione galenica sulla efficacia della nomenclatura, cf. p. es. *Tum.Pr.Nat.* VII 729,12 ss. K:

> "Poiché chiamano i tumori dei testicoli κῆλαι ('gobbe') scritto con η nella prima sillaba, e non con α come fanno gli Ateniesi. Come ciascuno dei nomi detti indica la malattia della parte di cui si parla, così anche κιρσοκήλη (varicocele), nome recente, dichiara l'affezione di cui si parla".[101]

in cui essi possono chiarire ciò che si vuole dire (ταυτὶ μὲν οὖν ἅπαξ εἰρήσθω μοι νῦν, ἀεὶ δὲ μέμνησο τοῦ σπουδάζειν ἐπὶ τοῖς ὀνόμασι τοσοῦτον, ὅσον εἰς σαφῆ δήλωσιν ὧν λέγομεν ἐξ αὐτῶν ἔστιν ὀνίνασθαι).

[101] Bisogna specificare che nei commenti considerazioni sul valore 'indicativo' delle parole non concernono solo i *kyria onomata* ma anche le figure come metafora o *katachresis*: anche le metafore infatti possono essere usate per la loro forte capacità indicativa e chiarificatrice, cf. p. es. *Hipp.Art.* XVIIIA 598, 18 ss. K. (sul valore di ἐκτεθηλυσμένον). Un caso analogo di metafora efficace in *Hipp.Fract.* XVIIIB 587,15 K: "(*Fract.* 31, p.94,12 Kühlewein: spesso le cose hanno affinità le une con le altre) ciò che siamo soliti dire 'si assimila' o 'è comune' o 'ha parentela', Ippocrate usa chiamarlo"è affratellato", indicando con la parola la stretta affinità e parentela delle cose. Infatti, poiché fra le molte cose che sono affini, nessuna potrebbe essere chiamata più propriamente affine, egli usa riferirsi

Non c'è dunque reale contraddizione fra l'ampio uso che Galeno fa dell'etimologia e il capitolo di *Sui termini medici*, da cui siamo partiti. Il fatto è che, all'epoca di Galeno, esistevano ormai molti modi diversi di fare etimologia, come ricorda Varrone nel *De lingua latina* 5, 7-10. Egli ne classifica quattro, di cui il primo è quello popolare alla portata di tutti, il secondo è quello dei grammatici come Aristofane di Bisanzio, che si occupa della derivazione delle parole poetiche, il terzo e il quarto pertengono invece al livello filosofico di influenza stoica.[102] Certamente è piuttosto il secondo tipo, rispecchiante la prassi dei filologi alessandrini, la base del modo con cui Galeno utilizza l'etimologia, mentre è totalmente assente, anzi viene da lui rigettato il 'modo' stoico. Tuttavia Varrone sembra dare dell'etimologia di tradizione alessandrina una visione riduttiva, limitata alla spiegazione delle parole poetiche.[103] In Galeno invece l'analisi delle parole ha un campo di applicazione molto vasto, che va da termini comuni a termini tecnici, a vere e proprie 'glosse' ippocratiche o poetiche.

Dunque, sia nella consapevolezza del linguaggio tecnico, anatomico o patologico, sia nella spiegazione di parole difficili nei

alla forte affinità che ha lo stesso valore di una sorta di fratellanza con il verbo ἠδελφίσθαι". Può esserci qui un'eco delle valutazioni sul valore e l'uso delle metafore, in relazione alla chiarezza, nel terzo libro della *Retorica* di Aristotele, p. es. 3, 2, 1404 b 1 ss., in particolare 1405 b 12 sul fatto che certe espressioni, più appropriate di altre, hanno il potere di ποιεῖν τὸ πρᾶγμα πρὸ ὀμμάτων. La matrice aristotelica dell'analisi di Galeno sulle metafore ippocratiche può essere rintracciata anche per la denominazione ippocratica di νεφέλαι per i sedimenti urinari, che Galeno chiama invece ἐναιωρήματα: cf. *Hipp.Prog.*, CMG V 9, 2, p.281,17 ss. Ippocrate, secondo Galeno, usa un'analogia fra urina e aria e ciò richiama il quarto tipo della classificazione delle metafore in ARIST. *Po.* 21, 1457 b 6 ss., cioè 1) genere-specie; 2) specie-genere; 3) specie-specie; 4) πρὸς τὸ ἀνάλογον. Sembra in parziale contraddizione con questo quadro il passo di *Diff.Puls.* VIII 675,3 ss. K in cui si afferma che l'uso di tropi non si addice all'istruzione scientifica primaria e che solo chi ha appreso già i *pragmata* può 'indicarli' con metafora e *katachresis*.

[102] Cf. BARWICK 1957, 57 ss.

[103] BARWICK 1957, 60 ss. Sulla critica di Sesto Empirico in *Math.* I 241-47 vd. *infra*.

commenti, l'etimologia ha in Galeno un ruolo più importante di quanto potesse sembrare, ma è solo uno dei fattori di indagine. La posizione di Galeno ha qualche affinità con l'atteggiamento di Quintiliano, *Inst.* 1, 6, 28-38, che riconosce all'etimologia un valore limitato ma positivo, soprattutto quando si tratti di individuare il significato di parole poco note.[104] Non è certo casuale che Galeno faccia analisi etimologica soprattutto di termini derivati (e non di πρῶτα ὀνόματα), per arrivare all'individuazione del significato di base, come p. es. *Hipp.Prog.*, CMG V 9, 2, p.260,12 ss. (κενεών) e *Hipp.Aph.* XVIIB 788 K (κραιπάλη), *Diff.Resp.* VII 753,1 ss. K (δύσπνοια).

Inoltre il particolare valore ermeneutico dell'etimologia risulta evidente nell'esegesi ippocratica specialmente in casi difficili come ἀλλοφάσσειν di *Prog.* 20 (*Hipp.Prog.*, XVIIIB 249,12 ss.; CMG V 9, 2, p.339,15 ss.):

> "La parola ἀλλοφάσσοντες (anch'essa compare nella frase), che non è affatto consueta, indica coloro che delirano o coloro che si agitano, cioè sono nauseati. Ma è migliore quanto è possibile congetturare dalla parola stessa in prima istanza, perché la parola è derivata da 'dire ora una cosa ora un'altra', ma alcuni sostengono che la parola sia derivata da 'cambiare lo sguardo ora in un modo ora in un altro', cioè (muovere) gli occhi (βέλτιον δ' ὅσον ἐξ αὐτῆς τῆς φωνῆς οἷόν τε τεκμαίρεσθαι τὸ πρότερον, ἵν' ᾖ γενόμενον τοὔνομα τὸ ἀλλοφάσσοντες ἐκ τοῦ ἄλλοτε φάσκειν ἄλλα, τινὲς δὲ ἀπὸ τοῦ μεταβάλλειν ἄλλοτε εἰς ἄλλο σχῆμα τὰ φάη, τουτέστι τοὺς ὀφθαλμούς, γεγονέναι φασὶ τὴν προσηγορίαν)".[105]

[104] Anche Aristotele aveva fatto uso molto limitato dell'etimologia, cf. SLUITER 1997, 163.

[105] Il termine è attestato anche in *Mul.* I 41, VIII p.100,8 L, in cui MV hanno la variante inferiore ἀλλοφρονήσει, probabilmente inserita per influsso delle glosse a *Prog.* di Erotiano (39,9 Nachmanson) o di Galeno (XIX 75,12 K), in cui prevale il significato di 'essere fuori di sé', 'delirare': la tradizione lessicografica testimonia anche altri significati, come 'cambiare colore' in Esichio, *s.v.* oppure περιορᾶν in Fozio *Lex.*, *s.v.* I due significati giudicati superiori da Galeno sulla base dell'analisi etimologica hanno riscontro uno in Eustazio *In Iliadem* 23, 698, 1324,10-12 οἱ δέ γε παρὰ τοῖς ἰατρικῶς ἰωνίζουσιν ἀλλοφάσσοντες οὐδέν τι ὅμοιον δηλοῦσιν, ἀλλὰ σημαίνουσι τοὺς ἄλλοτε ἄλλα φράζοντας καὶ μηδὲν ὅλως διασαφοῦντας (e quindi M. VAN DER VALK [Ed.], *Eustathii Commentarii ad Homeri Iiadem pertinentes*, IV, Leiden 1987, 814 ha torto a considerarlo un'invenzione di

Il caso può essere considerato esemplare: Galeno sembra conoscere due interpretazioni correnti, che egli però considera inferiori a quelle che possono risultare da un'analisi etimologica. L'indicazione che viene dalla parola stessa è però solo una via che permette di τεκμαίρεσθαι e non dà soluzioni certe, è una via tutta interna al sistema linguistico e non concerne i rapporti con la realtà; tuttavia sulla base della conoscenza dei sintomi Galeno può optare per una delle possibili soluzioni offerte dall'etimologia.[106]

Nei commenti a Ippocrate la considerazione del valore etimologico di una parola presenta caratteri interessanti specialmente quando vi siano contrasti fra la *lexis* ippocratica e il valore d'uso, la cosiddetta συνήθεια. In questi casi la riflessione sul significato acquista peso, ma l'esito dell'analisi etimologica per Galeno non prevale mai sul significato d'uso,[107] come si vede p. es. in *Hipp.Art.* XVIIIA 469,6 dove si analizza il significato di σητάνιος e ci si richiama alla συνήθεια. L'etimologia[108] è offerta con un certo distacco e deve trovare una conferma nell'uso: è uno dei numerosi passi in cui Galeno oppone ad una tradizione esegetica precedente (l'etimologia) un riferimento alla συνήθεια contemporanea dei Greci d'Asia. Un altro esempio significativo è l'analisi del significato di εὐήθης in Ippocrate, di cui parla in *Hipp.Fract.* XVIIIB 611,6 ss. K e *Hipp.Prog.*, CMG V 9, 2,

Eustazio), l'altro in *Etym.Magnum s.v.* ἀλλοφάσσειν (θορυβεῖσθαι, ἀλλαχοῦ τὰ φάη περιφέρειν).

[106] In modo analogo, l'evidenza della formazione di una parola che è *hapax* ippocratico, fornisce l'immediata comprensione dell'espressione ἀρβύλαι πηλοπατίδες "stivali per camminare nel fango" (*Art.* 62: *v.l.* πηλοβατίδες Γ), cf. *Hipp.Art.* XVIIIA 680,3 ss. K τοῦτο γὰρ γέγονε τὸ ὄνομα, εἰ μὲν διὰ τοῦ π γράφοιτο πηλοπατίδας διὰ τὸ πατεῖσθαι τὸν πηλὸν ὑπ' αὐτῶν, εἰ δὲ διὰ τοῦ β πηλοβατίδας, ἐπειδὰν βαίνειν ἀσφαλῶς ἐν πηλῷ δυνατόν ἐστι τοῖς ὑποδεδεμένοις τοιοῦτον ὑπόδημα. Attraverso l'etimologia si vede il significato primario e secondario: cf. κενεαγγεία *HVA*, CMG V 9, 1, p.208,4 ss. (ma influisce anche l'uso).

[107] Cf. *AA* 12, 2 (Garofalo 1991, 144), bisogna rispettare l'uso anche se inesatto, non solo per i nomi delle parti del corpo, ma in tutti i fatti della vita, con il solito richiamo alla coppia Ippocrate-Platone e al loro opposto Prodico.

[108] Εἰρῆσθαί φασι πρὸς αὐτοῦ τοὺς σῆτες ἐσπαρμένους, ὅπερ οἱ Ἀττικοὶ τῆτες ὀνομάζουσι.

p.331,23 ss. L'aggettivo è usato da Ippocrate nel suo senso etimologico e proprio "di buon carattere", ma tale significato è pressoché scomparso dall'uso, in cui prevale un senso eufemistico per "sciocco": questo contrasto, che era già oggetto di studio nella tradizione atticistica,[109] spinge Galeno a soffermarsi sulle denominazioni eufemistiche, ma anche a portare esempi concreti per il significato etimologico, in pratica a rintracciarne *un uso*, anche se sporadico e desueto.[110]

La stessa strategia è applicata in un altro caso in cui l'etimologia spiega un uso antico diverso da quello contemporaneo. In realtà si tratta di un uso catacrestico insolito di ὁμιλεῖν in Ippocrate *Art.* 1 (p.112,12 Kühlewein): l'articolazione del braccio è detta ὁμιλεῖν la cavità della scapola, con una estensione del senso di 'frequentare', 'avere contatto', 'essere vicino a', di solito riferito a persone. Galeno però ricorre ad un'analisi etimologica nata in realtà per il testo omerico, citando Omero *Il.* 18, 539, come esempio fra tutti gli antichi:

> *Hipp.Art.* XVIIIA 316,12 ss. K (con qualche correzione basata su L): "ὁμιλεῖν dicevano gli antichi per lo più non del parlare, come la maggioranza dei moderni, ma del radunarsi insieme e come 'avvinghiarsi l'un l'altro'. Anche Omero utilizza questa espressione, a proposito delle immagini incise da Efesto sullo scudo, dice"come uomini vivi si mescolavano"(Σ 539). Dice che il braccio è in contatto con la cavità della scapola obliquamente, quando l'arto è disteso lungo i fianchi, mostrando con la parola ὁμιλεῖν l'essere insieme e il toccarla (ὁμιλεῖν ἔλεγον οἱ παλαιοὶ τοὐπίπαν οὐκ ἐπὶ τοῦ διαλέγεσθαι, καθάπερ νῦν οἱ πολλοί, τὸ συνιέναι δὲ ἀλλήλοις καὶ οἷον ὁμοῦ εἱλεῖσθαι.[111] ταύτῃ προσηγόρευε τῇ φωνῇ καὶ Ὅμηρος (Σ 539), ἐπὶ τῶν κατὰ τὴν ἀσπίδα γεγραμμένων ὑπὸ τοῦ Ἡφαίστου φησίν "ὡμίλεον δ' ὥστε ζωοὶ βροτοί". τὸν βραχίονα τῷ κοίλῳ τῆς ὠμοπλάτης ὁμιλεῖν ἔφη

[109] Cf. MANETTI-ROSELLI 1994, 1575.

[110] Un procedimento analogo è seguito da Galeno per πρόνοια, che Ippocrate non usa nel senso comune degli Elleni (cf. *Hipp.Prog.*, XVIIIB 7,13 ss. K; CMG V 9, 2, p.201 ss.) e che gli offre il destro per una polemica contro gli Erofilei, che avrebbero forzato il significato di πρόνοια, distinguendola da πρόγνωσις, operando una νομοθεσία scorretta sui nomi.

[111] APOLLON.SOPH. *s.v.* ὅμιλος; *Etym.Magnum s.v.* ὅμιλος.

πλάγιον ὅταν παρὰ τὰς πλεύρας ἡ χεὶρ ᾖ παρατεταμένη, διὰ τοῦ ὁμιλεῖν ῥήματος δηλῶν τό τε ὁμοῦ εἶναι καὶ ψαύειν αὐτῆς)".

Ciò che risulta curioso è che Galeno, sulla scia di una tradizione grammaticale,[112] adatta a Ippocrate la soluzione che la tradizione esegetica aveva elaborato per spiegare il termine ὅμιλος in Omero e il suo particolare significato di 'mischia in battaglia', riferito a tutt'altro contesto, parallelo a quello del verbo ὁμιλέω come 'combatto' Ma la tradizione esegetica medica, testimoniata da Erotiano, *s.v.* ὁμιλίη, dava la stessa spiegazione di *Art.* 1 ("il verbo indica vicinanza, contiguità"), senza passare attraverso la mediazione omerica e quindi senza l'analisi etimologica.[113] Non era perciò necessario passare per l'etimologia per comprendere il valore dell'espressione ippocratica, ma ancora una volta l'etimologia serve ad avvicinare Ippocrate ad Omero, in altre parole ad identificare il contesto della συνήθεια antica di quest'espressione ippocratica, mentre la spiegazione alternativa l'avrebbe lasciata senza confronti. Si può forse osservare, come conclusione, che Galeno, nei fatti, condivide alcuni elementi della critica che Sesto Empirico rivolge all'etimologia in *Math.* 1, 241-247. Sesto svolge il suo attacco con argomentazioni specifiche (p. es. la possibilità di regresso all'infinito), ma in particolare afferma che l'etimologia o si risolve nell'uso ed è superflua o è del tutto dannosa. Anche per Galeno e per la sua impostazione esegetica, in fondo, l'etimologia — che non ha assolutamente un valore normativo per lo ἑλληνισμός e tantomeno può averne uno gnoseologico — è uno strumento che aiuta a ricostruire le opinioni degli antichi medici e per ciò stesso riporta a una συνήθεια: dunque in sostanza si dissolve nell'uso.

[112] Cf. p. es. HDN., *Gramm.Graeci* III 2, p.564,32 ss.

[113] La quale, se mai, veniva applicata a ὁμιλίη di *Aër.* 14,6, cf. EROT. *Voc.Hipp.Coll.* p.65,7 ss. Nachm.

BIBLIOGRAFIA

ARRIGHETTI, G. 1973. Epicuro. *Opere*, a cura di G. A. (Torino ²1973).

BARNES, J. 1991. "Galen on Logic and Therapy", in *Galen's Method of Healing*, ed. by F. KUDLIEN and R.J. DURLING (Leiden 1991), 50-102.

BARNES, J. 1993a. "Galen and the Utility of Logic", in *Galen und das hellenistische Erbe*, hrsg. von J. KOLLESCH und D. NICKEL, Sudhoffs Archiv Beihefte 32 (Stuttgart 1993), 33-52.

BARNES, J. 1993b. "A Third Sort of Syllogism. Galen and the Logic of Relations", in *Modern Thinkers and Ancient Thinkers. The Stanley Victor Keeling Memorial Lectures at University College London, 1981-1991* (Boulder, Colorado 1993), 172-194.

BARNES, J. 1997. "Logique et pharmacologie", in *Galen on Pharmacology*, Proc. of the Vth Intern. Galen Colloquium, Lille, 16-18 March 1995, ed. by A. DEBRU (Leiden 1997), 3-33.

BARWICK, K. 1957. *Probleme der stoischen Sprachlehre und Rhetorik*, Abh. Sächs. Akad. Wiss. zu Leipzig, Phil.-hist. Kl. 49,3 (Berlin 1957).

BONNER, S.F. 1939. *The Literary Treatises of Dionysius of Halicarnassus* (Cambridge 1939).

BOWERSOCK, G.W. 1969. *Greek Sophists in the Roman Empire* (Oxford 1969).

BRUNT, P.A. 1994. "The Bubble of the Second Sophistic", in *BICS* 39 (1994), 25-52.

BURNYEAT, M. 1994. "Enthymeme: Aristotle on the Logic of Persuasion", in *Aristotle's* Rhetoric. *Philosophical Essays*, ed. by D.J. FURLEY and A. NEHAMAS (Princeton 1994), 3-51.

CAVAZZA, F. 1981. *Studio su Varrone etimologo e grammatico* (Firenze 1981).

CLASSEN, C.J. 1959. *Sprachliche Deutung als Triebkraft platonischen und sokratischen Philosophierens*, Zetemata 22 (München 1959).

DAHLMANN, J.H. 1928. *De philosophorum Graecorum sententiis ad loquellae originem pertinentibus capita duo* (Weidae Thuringorum 1928).

DEBRU, A. 1995. "Les démonstrations médicales à Rome au temps de Galien", in *Ancient Medicine in its Socio-Cultural Context*, ed. by Ph.J. VAN DER EIJK — H.F.J. HORSTMANNSHOFF — P.H. SCHRIJVERS, I-II (Amsterdam1995), I 69-81.

DEICHGRÄBER, K. 1957. *Parabasenverse aus Thesmophoriazusen II des Aristophanes bei Galen*, Sb. Ak. Wiss. zu Berlin, Kl. für Sprachen, Literatur und Kunst 1956,2.

DE LACY, Ph. 1966. "Galen and the Greek Poets", in *GRBS* 7 (1966), 259-266.

EDLOW, R.B. 1977. *Galen on Language and Ambiguity* (Leiden 1977).

ERNOUT, A.-MEILLET, A. ^{4}1959. *Dictionnaire étymologique de la langue latine* (Paris ^{4}1959).

FREDE, M. 1977. "The origins of Traditional Grammar", in *Historical and Philosophical Dimensions of Logic, Methodology and Philosophy of Science*, ed. by R.E. BUTTS and J. HINTIKKA (Dordrecht-Boston 1977), 51-79.

FREDE, M. 1978. "Principles of Stoic Grammar", in *The Stoics*, ed. by J.M. RIST (Berkeley 1978), 27-75.

FREDE, M. 1981. "On Galen's Epistemology", in *Galen : Problems and Prospects*, ed. by V. NUTTON (London 1981), 65-86.

GAROFALO, I. (ed.). 1988. Erasistrati *fragmenta* (Pisa 1988).

GAROFALO, I. (ed.). 1991. Galeno. *Procedimenti anatomici*, I-III (Milano 1991).

GATZ, B. 1967. *Weltalter, goldene Zeit und sinnverwandte Vorstellungen*, Spudasmata 16 (Hildesheim 1967).

HANKINSON, R.J. 1991a. *Galen. On the Therapeutic Method. Books I and II*, Transl. with Intr. and Comm. by R.J. H. (Oxford 1991).

HANKINSON, R.J. 1991b. "Galen on the Foundation of Science", in *Galeno : obra, pensamiento e influencia*, ed. por J.A. LÓPEZ FÉREZ (Madrid 1991), 15-29.

HANKINSON, R.J. 1992. "Galen's Philosophical Eclecticism", in *ANRW* II 36, 5 (Berlin 1992), 3505-3522.

HANKINSON, R.J. 1994a. "Usage and Abusage: Galen on Language", in *Language*, ed. by S. EVERSON, Companions to Ancient Thought N.3 (Cambridge 1994), 166-187.

HANKINSON, R.J. 1994b. "Galen's concept of scientific progress", in *ANRW* II 37, 2 (Berlin 1994), 1775-1789.

HANKINSON, R.J. 1994c. "Galen's Anatomical Procedures: A Second-Century Debate in Medical Epistemology", in *ANRW* II 37, 2 (Berlin 1994), 1834-1855.

HANKINSON, R.J. 1994d. "Galen and the Logic of Relations", in *Aristotle in Late Antiquity*, ed. by L.P. SCHRENK, The Catholic University of America (Washington 1994), 57-75.

HELDMANN, K. 1982. *Antike Theorien über Entwicklung und Verfall der Redekunst*, Zetemata 77 (München 1982).

HERBST, W. 1911. *Galeni Pergameni de Atticissantium Studiis Testimonia*, Diss. Marburg (Leipzig 1911).

JOUANNA, J. 1992. *Hippocrate* (Paris 1992).

KOLLESCH, J. 1981. "Galen und die Zweite Sophistik", in *Galen: Problems and Prospects*, ed. by V. NUTTON (London 1981), 1-11.

KOTZIA PANTELE, P. 1995. *Ο Γαληνός για την ιατρική ορολογία και τη γλωσσα*, Aristoteleio Panepistimio Thessalonikis, Epistimoniké Epetirida 2, 5, 59-112.

KUDLIEN, F. 1991. "'Endeixis' as a Scientific Term: A) Galen's Usage of the Word", in *Galen's Method of Healing*, ed. by F. KUDLIEN and R.J. DURLING (Leiden 1991), 103-111.

LAUSBERG, H. 1973. *Handbuch der literarischen Rhetorik*, 2., durch einen Nachtrag vermehrte Aufl. (München 1973).

LONGO, O. 1994-95. "Il nome del cervello: Galeno contro Aristotele", in *AAPat* 107 (1994-1995), 131-134.

LÓPEZ FÉREZ, J.A. 1994. "Σαφήνεια en Galeno", in *Χάρις διδασκαλίας*. Homenaje a L. Gil, ed. por R.M. AGUILAR — M. LÓPEZ SALVÁ — I. RODRÍGUEZ ALFAGEME (Madrid 1994), 129-142.

LUZZATTO, M.J. 1993."Itinerari di codici antichi: un'edizione di Tucidide tra il II e il X secolo", in *MD* 30 (1993), 167-203.

MANETTI, D. 1995. "Commentarium in Hippocratis «De alimento»", in *Corpus dei Papiri Filosofici greci e latini* III (Firenze 1995), 39-51.

MANETTI, D. 1998. "Galeno e il significato di μακρολογία e μικρολογία (In Hipp. Fract., XVIII 2,518-19 e 526-27 K.)", in *RFIC* 126 (1998), 55-71.

MANETTI, D. 1999, "Il proemio di Erotiano e l'oscurità intenzionale di Ippocrate", in *I testi medici greci. Tradizione e ecdotica*, Atti del III Convegno Internazionale, Napoli 15-18 ottobre 1997, a cura di A. GARZYA e J. JOUANNA (Napoli 1999), 363-377.

MANETTI, D. — ROSELLI, A. 1994. "Galeno commentatore di Ippocrate", in *ANRW* II 37, 2 (Berlin 1994), 1529-1635.

MANSFELD, J. 1994. *Prolegomena. Questions to be settled before the study of an author, or a text*, Philosophia Antiqua 61 (Leiden 1994).

MANULI, P. 1984. "Lo stile del commento. Galeno e la tradizione ippocratica", in *La scienza ellenistica*, Atti delle tre giornate di studio

Pavia 14-16 Aprile 1982, a cura di G. GIANNANTONI e M. VEGETTI (Napoli 1984), 375-394.

MANULI, P. 1986. "Traducibilità e molteplicità di linguaggi nel *De Placitis* di Galeno", in *Storiografia e dossografia nella filosofia antica* (Torino 1986), 245-265.

MANULI, P. 1993. "Galen and Stoicism", in *Galen und das hellenistische Erbe*, hrsg. von J. KOLLESCH und D. NICKEL, Sudhoffs Archiv Beihefte 32 (Stuttgart 1993), 53-61.

MEYERHOF, M. — SCHACHT, J. 1931. Galen. *Über die medizinischen Namen.* Arabisch und Deutsch hrsg. Abh. Preuss. Akad. Wiss. 3 (Berlin 1931).

MILANESE, G. 1989. *Lucida carmina. Comunicazione e scrittura da Epicuro a Lucrezio* (Milano 1989).

MORETTI, G. 1995. *Acutum dicendi genus: brevità, oscurità, sottigliezze e paradossi nelle tradizioni retoriche degli Stoici* (Bologna 1995).

VON MÜLLER, I. 1895. *Über Galens Werk vom wissenschaftlichen Beweis*, Abh. der Kgl.Bayer.Akad.der Wiss., 1. Klasse, 20,2 (München 1895).

NOVARA, A. 1982-1983. *Les idées romaines sur le progrès d'après les écrivains de la République* I-II (Paris 1982-1983).

PEARCY, L.T. 1983. "Galen and Stoic Rhetoric", in *GRBS* 24 (1983), 259-272.

REARDON, B.P. 1971. *Courants littéraires grecs des IIe et IIIe siècles après J.-C.* (Paris 1971).

SCHIAPARELLI, A. 1999a. "L'ambiguità in Aristotele e in Galeno", in *Antiaristotelismo*, a cura di C. NATALI — S. MASO (Amsterdam 1999), 143-166.

SCHIAPARELLI, A. 1999b. "L'influenza della"Retorica" di Aristotele in età imperiale: l'importanza di essere chiaramente ambigui", in *Méthexis* 12 (1999), 53-75.

SCHIAPARELLI, A. 2002. *Galeno e le fallacie linguistiche. Il "De captionibus in dictione"*, Istituto Veneto di Scienze, Lettere e Arti, Memorie, Cl. di Sc.mor. ecc., 101 (Venezia 2002).

SCHRIJVERS, P.H. 1974. "La pensée de Lucrèce sur l'origine du langage (*DRN* 1019-1090)", in *Mnemosyne* 27 (1974), 337-364.

SIEBENBORN, E. 1976. *Die Lehre von Sprachrichtigkeit und ihre Kriterien. Studien zur antiken normativen Grammatik* (Amsterdam 1976).

SIMON, M. 1906. *Sieben Bücher Anatomie des Galen (H-IE)* I-II (Leipzig 1906).

SLUITER, I. 1995a. "The Embarrassment of Imperfection: Galen's Assessment of Hippocrates' Linguistic Merits", in *Ancient Medicine in its Socio-Cultural Context* (Amsterdam 1995), II 519-535.

SLUITER, I. 1995b. "The Poetics of Medicine", in *Greek Literary Theory after Aristotle*, A Collection of Papers in Honour of D.M. Schenkeveld, ed. by J.G.J. ABBENES, S.R. SLINGS, I. SLUITER (Amsterdam 1995), 193-213.

SLUITER, I. 1997. "The Greek Tradition", in *The Emergence of Semantics in Four Linguistic Traditions. Hebrew, Sanskrit, Greek, Arabic*, Amsterdam Studies in the Theory and History of Linguistic Science 82 (Amsterdam-Philadelphia 1997), 149-224.

SMITH, W.D. 1979. *The Hippocratic Tradition*, Cornell Publications in the History of Science (Ithaca-London 1979).

VON STADEN, H. 1995. "Science as Text, Science as History: Galen on Metaphor", in *Ancient Medicine in its Socio-Cultural Context* (Amsterdam1995), II 499-518.

VON STADEN, H. 1997. "Galen and the 'Second Sophistic'", in *Aristotle and After*, ed. by R. SORABJI, BICS Suppl. 68 (London 1997), 33-54.

VAN DER STOCKT, L. 1990. "Plutarch on Language", in *Le langage dans l'Antiquité*, sous la direction de P. SWIGGERS & A. WOUTERS (Leuven 1990), 180-196.

SWAIN, S. 1996. *Hellenism and Empire* (Oxford 1996).

VEGETTI, M. 1999. "Tradition and Truth. Forms of Philosophical-Scientific Historiography in Galen's *De placitis*", in *Ancient Histories of Medicine*, ed. by Ph.J. VAN DER EIJK (Leiden 1999), 333-357.

VEGETTI, M. 2001. "Il confronto degli antichi e dei moderni in Galeno", in *L'antico degli antichi*, a cura di G. CAJANI e D. LANZA (Palermo 2001), 87-100.

DISCUSSION

R.J. Hankinson: Thank you very much for that extremely interesting presentation. But I wondered whether perhaps more emphasis might have been placed on the fact that for Galen, at least officially, clarity is everything: He is prepared to accept solecisms in the interests of *saphêneia* even though of course he emphasizes his commitment to ordinary usage, and he says repeatedly he doesn't mind what you call things as long as you do so consistently (although he himself is often less than consistent, for instance in his use of the term *symptôma*); and the other thing that seems to me to matter is his rejection of adornment: it isn't functional, he says at *De sophismatibus* XIV 587,3 K, it's like carrying an ivory-handled sword or wearing eye make-up.

D. Manetti: Non credo affatto che Galeno, nel descrivere le caratteristiche dello stile ippocratico, si sia dimenticato di ciò che dice nel *De sophismatibus*: per lui la chiarezza resta sempre l'elemento più importante, come risulta chiaro anche dal proemio del commento a *Sulle fratture*, in cui definisce i criteri per giudicare l'oscurità, cioè il contrario della chiarezza. È piuttosto per ragioni apologetiche che Galeno connette la chiarezza di Ippocrate, per lui scontata sul piano generale, con altre determinate caratteristiche che lo inquadrano anche 'storicamente' e gli servono per difenderlo dalle accuse di altri commentatori. Non è infatti casuale che attribuisca ad Ippocrate proprio uno stile semplice e 'privo di ornamenti'.

G. Strohmaier: In the first chapter of Galen, *De partium homoeomerium differentiis* (ed. by G. Strohmaier, CMG, Suppl.Orient. III [Berlin 1970], 44-51) there is an interesting discussion about the somewhat misleading term ὁμοιομερής: Galen says that the parts of the so-called homoiomerous parts are in reality identical as to their *eidos*, therefore a better designation would be ταὐτομερής, but this would be awkward, and Galen does not use this word in what follows.

D. Manetti: Ringrazio per la citazione del passo, che conferma il grande interesse di Galeno per le ragioni della denominazione e per l'analisi semantica dei termini della scienza. Ma il giudizio che Galeno esprime sulla loro minore o maggiore adeguatezza allo standard scientifico, cui egli aspira, non intacca, come si vede, il ruolo privilegiato del linguaggio ereditato dalla tradizione.

M. Frede: If one wants to determine Galen's own position concerning the virtues of language and to situate it in the context of views concerning the virtues of language held in antiquity quite generally, of what relevance is it that Galen in *De captionibus* seems to claim that there is only one virtue, properly speaking, σαφήνεια?

D. Manetti: Galeno attribuisce alla chiarezza un ruolo privilegiato, non solo negli scritti teorici, ma anche nell'analisi del linguaggio ippocratico: il proemio del commento a *Sulle fratture* con la sua discussione sull'oscurità assoluta e relativa, dipende perciò dalle stesse premesse teoriche di *De captionibus*. Nei commenti cambia però il punto di vista, perchè Galeno deve fare i conti con un linguaggio dato, quello di Ippocrate, a cui egli deve attribuire la virtù della chiarezza per poter affermare la sua superiorità. Le strategie argomentative puntano dunque a relativizzare, a storicizzare la nozione di chiarezza, mettendola nel contesto preciso di una comunicazione a determinati destinatari, e ad esaminare i modi concreti messi in atto per raggiungerla. Per fare questo egli deve ricorrere anche all'analisi retorica.

M. Frede: You very persuasively point out that Galen thinks that we should follow current language (συνήθεια), in general and in medical writing, but that Hippocrates, rightly, was following the usage of his time, and that hence it takes learning of various kinds to determine what Hippocrates was saying in various places. Bur this raises various questions: 1) What is Galen referring to when he talks about present συνήθεια, current colloquial usage, current educated/cultivated usage in medical writing? 2) To the extent that he is referring to educated usage, this seems to raise a problem in that in Galen's time what counts as educated usage is very much determined by the classical authors and that is, at least supposedly, a usage of the past. 3) Is there any indication that Hippocrates was regarded as a classical author whose example helps to define what counts as good, educated current language?

D. Manetti: Sulla nozione di *synetheia* in Galeno bisognerebbe condurre un'analisi dettagliata, perché essa ha molta importanza ed egli ne usa di volta in volta diverse sfumature e specificazioni (principalmente greco colto della *paideia*, distinto dal linguaggio parlato, cf. *Diff.Puls.* VIII 582-583 K, ma anche il greco d'Asia, qualunque cosa ciò significhi): sul valore di *synetheia* vedi p. es. ciò che ne dice Swain 1996, cap.1, ma anche lo studio di K. Versteegh, "Latinitas, Hellenismos, Arabiyya", in *The History of Linguistics in the Classical Period*, ed. by D.J. Taylor (Amsterdam-Philadelphia 1987), 251-274, che giudica la nozione di *synetheia* del tutto estranea alla lingua parlata.

Per quanto riguarda il secondo punto Galeno, come dicevo, si riferisce all'uso colto di scuola, anche se in qualche caso fa riferimento alla '*synetheia* dei Greci d'Asia', che sembra definire perlomeno un ambito di greco parlato regionale: l'uso colto era largamente determinato da un certo canone di autori e in questo senso può coincidere con uso *del passato* (certamente c'è un'impostazione atticistica in senso generale), ma fino ad un certo punto. La lingua risultante dalla *paideia* era comunque la lingua riconosciuta come standard e *effettivamente* adoperata dalle classi colte del suo tempo: c'erano comunque diverse posizioni — come quelle degli atticisti radicali e di quelli moderati — e anche autori antichi e autorevoli esterni alla media delle letture scolastiche: credo quindi che Galeno avesse ragione a distinguere una *synetheia* antica da quella moderna.

Per il terzo punto, Ippocrate non aveva alcun ruolo fra gli autori 'classici' nella *paideia* generale. È menzionato solo una volta da Demetrio *De elocutione* (vd. n.29) con un giudizio negativo. L'operazione di inserire Ippocrate nel contesto degli scrittori 'classici' è operazione in larga parte galenica, anche se l'esegesi precedente (fin dal *Lessico* di Bacchio di Tanagra) aveva già cominciato ad analizzare i testi ippocratici con gli stessi strumenti di interpretazione usati per gli altri autori e quindi aveva di fatto già cominciato il processo di assimilazione.

G. Strohmaier: Galen offers an interesting remark about the expression "to be burnt by ice" in the commentary on Περὶ ἀέρων which I am going to publish. The passage is in Ms. Cairo, Ṭalʿat ṭibb 550, fol. 87v7-9 (the lemma) and fol. 87v10-12 (beginning of the commentary) and reads in my German translation:

[*De aere aquis locis* 20,3, p.70,17-19 Diller]: "Hippokrates sagt: Der Teint des Geschlechts der Türken ist rot wegen der kalten Beschaffenheit ihres Landes und weil die Sonne nicht mit ihrer Wärme über ihnen aufgeht. Wenn die weisse Farbe von der Kälte verbrannt wird, geht sie in die Röte über. Galen sagt: Alle Bewohner Asiens sagen bis auf den heutigen Tag, dass die Füsse verbrannt werden, wenn sie wegen starker Kälte gefühllos werden. Wegen dieses Umstandes und dieser Gewohnheit sagt auch Hippokrates, dass die weisse Farbe rot wird, wenn sie von der übermässigen starken Kälte verbrannt wird".

D. Manetti: La ringrazio della segnalazione. Si tratta di un passo molto importante, in cui Galeno sembra fare un confronto fra l'espressione ippocratica e il greco comune (in questo caso direi parlato) d'Asia.

J. Barnes: The breadth and wealth of your paper inclines me to reflexion rather than to interrogation. But let me raise one general point which the final section of your remarks suggests. Should we not distinguish between two — or more — sorts of etymology? Sometimes, in 'vulgar' etymologizing, we look at a compound word and think to decide its sense on the basis of the senses of its components. Galen frequently etymologizes in this fashion — and sometimes, as you have pointed out, remarks on the dangers of the procedure. Sometimes, however, etymologizing bears a more 'scientific' aspect — we might think of the rules of transformation most familiar from Varro, or of the theory of πάθη developed by the grammarians. This sort of etymologizing is often closer to fantasy than to fact: is it often used — or commented upon — by Galen?

D. Manetti: In effetti il tipo di etimologia regolato da criteri 'scientifici' è piuttosto di derivazione stoica (cf. sopra la distinzione fatta da Varrone e Barwick 1957, 58 ss.) e Galeno non sembra farne mai uso né lo commenta, al di là dei passi dedicati alla polemica con Crisippo in *PHP*. Il valore dell'etimologia per Galeno si rileva in maniera indiretta, come ho cercato di mostrare, e mi sembra faccia riferimento nella teoria alla tradizione platonica e nella prassi alla tradizione filologico-grammaticale alessandrina che già da tempo aveva incluso l'etimologia fra i suoi strumenti.

J. Jouanna: Dans votre communication très riche, dont la première partie porte sur le style d'Hippocrate vu par Galien, vous avez situé de façon éclairante cette analyse dans les autres théories contemporaines sur le style. Vous dites que la langue hippocratique se rappoche du *genus tenue*. Quel est le mot grec correspondant?

D. Manetti: La definizione greca del *genus tenue* o *subtile* è ἰσχνόν, cf. Quint. *Inst.* 12, 10, 58.

J. Jouanna: Quel rapport y-a-t-il entre ἰσχνός et σύντομος?

D. Manetti: ἰσχνός definisce un genere di scrittura, di cui la brevità (συντομία) è una delle caratteristiche, ma non la sola.

J. Jouanna: En ce qui concerne la βραχυλογία d'Hippocrate, vous avez bien montré ce que Galien pouvait approuver. Vous dites que cette concision mérite éloge parce qu'elle n'omet rien. En réalité Galien dit qu'elle n'omet rien des choses utiles (τῶν χρησίμων). N'y a-t-il pas une légère différence? Cette notion d'utilité est-elle à mettre en rapport avec les préoccupations particulières de la médecine dont le but est d'être utile?

D. Manetti: Che la brevità, per essere una virtù del discorso, non dovesse omettere cose 'utili' è già esplicitamente richiesto dai manuali di retorica, si veda per es. Dionigi di Alicarnasso nel definire lo stile breve di Lisia (*Lys*. 5,1), ma è certo che in Galeno la menzione degli 'elementi utili' si risemantizza immediatamente per la rilevanza che egli attribuisce nell'insegnamento medico a ciò che è utile per la τέχνη.

J. Jouanna: Vous avez bien montré que cette concision peut aussi dans certains cas aboutir à l'obscurité. Galien ne devait-il pas réagir contre une idée assez répandue sur l'obscurité d'Hippocrate?

D. Manetti: In effetti la fama di Ippocrate aveva prodotto reazioni opposte nel giudizio sui suoi scritti. Ci sono tracce evidenti che Ippocrate da molti era considerato oscuro e, come ho detto, tutta l'elaborazione galenica della brevità ippocratica ha sicuramente una matrice apologetica, ma di questo non ho esplicitamente trattato qui, rimandando semplicemente a quanto ho detto in un altro articolo (vedi n.8).

J. Jouanna: À propos de modèles concurrents, faut-il opposer une vision de la décadence des modernes par rapport aux anciens à l'idée que les progrès de la médecine ont entraîné aussi des progrès dans le langage ou est-il possible de les concilier en voyant dans le progrès du langage une continuation de ce que les Anciens ont fait?

D. Manetti: La visione della decadenza della medicina è funzionale alla polemica contro i rivali di Galeno, i 'sofisti' contemporanei, mentre la visione del progresso del linguaggio rimane tutta interna alla tradizione della medicina dogmatica di cui Galeno si sente erede e perfezionatore. In questo senso non sono modelli opposti ma complementari. Certamente Galeno vede se stesso su una linea di perfetta continuità con gli antichi, anche quindi sul piano del linguaggio, al di là delle divergenze dovute al progresso degli studi anatomici.

G. Strohmaier: A statement that the ancients were cleverer than the moderns and so it was not necessary to give long explanations occurs twice in the commentary on Περὶ ἀέρων:

1) "Der Rest der Rede des Hippokrates ist klar und deutlich, und auch das, was ich von diesen Dingen angeführt habe, ist deutlich für den, der nicht trägen Geistes ist. Jedoch bin ich gezwungen, bekannte Dinge zu erwähnen, weil ich sehe, wie stumpfsinnig unsere Zeitgenossen sind und wie wenig sie davon wissen und wie sie es verschmähen, sich damit zu befassen" (fol. 85v6-9; it belongs to the lemma 19,3: p.66,24-68,4 Diller).

2) "Galen sagt: Hippokrates hat uns über die Ursache unterrichtet, derentwegen die Türken ähnlich werden und einander gleichen. Er hat sie gut erklärt, und sie bedarf keiner Erläuterung. Er verfährt so an vielen Stellen dieses seines Buches, und das bedarf keiner Erläuterung, wenn der Leser einen Funken Verstand hat. Da jedoch jetzt die meisten, die mit der ärztlichen Kunst und der Wissenschaft der Philosophie beginnen, keine Bildung besitzen, müssen wir auch Dinge erklären, die klar und deutlich sind" (fol. 86v17-87r1; beginning after the lemma 19,9: p. 68,19-70,3 Diller).

D. Manetti: È una notizia molto interessante, che conferma alcune delle osservazioni fatte qui.

V. Barras: Vous mettez en lumière de façon très convaincante la tension, chez Galien, entre son admiration pour le texte 'bref' hippocratique et sa clarté d'une part et l'obligation pour lui de justifier l'enrichissement du vocabulaire, par exemple anatomique, dont sont redevables les progrès de l'anatomie. On pourrait même imaginer que Galien se trouve confronté au 'silence' hippocratique sur telle question où la médicine aurait non seulement 'fait des progrès' depuis Hippocrate, mais où elle aurait véritablement créé un nouveau champ de savoir, imposant une 'mise en texte' entièrement nouvelle (et non seulement des néologismes). Avez-vous connaissance de telles situations dans lesquelles Galien se verrait poussé à justifier l'apparition des textes nouveaux?

D. Manetti: Per quanto so, Galeno tende a diminuire le differenze all'interno della tradizione dogmatica e dunque a riportare tutto ad un progressivo correggersi e interpretarsi meglio. Ritengo dunque che Galeno non sia disposto ad ammettere davvero 'silenzi' di Ippocrate così importanti come lei suppone. In questo senso il silenzio degli antichi può riguardare, per Galeno, solo la loro differenza rispetto alle chiacchiere imbroglione dei suoi avversari; un silenzio giusto, dunque, che è prova della loro disonestà.

VI

Jacques Jouanna

LA NOTION DE NATURE CHEZ GALIEN

Galien nous dit lui-même qu'il avait traité du sens du mot 'nature'. C'est dans un traité perdu. Il s'agit de son ouvrage intitulé *Sur les termes médicaux*, exactement au Ve livre.[1] On ne peut que regretter cette perte. Elle peut toutefois être compensée par les discussions partielles des sens du terme que Galien a l'occasion d'analyser, notamment quand il le rencontre dans les textes hippocratiques qu'il commente.

C'est le Galien philologue que nous aborderons donc dans une première partie en examinant des passages fondamentaux où il discute du sens de φύσις ou de l'expression κατὰ φύσιν.

Nous verrons ensuite, dans une seconde partie, le Galien historien de la recherche sur la nature, à partir du texte fondamental servant de prologue à son *Commentaire* du traité de la *Nature de l'homme* d'Hippocrate.

Nous terminerons par le Galien φυσικός, observateur des œuvres de la nature, en prenant pour base de réflexion un texte du *Sur les facultés naturelles*, où Galien reconnaît chez Hippocrate le premier des philosophes et des médecins qui aient étudié les œuvres de la nature.

Comme on le constate d'après cette annonce, notre propos n'est pas de faire une synthèse de l'extérieur sur la nature chez Galien, ce qui s'impose d'autant moins que l'on dispose de

[1] L'indication est donnée par Galien, *In Hippocratis De natura hominis* (=*HNH*) 1, Prooemium (CMG V 9, 1, p.6,9 sq. = XV 7,7 sq. K).

l'étude très récente de Franjo Kovacic.[2] L'intention est autre: elle est d'essayer de cerner, de l'intérieur, la vision de Galien sur la nature, en suivant des pistes à partir de textes qui ne sont pas toujours les plus connus, mais dont le choix tout à fait personnel, et par conséquent contestable, a été guidé par une évidence qui s'est imposée au cours de la recherche, à savoir l'extraordinaire importance de la figure d'Hippocrate — d'un Hippocrate évidemment recomposé — dans la pensée de Galien dès qu'il parle de la nature, et cela à tous les niveaux, que ce soit pour les sens du mot, pour l'histoire de la recherche sur les éléments premiers, ou pour la conception des œuvres de nature.

*
* *

Commençons par examiner les discussions de Galien sur le sens de φύσις. Nous partirons de l'examen conjoint de deux passages du *Commentaire aux Aphorismes*. Le premier est le commentaire à l'aphorisme 2, 34, où il est dit que le danger est moins grand "quand la maladie est conforme à la nature (τῆς φύσιος) du malade",[3] et le second commente l'aphorisme 3, 2, où il est dit que "parmi les natures (τῶν φυσίων) les unes sont bien ou mal disposées pour l'été, les autres pour l'hiver".[4] Ces deux passages sont liés déjà dans l'esprit de Galien, car il fait référence au premier passage dans le second.[5] Ces deux passages seront donc commentés conjointement. Le terme φύσις a plusieurs sens, dit Galien.[6] Et entre ces différents sens qu'il n'énumère pas, Galien

[2] *Der Begriff der Physis bei Galen vor dem Hintergrund seiner Vorgänger* (Stuttgart 2001), 320 p., avec une abondante bibliographie à laquelle je renvoie. Voir en particulier P. Moraux, "Galien comme philosophe: la philosophie de la nature", in *Galen. Problems and Prospects,* ed. by V. Nutton (London 1981), 87-116.

[3] Hipp. *Aph.* 2, 34: οἷσιν ἂν οἰκείη τῆς φύσιος … ἡ νοῦσος ᾖ = Gal. *Hipp.Aph.* XVIIB 529-532 K.

[4] Hipp. *Aph.* 3, 2: τῶν φυσίων αἱ μὲν πρὸς θέρος, αἱ δὲ πρὸς χειμῶνα εὖ ἢ κακῶς πεφύκασιν = Gal. *Hipp.Aph.* XVIIB 565-566 K.

[5] Gal. *Hipp.Aph.* XVIIB 565 K: ἐλέγομεν δ' ἐν τοῖς ἔμπροσθεν.

[6] Gal. *Hipp.Aph.* XVIIB 529 K: τῆς φύσεως πολλαχῶς λεγομένης.

établit une hiérarchie et un ordre. Car il est un sens qui, selon ses propres mots, est "le plus important et le premier".[7] C'est le sens, dit Galien, qu'Hippocrate utilise dans plusieurs de ses ouvrages, et en particulier dans tout son traité de la *Nature de l'homme.*[8] On voit poindre déjà ici le rôle de référence qu'a le traité de la *Nature de l'homme* dans l'esprit de Galien. Ce sens est le plus important et le premier selon Galien, car il est le plus conforme à l'οὐσία de la nature, prise en elle-même.[9] Il définit ce sens comme étant le mélange ou tempérament des éléments premiers,[10] le mélange des quatre éléments, à savoir le chaud, le froid, le sec et l'humide.[11] Galien fait alors référence à son traité *Sur les tempéraments,* pour rappeler que si le bon mélange est unique, il y a huit mélanges mauvais, quatre selon qu'une seule qualité domine, et quatre autres selon que deux qualités l'emportent.[12] Il est inutile de signaler, tellement la chose est évidente, que cette reconstruction galénique procède d'une pensée systématique qui n'a plus rien d'hippocratique.

À côté de ce sens principal et premier, qui se trouve dans les deux passages, Galien signale dans la discussion du premier un autre sens, en se référant à un passage des *Épidémies I* où il est dit que "mouraient surtout ceux pour qui la nature penchait vers le phtisique".[13] Galien dit que φύσις n'a pas là le sens de 'mélange des éléments', mais celui de 'forme du corps' (τὴν τοῦ σώματος ἰδέαν), et il ajoute: "parfois, en effet, on appelle φύσις

[7] GAL. *Hipp.Aph.* XVIIB 565 K: τὸ κυριώτατόν τε καὶ πρῶτον σημαινόμενον.

[8] GAL. *Hipp.Aph.* XVIIB 529 K.

[9] GAL. *Hipp.Aph.* XVIIB 565 K.

[10] GAL. *Hipp.Aph.* XVIIB 529 K: κρᾶσις ... τῶν πρώτων στοιχείων.

[11] À cette discussion sur le sens de φύσις il faudrait joindre celle qui est dans *In Hippocratis de acutorum morborum victu* (= *HVA*), CMG V 9, 1, p.189,22-24 Helmreich = XV 570,1-4 K, où φύσις chez Hippocrate est entendu au sens de κρᾶσις. L'intérêt du passage est qu'il donne à côté de φύσις/κρᾶσις l'explication de ἕξις par τῶν μορίων κατασκευή.

[12] GAL. *Hipp.Aph.* XVIIB 565 K. Selon qu'une seule qualité domine, les quatre mauvais tempéraments sont le chaud, le froid, le sec, l'humide; et selon que deux qualités l'emportent, les quatre autres mauvais tempéraments sont le chaud et sec, l'humide et chaud, le froid et humide, le froid et sec.

[13] *Epid. I,* 1, 2, II p.604,7 sq. Littré.

aussi cela".[14] Or, par l'explication que Galien donne, en disant que la nature de celui qui penche vers le phtisique est celui qui a un thorax étroit (στενόθωραξ),[15] il est clair que le mot dans l'esprit de Galien a le sens concret de forme visible du corps, ou peut-être de disposition des parties.

Si j'ai choisi ces deux passages du *Commentaire des Aphorismes* distinguant deux sens de φύσις, c'est en partie pour montrer que la discussion sur les sens du mot ne sert pas seulement à une élucidation ponctuelle dans ce que l'on pourrait appeler un but purement philologique, mais qu'elle prend sa place dans la stratégie de Galien visant à l'apologie d'Hippocrate, au sens étymologique du terme, c'est-à-dire à la défense d'Hippocrate contre des critiques. Si Galien distingue ces deux sens du mot φύσις, c'est en effet pour montrer que des contradictions apparentes relevées par des commentateurs entre certains passages d'Hippocrate viennent en réalité de ce qu'ils ne tiennent pas compte de la diversité du sens que peut avoir le mot φύσις chez lui. Galien reproche ainsi à ces commentateurs de commettre une faute "et sur la vérité des choses et sur la pensée d'Hippocrate".[16] On connaît l'agacement de Galien, qui n'aime pas perdre son temps dans des discussions oiseuses sur le choix de mots différents mais synonymes désignant la même réalité; mais il y a des mots avec lesquels on ne badine pas; et le mot φύσις en fait partie, lui qui peut désigner des aspects de la réalité aussi distincts que la texture invisible des corps ou un aspect visible de leur forme.

Le choix de ces deux passages du *Commentaire aux Aphorismes*, où sont signalés ces deux sens distincts du mot φύσις, est motivé aussi par l'importance historique qu'ils revêtent pour la réflexion sur les sens de φύσις dans la postérité d'Hippocrate vu à travers Galien. Ce sont, en effet, les deux premiers sens distingués par les commentateurs alexandrins d'Hippocrate et de

[14] GAL. *Hipp.Aph.* XVIIB 532,6-8 K.

[15] GAL. *Hipp.Aph.* XVIIB 532,10 K. Sur le mot στενόθωραξ, voir *infra*, p.233.

[16] GAL. *Hipp.Aph.* XVIIB 532,15 sq. K: καὶ περὶ τῆς τῶν πραγμάτων ἀληθείας καὶ τῆς Ἱπποκράτους γνώμης.

Galien aux VIe/VIIe siècles après J.-C., lorsqu'ils exposent les différents sens de φύσις.[17] Ils définissent le premier sens par 'mélange' (κρᾶσις) et le second par 'disposition des parties' (μορίων κατασκευή). Et nous sommes sûrs que la source de leur enseignement est bien ces deux passages précis du *Commentaire* de Galien aux *Aphorismes*; car, pour illustrer chacun de ces deux sens, ils choisissent comme exemple, pour le premier, l'aphorisme 3, 2, où justement Galien dans son commentaire définit φύσις par κρᾶσις, et pour le second, l'exemple pris par Galien dans son commentaire de l'aphorisme 2, 34, à savoir de l'homme au thorax étroit (στενόθωραξ). Or le terme στενόθωραξ est extrêmement rare dans la littérature grecque. En dehors de deux attestations chez Galien, il n'est employé que par les commentateurs alexandrins, justement dans leur définition de la φύσις chez Hippocrate et chez Galien.[18] Il est donc assuré que la réflexion des commentateurs médicaux de la seconde renaissance alexandrine sur φύσις prend sa source dans le *Commentaire* de Galien au texte le plus connu d'Hippocrate, les *Aphorismes*.

Il reste que ces commentateurs ne s'arrêtent pas aux deux sens signalés par Galien dans son *Commentaire*. Ils en ajoutent deux autres, car ils distinguent quatre sens: le troisième sens est "faculté organisatrice" (τὴν διοικοῦσαν τὰ σώματα) et le quatrième sens est "impulsion des âmes" (τὴν ὁρμὴν τῶν ψυχῶν). Pour illustrer ces deux derniers sens, ils prennent en exemple deux phrases d'Hippocrate: pour le troisième sens, c'est une

[17] Les cinq textes exposant ces sens ont été commodément mis en parallèle par I. GAROFALO dans "La nature d'Hippocrate chez les Alexandrins", in *Le normal et le pathologique dans la Collection hippocratique.* Actes du Xème Colloque International Hippocratique, oct. 1999, éd. par A. THIVEL (Nice 2002), 753-765, surtout 755-757. Il s'agit de Stephanus Alex., *In Gal. Ad Glauc.* (avec son sommaire en arabe); Palladius Alex., *In Epid. VI* 5,1; Ioannes Alexandrinus, *In Epid. VI* 4, 13; Agnellus iatrosophista, *In Gal. De sectis.*

[18] Le LSJ ne signale qu'une seule attestation chez Galien, justement notre passage (XVIIB 532 K). Il faut ajouter XVIIB 34,13 sq. Voir Stephanus Alex. (*In Gal. Ad Glauc.* 22, 8 Dikson = I p.234,17 Dietz) et Palladius Alex. (*In Hipp.Epid. VI*, II p.127,1 Dietz) dans la définition de la φύσις; cf. Theophilus, *In Hipp.Aph.* II p.361,18 et II p.361,30 Dietz.

phrase d'*Épidémies VI* "Les natures sont les médecins des maladies",[19] et pour le quatrième, une phrase du traité intitulé *Aliment* "Les natures des êtres vivants sont non-instruites".[20] La source de la troisième définition des Alexandrins doit être cherchée dans le très long et très riche commentaire que Galien a consacré dans son *Commentaire aux Épidémies VI* à la célèbre phrase qu'ils ont pris comme exemple de la définition. Galien y précise le sens de nature en disant: "Il convient d'entendre ici par le mot φύσις la faculté (δύναμιν) résidant dans les corps eux-mêmes qui sont organisés par elle (ἐνοικοῦσαν αὐτοῖς τοῖς σώμασι τοῖς διοικουμένοις ὑπ' αὐτῆς)".[21] C'est la fin de la phrase qui a été retenue comme définition par les commentateurs alexandrins, car ce qui les intéressait ce n'était pas la faculté naturelle résidant dans les corps, mais la nature organisatrice, et c'est évidemment l'un des sens les plus importants chez Galien. Je n'ai pas déterminé, en revanche, la source de la formulation de la quatrième définition des Alexandrins, mais la phrase d'Hippocrate qui l'illustre fait partie, comme la précédente, des citations-phares que Galien reprend à Hippocrate sur la nature, ou, si l'on préfère, des perles d'Hippocrate sur la nature que Galien a retenues dans le coffret à bijoux de sa mémoire.

De l'explication sur le mot φύσις que l'on trouve dans le premier passage du *Commentaire aux Aphorismes*, je voudrais rapprocher une explication de l'expression κατὰ φύσιν que l'on rencontre dans un passage plus complexe du livre VI du *Sur les opinions d'Hippocrate et de Platon*:

> "L'expression κατὰ φύσιν se disant en plusieurs sens, il faut entendre ceci maintenant: ce qui se produit κατὰ πρῶτον λόγον par la nature. Nous disons que se produit κατὰ

[19] Hipp. *Epid.* 6, 5, 1, p.100,7 Manetti-Roselli (= V p.314,5 Littré).

[20] Hipp. *Alim.* 39, p.145,12 Joly (= IX p.112,3 Littré): le texte présente une variante par rapport à la tradition directe: "les natures des êtres vivants", au lieu de: "les natures de toutes choses".

[21] Gal. *Hipp.Epid. VI*, 5, 1, CMG V 10, 2, 2, p.253,19-21 = XVIIB 223, 6-8 K): δύναμιν δὲ προσήκει νῦν ἀκούειν ἐκ τοῦ φύσεως ὀνόματος ἐνοικοῦσαν αὐτοῖς τοῖς σώμασι τοῖς διοικουμένοις ὑπ' αὐτῆς.

> πρῶτον λόγον par la nature ce qu'elle revendique comme but (σκοπῶν) et non des choses qui suivent nécessairement d'autres choses. Un tel mouvement κατὰ φύσιν existe, que ce qui est mû le soit de lui-même ou qu'il le soit du fait d'un autre".[22]

Le rapprochement entre les deux passages se fait de lui-même, car ils commencent exactement de la même manière. Dans le commentaire aux *Aphorismes*, la première phrase de l'explication sur φύσις commmençait par "φύσις se disant en plusieurs sens" (τῆς φύσεως πολλαχῶς λεγομένης);[23] dans le *Sur les opinions d'Hippocrate et de Platon*, l'explication sur l'expression κατὰ φύσιν commence aussi par un génitif absolu analogue "κατὰ φύσιν se disant en plusieurs sens" (πολλαχῶς δὲ τοῦ κατὰ φύσιν λεγομένου). Vient ensuite, dans les deux passages, une proposition principale analogue qui précise le sens qui convient pour le moment. On comparera dans le premier passage "On doit entendre maintenant selon ce sens" (ἀκουστέον νῦν ἐστιν αὐτῆς κατ' ἐκεῖνο τὸ σημαινόμενον), et dans le second "Il faut entendre maintenant ceci" (τοῦτ' ἀκούειν χρὴ νῦν). Les démonstratifs annoncent, dans les deux cas, l'explication du sens.

L'explication du sens de κατὰ φύσιν donnée dans le *Sur les opinions d'Hippocrate et de Platon* ne ne se comprend que par référence au contexte. Galien se livre à une explication de mots, comme il le dit lui-même (τὴν τῶν ὀνομάτων ἐξήγησιν).[24] L'explication de κατὰ φύσιν s'insère, comme une poupée gigogne, dans une autre explication de mots, la définition de ἐνέργεια et de πάθος. Un premier sens de ces deux termes a été donné: l'ἐνέργεια est un mouvement (κίνησις) qui vient

[22] GAL. *PHP* 6, 1, 8-9, II p.362,5-9 De Lacy (= V 507,12-18 K): Πολλαχῶς δὲ τοῦ κατὰ φύσιν λεγομένου, τοῦτ' ἀκούειν χρὴ νῦν ὁ κατὰ πρῶτον λόγον ὑπὸ τῆς φύσεως γίγνεται. Κατὰ πρῶτον δὲ λόγον ἐκεῖνα γίγνεσθαί φαμεν ὑπὸ τῆς φύσεως, ὧν ὥσπερ σκοπῶν ἀντιποιεῖται καὶ μὴ δι' ἀκολουθίαν τινὰ ἑτέροις ἐξ ἀνάγκης ἕπεται. Ἡ τοιαύτη κίνησις κατὰ φύσιν, εἴτ' ἐξ αὑτοῦ κινοῖτο τὸ κινούμενον εἴθ' ὑφ' ἑτέρου.

[23] Voir *supra*, p. 230 et n.6.

[24] GAL. *PHP* 6, 1, 3, II p.360,13 sq. De Lacy (= V 506,6 sq. K).

de ce qui est mû, tandis que le πάθος est un mouvement venant d'autre chose que ce qui est mû. Dans la suite de l'explication, Galien expose ce qu'est l'autre sens de ces deux mots. Et c'est dans cette seconde définition qu'interviennent les expressions κατὰ φύσιν et παρὰ φύσιν. L'ἐνέργεια est définie comme un mouvement κατὰ φύσιν et le πάθος comme un mouvement παρὰ φύσιν. C'est alors que Galien donne la définition de κατὰ φύσιν qu'il retient et que je viens de citer: ce qui est du fait de la nature (ὑπὸ φύσεως) κατὰ πρῶτον λόγον. Et comme l'expression peut paraître obscure, il ajoute ce qu'il entend par là. C'est ce que la nature recherche comme fin et non ce qui découle par nécessité d'autres choses. Galien estime après cette définition que le lecteur est éclairé, mais il rendra les choses encore plus claires en donnant des exemples concrets.

On peut s'étonner que Galien ait donné cette définition sans autre commentaire, car cette expression κατὰ πρῶτον λόγον ὑπὸ τῆς φύσεως se rencontre dans d'autres ouvrages de Galien. Il y aurait toute une étude à faire sur l'expression.[25] Je ne prendrai que quelques exemples; mais ce détour, assez long, me paraît nécessaire, non seulement pour éclairer l'expression, mais surtout pour juger de la manipulation que Galien opère sur le sens de l'expression usuelle κατὰ φύσιν. On a un passage tout à fait parallèle à celui-ci dans le *Sur les tempéraments.*[26] Galien oppose aux cheveux les sourcils et les cils. La pousse (γένεσις) des cheveux varie, d'une part suivant les φύσεις du corps définies comme κράσεις (c'est la définition de φύσις que l'on a vue dans le *Commentaire aux Aphorismes* avec référence au *Sur les tempéraments* — ainsi la boucle se referme), d'autre part suivant l'âge et suivant les lieux. Au contraire, les sourcils et les cils existent dès l'enfance. Galien définit la pousse des sourcils et des cils

[25] Dans ses notes au passage du *De placitis*, Phillip DE LACY se contente, pour l'expression κατὰ πρῶτον λόγον, d'un rapprochement avec Némésius d'Émèse, *De natura hominis*, 7.

[26] GAL. *Temp.* 2, 5, I 619,8 sqq. K.

avec des termes qui correspondent à la définition du κατὰ φύσιν dans le *Sur les opinions d'Hippocrate et de Platon*:

> "La pousse chez ceux-ci (*sc.* sourcils et cils) ne ressemble pas à celle des herbes, mais à celle des plantes, étant donné qu'ils (*sc.* les sourcils et les cils) sont faits par la nature κατὰ πρῶτον λόγον et ne dépendent pas nécessairement des tempéraments, comme il est montré dans le *Sur l'utilité des parties.*"[27]

Le rapprochement des deux textes, avec la même expression positive (κατὰ πρῶτον λόγον ὑπὸ φύσεως) ou négative (μὴ … ἐξ ἀνάγκης ἕπεται / οὐκ ἐξ ἀνάγκης ἑπομέναις), montre la cohérence remarquable de l'écriture de Galien, et aussi de sa représentation de la φύσις. C'est la nature démiurge qui est à l'œuvre (φύσις), et non pas les phénomènes naturels qui résultent nécessairement des différentes constitutions (φύσεις = κράσεις). Cependant le passage du *Sur les tempéraments* est plus concret dans sa formulation que celui du *Sur les opinions d'Hippocrate et de Platon*, comme l'indique la comparaison avec les plantes, et non avec les herbes. Or, la comparaison renvoie à un autre ouvrage que Galien rapproche lui-même, le *Sur l'utilité des parties.* C'est effectivement dans cette œuvre[28] que l'on rencontre, sous une forme développée, la comparaison qui est simplement allusive dans le *Sur les tempéraments* et qui risque d'être obscure pour un lecteur non averti. L'apologue développé dans le *Sur l'utilité des parties* du champ labouré où poussent des graines semées par le laboureur (φυτά), opposé à une partie non cultivée où pousse de l'herbe sauvage (πόαι), éclaire ce que Galien veut dire dans le *Sur les tempéraments.* La pousse des cils et des sourcils est l'œuvre de la φύσις, comme la pousse des plantes est l'œuvre du laboureur.[29] Certes, l'apologue du *Sur l'utilité des*

[27] GAL. *Temp.* 2, 5, I 619,10-14 K: γένεσις γὰρ δὴ ταύταις, οὐχ οἷα ταῖς πόαις, ἀλλ' οἷα τοῖς φυτοῖς, κατὰ πρῶτον λόγον ὑπὸ τῆς φύσεως ἀπειργασμέναις, καὶ οὐκ ἐξ ἀνάγκης ἑπομέναις ταῖς κράσεσιν, ὡς κἀν τοῖς περὶ χρείας μορίων δείκνυται.

[28] GAL. *UP* 11, 14, II p.159,21sqq. Helmreich = III 907,8 sqq. K.

[29] Toutefois on observe un décalage entre les deux traités: dans le *De usu partium*, l'opposition est entre les cils, les sourcils et les cheveux d'un côté et de

parties ne présente pas la formule κατὰ πρῶτον λόγον ὑπὸ τῆς φύσεως. Toutefois cette formule apparaît à plusieurs reprises dans le traité, et elle a même, dans un passage, une fonction programmatique. En effet, elle définit les limites du sujet de son ouvrage:

> "Nous expliquons dans ce traité non pas les choses qui sont la conséquence nécessaire de celles qui sont en vue d'un but (ἕνεκά του), mais celles qui sont produites par la nature κατὰ πρῶτον λόγον."[30]

L'intention de Galien dans le *Sur l'utilité des parties* est de traiter des parties produites par la nature en vue d'une utilité, et non de celles qui, comme le jejunum, ne présentent pas d'utilité en elles-mêmes, mais sont une conséquence nécessaire d'autres parties qui sont créées, elles, en vue de l'utilité. On retrouve ici les expressions positives (τῶν κατὰ πρῶτον λόγον ὑπὸ τῆς φύσεως δεδημιουργημένων) ou négatives (Οὐ ... τῶν ἐξ ἀνάγκης ἑπομένων) rencontrées dans le *Sur les opinions d'Hippocrate et de Platon* ou le *Sur les tempéraments* et l'affirmation, formulée dans

l'autre les poils des aisselles et du reste du corps, alors que dans le *De temperamentis* elle est entre la pousse des cheveux d'un côté et celle des cils et des sourcils de l'autre. Un troisième texte concernant la pousse des poils doit être rapproché, c'est l'introduction du *De compositione medicamentorum secundum locos* (= *Comp.Med.Loc.*) 1, 4, XII 379,8-380,9 K, qui fait précisément référence au *De temperamentis*. On y retrouve: 1) la comparaison avec les plantes; 2) l'opposition entre les plantes qui poussent par l'art et la décision préalable du cultivateur (κατὰ τὴν τέχνην καὶ προαίρεσιν τοῦ γεωργοῦ) et celles qui poussent pour des causes naturelles (κατὰ τὰς φυσικὰς αἰτίας); 3) l'opposition comparable des poils qui poussent sur la tête et de ceux qui poussent sur le reste du corps. "Ces derniers, ce n'est pas κατὰ πρῶτον λόγον que la nature a l'habitude de les faire pousser, mais selon quelque accident. Les poils aux paupières et aux sourcils ont montré qu'ils offraient une utilité qui n'est pas petite aux êtres vivants, alors que les poils au menton et aux parties génitales semblent exister pour une utilité plus petite" (380,1-4: οὐ γὰρ κατὰ πρῶτον λόγον ἡ φύσις αὐτὰς εἴωθε γεννᾶν, ἀλλὰ κατά τι συμβεβηκός· αἵ γε μὴν κατά τε βλέφαρα καὶ τὰς ὀφρῦς ἐδείκνυντο χρείαν οὐ μικρὰν παρέχουσαι τοῖς ζώοις· αἱ δ' ἐπὶ τῶν γενείων τε καὶ τῶν αἰδοίων ἕνεκα μικροτέρων χρειῶν γεγονέναι δοκοῦσι).

[30] GAL. *UP* 5, 3, I p.257,4-8 Helmreich = III 350,16-351,2 K: Οὐ γὰρ τῶν ἐξ ἀνάγκης ἑπομένων τοῖς ἕνεκά του γεγονόσιν, ἀλλὰ τῶν κατὰ πρῶτον λόγον ὑπὸ τῆς φύσεως δεδημιουργημένων ἐξήγησιν ἐν τοῖσδε τοῖς ὑπομνήμασι ποιούμεθα.

le *Sur les opinions d'Hippocrate et de Platon*, que la nature agit en vue d'un but.[31]

Jusqu'à présent je n'ai pas traduit l'expression κατὰ πρῶτον λόγον. Cette expression est tout à fait remarquable, car elle n'apparaît pas, à ma connaissance, dans la littérature grecque avant Galien, où elle est employée treize fois et, parmi ces treize fois, sept fois avec ὑπὸ τῆς φύσεως comme complément d'agent ou φύσις comme sujet. Daremberg, dans le passage du *Sur l'utilité des parties* que je viens de citer, traduit par "(les choses qui ont été créées par la nature) dans un dessein primitif". Mais quand il rencontre la même expression plus loin, il traduit "dans un but principal" (X 14),"par un premier calcul" (XI 13) et "en premier lieu" (XV 8).[32] Il y a là, au moins, un manque de cohérence. Que l'on donne à l'expression un sens plein ("en premier calcul", "en première intention") ou un sens adverbial ("de premier rang" "primordialement"), l'expression désigne ce qui est premier, primordial, principal, essentiel, par opposition à ce qui est secondaire, accidentel ou accessoire, car il est des passages où l'expression chez Galien s'oppose soit à "de second rang" (κατὰ δεύτερον λόγον) soit à "par accident" (κατὰ συμβεβηκός) ou toute autre expression comparable.[33] L'œuvre de la nature relève donc fondamentalement de ce qui est premier et primordial.

Après cet assez long détour, on peut revenir au texte du *Sur les opinions d'Hippocrate et de Platon* où Galien précise le sens qu'il donne à κατὰ φύσιν. On peut souligner maintenant ce qu'il

31 Comparer dans le *PHP* σκοπῶν et ici ἕνεκά του.

32 Ch. Daremberg (éd.), *Œuvres anatomiques, physiologiques et médicales de Galien* (Paris 1854), I p.342, 648 et II p.156.

33 Pour l'opposition κατὰ πρῶτον λόγον / κατὰ συμβεβηκός, voir par exemple le texte cité à la note 29 (*in fine*). On trouve même l'expression κατὰ τρίτον λόγον trois fois dans le *De anatomicis administrationibus* (= *AA*) 6, 1, II p.349,11 et p.351,3 Garofalo (= II 542,13 et 543,17 K) et 6, 3, II p.351,29 Garofalo (= II 545,6 sq. K). Les passages sont fort intéressants, car ils établissent, à propos des organes (de la nourriture) une hiérarchie plus élaborée comprenant trois niveaux: ceux qui sont "de premier rang du fait de la nature" (πρῶτον λόγον ὑπὸ τῆς φύσεως), ceux qui sont "de second rang" et ceux qui sont de "troisième rang".

y a d'étonnant. Galien donne à cette expression adverbiale bien connue, désignant usuellement la conformité à un ordre naturel ou normal, un sens tout à fait exceptionnel qu'il est probablement le seul à donner, en réinterprétant l'expression par sa conception de la nature-démiurge produisant de façon primordiale les différentes parties du corps en vue d'un but précis, leur utilité.

La définition que Galien donne de κατὰ φύσιν dans le *Sur les opinions d'Hippocrate et de Platon*, tout en ayant pour but avoué la clarté pour éviter toute méprise de la part du lecteur, devient un outil de manipulation du langage pour plier le sens usuel des mots à ses propres conceptions de la nature et pour réduire ainsi de façon significative l'extension de ce qui était κατὰ φύσιν dans l'usage courant, et par voie de conséquence, pour étendre le domaine du παρὰ φύσιν. Il va de soi que Galien ne s'en tient pas toujours à ce sens que je qualifierais de technique, et qu'il sait jouer avec la pluralité des sens, comme on le voit parfaitement dans sa discussion sur le problème de savoir si la vieillesse est ou non κατὰ φύσιν, dans son traité *Sur le marasme.*[34] Il n'ose pas heurter le sens commun au point de dire que la vieillesse, qui est pourtant un πάθος ἐξ ἀνάγκης ἑπόμενον, est παρὰ φύσιν, ce qu'il devrait dire selon son sens technique. Il préfère interrompre la discussion qu'il a entreprise sur les sens de κατὰ φύσιν, en acceptant de dire, conformément à l'usage, que la vieillesse est κατὰ φύσιν, dans la mesure où elle est conforme à l'ordre naturel de l'évolution de tout être vivant.[35]

[34] Gal. *De marcore* (= *Marc.*) 2, VII 669,6 sqq. K. Là, Galien reconnaît que κατὰ φύσιν a plusieurs sens et il semble composer avec un sens plus proche de l'usage courant. En effet, tout en affirmant que la vieillesse n'est pas une œuvre de nature, mais un *pathos* qui suit nécessairement les œuvres de nature (τὸ γῆρας δὲ οὐκ ἔργον [*sc.* τῆς φύσεως], ἀλλὰ πάθος ἐξ ἀνάγκης ἑπόμενον), il accepte de l'appeler κατὰ φύσιν et ne juge pas nécessaire de continuer à examiner les autres sens de l'expression. Il accepte donc d'appeler dans ce passage κατὰ φύσιν ce qui suit nécessairement les œuvres de la nature, ce qui n'est pas le cas dans le *De placitis*.

[35] Une indécision analogue est décelable même à propos de l'emploi de l'expression κατὰ πρῶτον λόγον. Alors que l'œuvre de nature s'arrête à ce qui est κατὰ πρῶτον λόγον dans le *De placitis*, elle s'étend aussi à ce qui est κατὰ συμβεβηκός

Je n'insisterai pas non plus sur d'autres sens plus usuels de ce qui est κατὰ φύσιν et παρὰ φύσιν. L'un d'entre eux, toutefois, mérite d'être mentionné. Il concerne l'opposition entre le normal et le pathologique. Par exemple, dans l'*Art médical*, il est dit que "tout est selon la nature (κατὰ φύσιν) pour les corps en bonne santé, alors que tout est contre nature (παρὰ φύσιν) pour les corps malades, dans la mesure où ils sont malades".[36] Ce lien était déjà en germe dans la prose des médecins hippocratiques. Ainsi, dans le traité du *Pronostic*, le rythme du sommeil, qui est habituel dans l'état sain (κατὰ φύσιν), sert de critère pour mesurer la plus ou moins grande gravité de l'état du malade;[37] et dans la *Nature de l'homme,* il est dit que la cause des maladies est l'état contre nature (παρὰ φύσιν) des éléments constitutifs du corps.[38] Cependant, dans les traités hippocratiques, aucune formulation de l'opposition n'est aussi nette que chez Galien, sans compter que le médecin de Pergame introduit un état intermédiaire à la frontière (ἐν μεθορίῳ) entre le κατὰ φύσιν et le παρὰ φύσιν, ce qui fait appel à un concept de l'entre-deux inconnu des médecins hippocratiques.[39]

Avec ce premier groupe de textes où Galien aborde en philologue la discussion du sens du mot φύσις ou de l'expression κατὰ φύσιν, mais où l'on voit poindre déjà les options les plus profondes de Galien sur la nature, j'ai voulu montrer, d'une part, que Galien est conscient de l'enjeu de la diversité des sens du

dans le *De compositione* (pour le texte, voir n.29 *in fine*), dans la mesure où l'on peut déceler une certaine utilité dans ce qui est κατὰ συμβεβηκός, même si elle est plus faible que dans ce qui est κατὰ πρῶτον λόγον. L'opposition de nature est donc parfois envisagée comme une question de degré.

36 GAL. *Ars med.* 21, 1, p.337,6-8 Boudon (= I 358,7-9 K).

37 HIPP. *Prog.* 10, p.205,9 Alexanderson (= II p.134,5 Littré).

38 HIPP. *Nat.hom.* 2, p.168,7 sq. Jouanna (= VI p.36,2-4 Littré).

39 La notion de ἐν μεθορίῳ, qui est exprimée aussi par l'expression ἐν τῷ μεταξύ, désigne chez Galien l'espace frontière situé entre deux états (opposés) qui peuvent mutuellement se transformer l'un dans l'autre, de telle façon qu'il participe modérément à l'un comme à l'autre; voir pour cette définition *De compositione medicamentorum per genera* (*Comp.Med.Gen.*) 7, 1, XIII 950,10-12 K: "Comme dans tout ce qui est de nature à se transformer l'un dans l'autre, il y a un espace frontière qui participe modérément de l'un et de l'autre à la fois".

mot et des registres plus ou moins techniques dont la méconnaissance risque d'entraîner chez les interprètes ou les lecteurs des erreurs de jugement, et d'autre part, que la φύσις est liée chez lui, en dernière analyse, à la notion unifiante de primordial et de fondamental.

*

* *

J'en viens maintenant au texte essentiel où Galien discute du sens de φύσις, le préambule au *Commentaire* du traité de *La nature de l'homme* d'Hippocrate.[40] Mais avec ce texte, j'aborde ma seconde partie qui est consacrée à la vision que Galien a de l'histoire de la recherche philosophique sur la nature. Car Galien parle maintenant du sens du mot φύσις dans la recherche des philosophes dont les ouvrages sont intitulés *Sur la nature*, et surtout il dépasse le point de vue philologique en liant cette recherche à une méthode d'analyse de la φύσις. Galien devient historien de la philosophie. Mais l'on verra dans quelle mesure cette histoire de la philosophie est vue par un médecin.

Galien commence, dans ce préambule, par donner le sens du mot φύσις dans la recherche des philosophes:

> "Le premier point consiste à dire ce que peut bien signifier le terme de φύσις, à partir duquel certains des philosophes anciens ont tiré leur nom et ont été appelés φυσικοί. La raison pour laquelle je dis cela vous paraîtra évidente si vous lisez leurs écrits Περὶ φύσεως. Car il est clair qu'ils exposent ce qu'est la substance première (τὴν πρώτην οὐσίαν), substance qu'ils disent non engendrée et éternelle à la base de tous les corps susceptibles d'être engendrés et détruits, et ce

[40] Voir déjà J. Jouanna, "La lecture du traité hippocratique de la *Nature de l'homme* par Galien. Les fondements de l'hippocratisme de Galien", in *Le commentaire entre tradition et innovation*, éd. par M.-O. Goulet-Cazé (Paris 2000), 273-292.

que sont les éléments qui de façon propre (κατὰ τὸν ἴδιον λόγον)[41] sont constitutifs de chacun des êtres engendrés et détruits, éléments qui, une fois connus, entraînent aussi la connaissance de tout ce qui arrive d'une façon qui n'est pas propre (οὐ κατὰ τὸν ἴδιον λόγον) à chacune des substances prises tour à tour. C'est ainsi donc que devient complet l'enseignement sur la nature de chacun des étants, même si l'on n'expose qu'un seul ou deux principes constitutifs d'une chose."[42]

Cette définition de la nature selon les philosophes est comparée, de façon qui peut paraître paradoxale, à celle du poète par excellence, Homère, dont il cite un vers de l'*Odyssée* (10, 303). C'est le vers offrant, comme on le sait, la première attestation dans la littérature grecque du mot φύσις. Il s'agit de la φύσις d'une plante définie par le poète comme ayant une racine noire et une fleur blanche. Galien caractérise cette nature dégagée par le poète, et après lui par les botanistes, comme la nature sensible (τὴν αἰσθητὴν φύσιν), et l'oppose à la nature première des philosophes (ἡ δὲ τούτων ἀνωτέρω καὶ πρώτη).[43] Au cours de son analyse de la recherche sur la φύσις, il cite des philosophes grecs de l'époque archaïque, de l'époque classique et de l'époque hellénistique. Parmi les philosophes présocratiques qu'il appelle "les anciens philosophes" (τῶν παλαιῶν φιλοσόφων), il fait allusion à cinq d'entre eux qu'il cite dans l'ordre suivant: Empédocle,

[41] L'expression κατὰ τὸν ἴδιον λόγον est dans une certaine mesure comparable à κατὰ τὸν πρῶτον λόγον, car elle va aussi avec l'idée de premier et s'oppose à κατὰ τὸ συμβεβηκός; voir par exemple *Ad Thrasybulum utrum medicinae sit an gymnasticae hygiene* 17, *Scripta min.* III p.55,1 sq. = V 836,15 sq. K: κατά τι συμβεβηκός, οὐ πρώτως οὐδὲ κατὰ τὸν ἴδιον λόγον. C'est ce qui est premier et ne découle pas par accident.

[42] Éd. J. Mewaldt, CMG V 9, 1, p.3,20-4,7.

[43] Il ne paraît pas qu'une telle expression de nature sensible, c'est-à-dire perceptible par les organes des sens, se retrouve ailleurs chez Galien. C'est vraisemblablement le désir d'intégrer l'emploi homérique dans la continuité de la recherche sur la φύσις, tout en le distinguant de l'emploi philosophique, qui a amené Galien à le qualifier ainsi.

Parménide, Mélissos, Alcméon et Héraclite.[44] La présence de Mélissos de Samos dans cette liste ne doit pas étonner, car Mélissos est cité dans le début du traité de la *Nature de l'homme* d'Hippocrate qui est l'objet du commentaire.[45] Concernant la période classique, Galien mentionne Platon et Aristote. La philosophie hellénistique n'est représentée que par un nom, Épicure. Il n'est pas question des Stoïciens, ce qui peut paraître étonnant, car Galien voit dans leur philosophie de la nature un héritage indirect d'Hippocrate.[46] Pour terminer avec sa vision de l'histoire de la philosophie de la nature, on signalera que Galien fait une distinction de vocabulaire sur la façon dont les philosophes anciens et leurs successeurs ont désigné les éléments. Il a noté que le terme στοιχεῖον n'était pas employé par les Anciens, alors qu'il est devenu usuel chez les successeurs.[47] Il sait aussi que les homéomères sont une appellation aristotélicienne. On appréciera donc, grâce à ce développement sur la φύσις dans la philosophie grecque, l'attention extrême de Galien à l'histoire de la langue philosophique et à l'apparition de certains termes au cours de cette histoire. Cette attention n'est toutefois pas systématique, car tout en rappelant que les traités philosophiques étaient connus sous le titre de Περὶ φύσεως "Sur la nature", Galien emploie le terme de φυσιολογία pour désigner la recherche philosophique sur la nature, sans signaler que c'est, là aussi, un terme récent. En effet, les Anciens parlaient de περὶ φύσεως ἱστορία, comme le Socrate du *Phédon*;[48] le terme φυσιολογία n'est devenu usuel, pour désigner cette recherche, qu'à partir de la philosophie hellénistique, notamment chez Épicure.[49]

[44] Comparer la liste du *De elementis* (= *Hipp.Elem.*) 1, 9, 27, CMG V 1, 2, p.134,17-19 De Lacy = I 487,12-14 K: les mêmes sauf Héraclite, mais en plus Gorgias et Prodicos.

[45] HIPP. *Nat.hom.* 1, p.166,11 Jouanna (= VI p.34,6 Littré).

[46] Voir *infra*, p. 246.

[47] Voir aussi *Hipp.Elem.* 1, 9, 25, p.134,13 sqq. De Lacy = I 487,8 sqq. K.

[48] PL. *Phaedo* 96 a 5 sqq.("Moi, quand j'étais jeune, j'étais passionné de façon ô combien étonnante pour cette science que l'on appelle recherche sur la nature").

[49] C'est chez Épicure que l'on rencontre pour la première fois dans les textes conservés φυσιολογία au sens général de 'science de la nature'; voir *Lettre à*

Il est vrai que, dans ce panorama de la recherche philosophique sur la nature, Galien s'attache moins, comme il le dit lui-même, aux mots qu'aux réalités. Ce qui est plus important que les mots, c'est la méthode pour connaître la nature première. Galien en trouve la formulation chez Platon, non pas dans le *Timée*, comme on pourrait s'y attendre, mais dans le *Phèdre*, où Platon, cherchant la méthode pour connaître la nature de l'âme, se réfère à la méthode d'Hippocrate pour connaître la nature du corps.[50] Cette méthode platonicienne consiste à diviser l'objet dont on cherche la nature en ses éléments simples et, après dénombrement, à déterminer leurs propriétés naturelles relativement à l'agir et au pâtir. Or Galien, dans la suite de son commentaire de la *Nature de l'homme*, voit dans la première partie du traité hippocratique le livre du maître auquel Platon se réfère dans l'exposé de sa méthode.[51] La conséquence, qui peut paraître paradoxale, est que Galien en vient à présenter Platon, comme un "imitateur", "un zélote" d'Hippocrate, dans sa méthode de recherche sur la nature.[52] Dès lors, on comprend la place tout à fait prééminente que Galien attribue à Hippocrate dans l'histoire de l'étude sur la nature non seulement chez les médecins, mais aussi chez les philosophes. Il va même jusqu'à affirmer dès le *De elementis* qui est antérieur au commentaire de la *Nature de l'homme*:

Hérodote, éd. J. BOLLACK, 37,2 et 3 et 78,2. Cependant, les deux composés de la même famille, le substantif φυσιόλογος et le verbe φυσιολογέω sont déjà fréquents chez Aristote. Les φυσιόλογοι y désignent ceux qui ont écrit des ouvrages sur la nature, tels Empédocle et Démocrite. En revanche, φυσιολογία n'est attesté qu'une fois chez Aristote dans un emploi particulier à la recherche sur les plantes (*De sensu* 442 b 25: ἐν τῇ φυσιολογίᾳ τῇ περὶ τῶν φυτῶν). Aucun de ces trois composés n'apparaît encore chez Platon.

50 PL. *Phaedr.* 270 c.

51 Déjà dans le *De elementis*, qui est, on le sait, un commentaire synthétique du traité de la *Nature de l'homme*, Galien attribue la méthode de la découverte de la nature par le dénombrement à Hippocrate, mais il le fait sans mentionner Platon (1, 2, 1-2, p.58,6-10 De Lacy = I 415,4-10 K).

52 GAL. *HNH* 1, 42, CMG V 9, 1, p.54,10 Mewaldt = XV 103,11 K: μιμεῖσθαι; cf. *UP* 1, 8, I p.11,21-23 Helmreich = III 16, 7-9 K: "Platon étant un partisan (ζηλωτής) s'il en fut, et ayant repris de lui les plus importantes de ses doctrines".

> "Hippocrate est manifestement le premier de tous à avoir découvert les éléments de la nature des étants et le premier à les démontrer de façon satisfaisante."[53]

La répétition du mot "premier" est significative. Hippocrate est le premier découvreur de la science de la nature, car il a trouvé non seulement les résultats (à savoir les éléments premiers de la nature des étants), mais aussi la méthode pour y parvenir. Galien emploie dans le même traité une expression très caractéristique, c'est celle de "science de la nature hippocratique" (τὴν Ἱπποκράτειον φυσιολογίαν).[54]

Ce n'est pas seulement Platon qui est le continuateur d'Hippocrate, mais aussi Aristote et Théophraste. Voici en effet ce que l'on peut lire dans le *Sur les facultés naturelles*:

> "Si l'on étudie les écrits d'Aristote et de Théophraste, on croirait y trouver les commentaires de la théorie d'Hippocrate sur le chaud, le froid, le sec, l'humide, sur leur action mutuelle, le chaud étant parmi ces qualités élémentaires le plus actif, et le froid venant après lui pour la puissance; toutes ces considérations sont faites par Hippocrate en premier, et en second par Aristote."[55]

Cette citation n'est que le début d'un assez long développement où Galien montre en quoi Aristote est le continuateur d'Hippocrate. Mais je n'ai retenu que ce qui concerne la science de la nature proprement dite. Et dans le même passage, un peu plus loin, Galien poursuit la filiation en y ajoutant les Stoïciens. Il parle en effet des doctrines sur la nature:

> "qui sont d'Hippocrate en premier, d'Aristote en second, et en troisième des Stoïciens, avec une seule modification, à savoir que pour eux les qualités sont des corps."[56]

[53] GAL. *Hipp.Elem.* 1, 9, 25-27, p.134,13 sqq. De Lacy = I 487,8-9 K.
[54] GAL. *Hipp.Elem.* 1, 9, 21, p.134,3 sq. De Lacy = I 486,10 sq. K.
[55] GAL. *Nat.Fac.* 2, 4, *Scripta min.* III p.165,12-19 Helmreich = II 88,14-89,4 K.
[56] GAL. *Nat.Fac.* 2, 4, p.168, 11-13 Helmreich = II 92,14-16 K.

Dans toute cette problématique sur la recherche des éléments premiers de la nature des étants, si Hippocrate est le premier découvreur, c'est toujours par référence au traité de la *Nature de l'homme*.

Dans son opuscule sur *Que le meilleur médecin est aussi philosophe*, Galien revient sur cette méthode hippocratique de connaissance de la *physis* qu'il qualifie de méthode logique et il distingue clairement trois niveaux, ce qu'il ne faisait pas dans son commentaire de la *Nature de l'homme*:

> "Cette même méthode enseigne aussi ce qu'est la nature (φύσις) du corps elle-même, celle qui provient des éléments premiers qui sont en totalité mêlés entre eux, celle des éléments seconds, les sensibles que l'on appelle aussi les homéomères et la troisième, en plus de ces deux-là, celle qui provient des parties organiques."[57]

Ces trois niveaux sont, bien entendu, galéniques et non pas hippocratiques.

Mais Hippocrate est aussi pour Galien le premier des médecins et des philosophes qui a étudié les "œuvres de nature" (τὰ τῆς φύσεως ἔργα). C'est ce qu'il dit aussi dans le traité *Sur les facultés naturelles.*[58] Sans doute Galien ne voit-il aucune discontinuité entre les deux affirmations, bien que l'on passe à un sens fort différent de φύσις, du sens de "constitution première des êtres" à celui de "nature agissante". Mais là où Galien ne voit aucune discontinuité, les traités hippocratiques qui lui servent de modèle de référence sont différents, et cette différence est là comme critère pour montrer que la représentation de la nature, au départ, est autre.

*
* *

[57] GAL. *Opt.Med.* 3, *Scripta min.* II p.6,14-19 Mueller = I 60,2-6 K.

[58] GAL. *Nat.Fac.* 1, 13, p.128,23 sqq. Helmreich = II 38,10 sqq. K. Pour le texte de ce passage avec apparat critique, voir A. ANASTASSIOU/D. IRMER, *Testimonien zum Corpus Hippocraticum* II 2 (Göttingen 2001), 38.

Venons-en donc aux œuvres de nature (τὰ τῆς φύσεως ἔργα) chez Galien, en prenant pour base de la réflexion ce passage du *Sur les facultés naturelles*, où il reconnaît chez Hippocrate le premier des philosophes et des médecins qui ait étudié les œuvres de nature. Voici le texte; il s'inscrit dans une polémique contre Asclépiade sur la manière dont l'urine parvient à la vessie:

> "Si quelqu'un veut faire par lui-même ces expériences sur l'animal, il condamnera sévèrement, j'en ai l'assurance, la témérité d'Asclépiade. S'il se rend compte de la cause pour laquelle rien ne remonte de la vessie dans les uretères, cet examen seul lui suffira, je pense, pour se convaincre de la prévoyance et de l'art de la nature (πρόνοιάν τε καὶ τέχνην τῆς φύσεως) à l'égard des êtres vivants. Hippocrate, le premier des médecins et des philosophes que nous connaissions, et le premier qui ait reconnu les œuvres de la nature (τὰ τῆς φύσεως ἔργα), l'admire (θαυμάζει) et la célèbre continuellement (διὰ πάντος ταύτην ὑμνεῖ), l'appelant juste (δικαίαν = *Fract.* 1, III p.414,1 Littré), et il dit qu'elle suffit, à elle seule, en tout, pour les êtres vivants (καὶ μόνην ἐξαρκεῖν εἰς ἅπαντα τοῖς ζῴοις φησίν = *Alim.* 15, IX p.102,16 Littré), elle qui fait d'elle-même, sans avoir appris tout ce qui convient (αὐτὴν ἐξ αὑτῆς ἀδιδάκτως = *Alim.* 9, IX p.102,3 Littré πράττουσαν ἅπαντα τὰ δέοντα = *Epid. VI* 5, V p.314,8 Littré). La nature étant telle, il a aussitôt supposé qu'elle possédait des facultés, l'une attractive de ce qui est familier, l'autre expulsive de ce qui est étranger, et il pensait que la nature forme et accroît les êtres vivants et qu'elle juge les maladies avec ces facultés; et c'est la raison pour laquelle il dit que, dans nos corps, il y a une communauté de flux, une communauté d'air, et que tout est en sympathie (σύμπνοιάν τε μίαν εἶναί φησι καὶ σύρροιαν καὶ πάντα συμπαθέα = *Alim.* 23, IX p.106,6 Littré). Au contraire, selon Asclépiade, rien n'est en sympathie avec rien, étant donné que toute la subtance est divisée par

nature et scindée en éléments insécables et en particules délirantes."[59]

La citation est longue, mais il est impossible de la tronquer, car elle contient une présentation par Galien de ce qu'Hippocrate pensait sur la nature et ses œuvres. Une analyse détaillée de ce passage me paraît essentielle pour dégager, de l'intérieur, la façon dont Galien reconstruit cet Hippocrate qui est pour lui au fondement de l'idée de nature, non seulement, comme nous l'avons vu dans la partie précédente, par la méthode qui remonte jusqu'à la nature première des êtres et qui a servi de modèle à Platon, mais même par sa conception d'une nature organisatrice structurant le vivant.

Avant d'introduire Hippocrate dans ce passage, Galien dégage, de l'observation de la physiologie de l'urine qui ne remonte pas dans les uretères, un indice, parmi bien d'autres, de "la prévoyance et de l'art de la nature". L'idée et l'expression sont bien galéniques. C'est un leitmotiv qui s'épanouit tout particulièrement dans le *Sur l'utilité des parties*, où l'on trouve évoquée, près de soixante-dix fois, la prévoyance de la nature ou, beaucoup plus rarement, la prévoyance du démiurge, mot qui se substitue parfois à celui de φύσις sans désigner une réalité différente. Et quand le mot "prévoyance" (πρόνοια) forme un couple avec un autre mot, c'est, dans la très grande majeure partie des cas, avec le mot "art" (τέχνη). On rencontre ce couple pas moins de seize fois dans le *Sur l'utilité des parties*, ce qui est considérable.[60] Je donne un seul exemple.[61] Lorsque Galien traite de la distribution des veines et des artères, il déclare: "En tout cela, il est clair

[59] GAL. *Nat.Fac.* 1, 13, p.128,17-129,12 Helmreich = II 38,4-39,6 K). Un autre texte devrait être joint et comparé à celui-ci, c'est le passage du *PHP* 9, 8, 26-27, p.596,21-29 De Lacy = V 790,16-791,8 K, où Galien rassemble des citations d'Hippocrate qui font de lui le chantre de la nature-démiurge. Certaines citations sont communes aux deux textes.

[60] On rencontre plus rarement le couple σοφία/πρόνοια et encore plus rarement le couple σοφία/δικαιοσύνη.

[61] GAL. *De usu partium* 16, 14, II p.435,10 sqq. Helmreich = IV 343,12 sq. K.

que la nature a agi avec prévoyance” (προνοητικῶς ἡ φύσις ἐργασαμένη),[62] puis, en observant en particulier le trajet de la veine cave, il remarque: “Je sais qu’il vous apparaîtra, en cela aussi, que l’art et la prévoyance de la nature (τέχνη τε καὶ πρόνοια) ne sont pas petites”. C’est donc la même expression employée ici en chiasme. Dans l’esprit de Galien, c’est bien de cette nature prévoyante et artiste qu’Hippocrate est le découvreur.

Or si on lit maintenant les traités hippocratiques en eux-mêmes, et non plus avec les yeux de Galien, on constatera le décalage absolu sur l’emploi du terme πρόνοια. Le mot ne s’y rencontre que deux fois, si l’on ne tient pas compte des *Lettres* apocryphes, et c’est dans un sens tout à fait différent: il s’agit de la πρόνοια du médecin au sens de “pronostic” et non de “prévoyance”. C’est au début du *Pronostic* que l’on rencontre ces deux emplois. “Le meilleur médecin, est-il dit dans la première phrase du traité, est celui qui sait pratiquer le pronostic (πρόνοιαν)”.[63] Le décalage n’est pas moins grand pour les relations de φύσις et de τέχνη. Il n’est jamais question, dans les écrits hippocratiques anciens, de l’art de la nature; c’est toujours l’art du médecin. Nature et art sont deux ordres qui ne se confondent pas et les rapports de l’art et de la nature peuvent même être conflictuels; de plus, quand il y a parallélisme entre les deux, ce sont les arts des hommes qui sont à l’imitation de la nature.[64] Le vocabulaire des activités humaines n’est pas encore transféré à la nature.

Et pourtant Galien nous présente Hippocrate comme celui qui a compris le premier les travaux de la nature, qu’il admire (θαυμάζει). Cette phraséologie, totalement absente du corpus

[62] L’adverbe προνοητικῶς est attesté huit fois chez Galien, et de façon remarquable sept fois sur huit avec la nature: *AA* 5, 4, II 502,9 K = II p.299, 21 Garofalo; *UP*, outre notre passage, 6, 21, I p.372,7 Helmreich = III 511,13 K; 7, 22, I p.441,13 Helmreich = III 607,13 K; *At.Bil.* 7, V 131,12 K; *Hipp.Epid.VI* 5, 3, CMG V 10, 2, 2, p.264,6 Wenkebach = XVIIB 240,12 K, et 5, 25, p.304,4 sq. Wenkebach = XVIIB 287,7 K.

[63] HIPP. *Prog.* 1, p.193,1 Alexanderson = II p.110,1 Littré.

[64] Voir HIPP. *Vict.* 11, p.134,21 sq. Joly = VI p.486,13 sq. Littré: “Alors que les hommes usent d’arts semblables à la nature humaine, ils ne le comprennent pas”.

hippocratique, est en revanche tout à fait galénique. En parlant d'Hippocrate, Galien nous renseigne beaucoup sur lui-même. Ce qui est tout à fait caractéristique de Galien, c'est ce sentiment d'admiration pour la nature. Le vocabulaire de l'admiration, en relation avec celui de la nature, est constant, notamment dans le *Sur l'utilité des parties*. Galien parle, en un passage, de la prévoyance admirable de la nature (θαυμαστήν τινα πρόνοιαν);[65] en un autre, de son art admirable (τέχνην θαυμαστήν).[66] Il engage son lecteur à admirer la nature, ainsi que les médecins et les philosophes qui admirent la nature, tels Hippocrate et Platon, ou encore Aristote, mais il fustige les philosophes et les médecins qui, au lieu d'admirer l'art de la nature, l'injurient,[67] c'est-à-dire les atomistes parmi lesquels Asclépiade et ses disciples sont particulièrement visés dans notre passage de base. Hippocrate, selon Galien, non seulement admire la nature, mais la célèbre constamment (διὰ πάντος ὑμνεῖ ταύτην). On serait bien en peine de trouver ce verbe ὑμνεῖν dans la *Collection hippocratique*. C'est là encore un vocabulaire galénique. Galien voue à la nature personnifiée et presque divinisée une admiration religieuse. Sans doute ne faut-il pas forcer le sens du verbe ὑμνεῖν qui est, chez Galien, un intensif de ἐπαινεῖν, avec le sens de "louer fortement"; mais certains passages montrent que la connotation religieuse n'est pas toujours absente, surtout quand c'est le substantif ὕμνος qui est employé. Le passage le plus célèbre se situe dans le *Sur l'utilité des parties*, où Galien, à propos de la disposition du pied, se livre à un hymne sur le démiurge organisateur du macrocosme et du microcosme, démiurge qui n'est autre que la nature.[68] Il compose un hymne véritable (ὕμνον ἀληθινὸν συντίθημι) en l'honneur du démiurge, et il considère que c'est la forme authentique de la piété (τὴν ὄντως εὐσέβειαν).[69] Une

[65] *UP* 4, 13, I p.221,3 Helmreich = III 301,3 K.
[66] *UP* 2, 8, I p.89,10 Helmreich = III 122,2 K.
[67] *UP* 7, 14, I p.415,22 Helmreich = III 572,2 K.
[68] Gal. *UP* 3, 10, I p.174,7 Helmreich = III 237,11 K.
[69] Voir aussi l'extrême fin du *De usu partium* avec l'allusion à l'épode des poètes méliques chantant les dieux (ὑμνοῦντες τοὺς θεούς) devant les autels.

telle attitude du médecin, face à la nature, est totalement absente des écrits anciens de la *Collection hippocratique*.

Comment Galien peut-il donc justifier qu'Hippocrate célèbre constamment la nature? La suite de son exposé sur la nature chez Hippocrate va nous permettre de repérer les points d'ancrage dans les textes hippocratiques, et de mesurer les divers degrés de réinterprétation. Car Galien fait ensuite allusion à des expressions repérables ou à des citations. Quand il dit qu'Hippocrate qualifie φύσις de δικαία (en réalité δικαίη en ionien), c'est exact. L'adjectif, soit au positif, soit au comparatif, soit au superlatif, qualifie cinq fois le mot φύσις dans les traités chirurgicaux *Fractures* et *Articulations*. Mais cette remarque, formellement juste, est utilisée de manière abusive et dans un sens qui s'écarte du texte hippocratique. D'abord elle est utilisée de manière abusive, car Galien donne l'impression, non seulement ici, mais aussi ailleurs,[70] que l'appellation est fréquente chez Hippocrate. Or, l'expression n'est employée que cinq fois dans un seul groupe de traités, ou plus exactement dans un seul traité, s'il est vrai que *Fractures* et *Articulations* ne font qu'un seul grand ensemble. Galien, en revanche, ne cesse de rappeler qu'Hippocrate qualifie la nature de juste: dans un seul traité, le *Sur l'utilité des parties*, il le rappelle six fois, donc plus souvent que le mot n'est employé par Hippocrate. Il y a là une technique de publicité ou d'auto-persuasion assez étonnante. Mais surtout Galien change considérablement la portée du sens hippocratique. Alors que l'expression a un emploi technique restreint dans le traité chirurgical et désigne la position normale et correcte d'un membre, Galien réinsère l'expression dans sa représentation de la nature organisatrice du vivant, comme l'indique par exemple cette proposition importante du *Sur l'utilité des parties* à propos des deux muscles de la jambe qui sont de longueur inégale: "La nature, juste en tout point, a mesuré la grandeur de ces muscles à l'utilité de la fonction que chacun devait

[70] Voir *UP* 1, 22, I p.59,21 Helmreich = III 81,10 sq. K: δικαία ἡ φύσις, ὡς πολλάκις αὐτὴν Ἱπποκράτης εἴωθεν ὀνομάζειν.

remplir".[71] L'équité de la nature consiste ici dans une juste proportion entre la taille de l'organe et sa fonction. Pour Galien, "la nature a tout organisé avec équité" (δικαίως ἡ φύσις ἅπαντα διέταξεν); cela rappelle le principe organisateur d'Anaxagore. Galien ne se contente pas d'utiliser librement les passages hippocratiques sur la δικαίη φύσις, mais il attribue clairement à Hippocrate lui-même le sens qu'il a réinterprété. En effet, reprenant dans le *Sur l'utilité des parties* la référence à Hippocrate que l'on a vu dans le *Sur les facultés naturelles*, Galien fait un pas supplémentaire dans l'appropriation en parlant d'Hippocrate "qui célèbre continuellement la justice de la nature et sa prévoyance à l'égard des êtres vivants" (διὰ παντὸς ὑμνοῦντι τὴν δικαιοσύνην αὐτῆς καὶ τὴν εἰς τὰ ζῷα πρόνοιαν).[72] De nature appelée juste on passe, par un glissement significatif, à la justice de la nature, et cette justice est mise sur le même plan que la prévoyance. L'Hippocrate qui sert de modèle à Galien est, à la faveur du détournement d'un sens technique, et d'un glissement apparemment anodin du vocabulaire, parfaitement galénisé.[73]

Voyons maintenant, toujours à partir de notre passage de base, comment Galien utilise des citations d'Hippocrate pour conforter la conception de la nature qu'il lui attribue. Il emploie deux fois le verbe "il dit" (φησι), en citant Hippocrate sous la forme du discours indirect. Voici la première phrase: "Il dit qu'elle (*sc.* la nature) suffit à elle seule, en tout, pour les êtres vivants, elle qui fait d'elle-même, sans avoir appris, tout ce qui convient".[74] Ce sont en réalité deux citations prises dans le même traité, l'*Aliment*, mais à deux endroits différents. La première

[71] GAL. *UP* 3, 10, I p.171,8 Helmreich = III 233,10-11 K.

[72] GAL. *UP* 3, 10, I p.172,15-17 Helmreich = III 235,6-8 K.

[73] Sur la réinterprétation de la δικαίη φύσις d'Hippocrate par Galien, voir A. ROSELLI, "Dalla δικαίη φύσις dei trattati chirurgici alla δικαιοσύνη τῆς φύσεως di Galeno", in *Le normal et le pathologique dans la Collection hippocratique*, Actes du Xème Colloque International Hippocratique, éd. par A. THIVEL et A. ZUCKER (Nice 2002), II 731-752.

[74] Voici le texte grec: καὶ μόνην ἐξαρκεῖν εἰς ἅπαντα τοῖς ζῴοις φησίν, αὐτὴν ἐξ αὐτῆς ἀδιδάκτως πράττουσαν ἅπαντα τὰ δέοντα.

correspond au texte hippocratique suivant: “La nature suffit en tout pour tout” (φύσις ἐξαρκεῖ πάντα πᾶσιν)[75] et la seconde à: “Les natures sont, en tout point, sans maître” (φύσιες πάντων ἀδίδακτοι).[76] Toutefois Galien amalgame très habilement cette seconde citation tirée de l'*Aliment* avec une phrase d'*Épidémies VI*: “La nature, sans être instruite et sans avoir appris, fait ce qu'il convient” (ἀπαίδευτος ἐοῦσα καὶ οὐ μαθοῦσα τὰ δέοντα ποιεῖ).[77] Le collage se fait à la faveur de la synonymie des deux adjectifs ἀδίδακτος et ἀπαίδευτος et par le remplacement du pluriel φύσιες par le singulier φύσις dans la citation de l'*Aliment*. La perfection de ce collage tient à l'identité du contenu, et aussi à la forme aphoristique des deux passages, formant deux maximes indépendantes de tout contexte. Voilà donc trois citations de deux ouvrages différents données dans la proposition infinitive sous le premier “il dit” (φησι). Le second φησι introduit la proposition infinitive suivante: “Il dit que dans nos corps il y a une communauté de flux, une communauté d'air, et que tout est en sympathie.”[78] C'est à nouveau une citation de l'*Aliment*.[79] À propos de cette citation, il convient de remarquer que la phrase choisie par Galien est, au moins par sa formulation, tout à fait exceptionnelle dans la *Collection hippocratique*. Aucun des trois termes composant cet aphorisme (σύρροια, σύμπνοια, συμπαθής) ne se retrouve ailleurs dans les traités hippocratiques. En revanche, c'est une formulation qui, pour deux termes sur trois, est caractéristique du stoïcisme. On peut comparer le passage de Plutarque résumant dans son *De fato* 11 (574 E) la doctrine

[75] Hipp. *Alim.* 15, p.141,24 Joly = IX p.102,16 Littré.

[76] Hipp. *Alim.* 39, p.145,12 Joly = IX p.112,3 Littré.

[77] Hipp. *Epid.* 6, 5, 1, p.102,1-2 Manetti-Roselli = V p.314,7-8 Littré.

[78] Voici le texte grec: ἐν τοῖς σώμασιν ἡμῶν σύμπνοιάν τε μίαν εἶναί φησι καὶ σύρροιαν καὶ πάντα συμπαθέα.

[79] Hipp. *Alim.* 23, p.143,1 Joly = IX p.106,6 Littré: σύρροια μία, σύμπνοια μία, συμπαθέα πάντα. La suite de cet aphorisme (“Pour la totalité tout est en sympathie et pour les parties, les parties dans chaque partie en vue d'une fonction”), cité et explicité, sert de base à Galien, dans le début du *De usu partium* 1, 8, I p.12,23 sqq. Helmreich = III 17,14 sqq. K), pour exposer sa méthode de recherche de l'utilité des parties.

de Chrysippe: "Ce cosmos-ci est régi par la nature de telle façon qu'il y a en lui-même communauté de souffle et sympathie (σύμπνουν καὶ συμπαθῆ αὐτὸν αὑτῷ ὄντα)". Le parallélisme formel est notable. Aussi considère-t-on actuellement que le traité hippocratique *Aliment*, malgré son style héraclitéen, est récent et postérieur au stoïcisme. S'il en est ainsi, Galien reconstituerait à son insu un Hippocrate teinté de stoïcisme. Ce qui semble indéniable, en tout cas, c'est que la conception de la nature organisatrice et d'un organisme où toutes les parties sont solidaires, par l'agir comme par le pâtir, sont plus proches de la conception de la nature des Stoïciens que de celle qui peut ressortir des traités de la *Collection hippocratique* ayant chance d'être d'Hippocrate ou contemporains du médecin de Cos. Mais à la décharge de Galien, il faut reconnaître qu'il n'est pas le seul, dans l'Antiquité, tant s'en faut, à considérer que l'*Aliment* est une œuvre d'Hippocrate.[80]

Sans pouvoir entrer dans plus de détails dans l'analyse de la suite de ce passage où Galien expose ce qu'est la conception de la nature chez Hippocrate, on peut en conclure qu'il reconstruit la théorie de la nature chez Hippocrate à partir de matériaux divers qu'il assemble avec beaucoup d'intelligence et d'habileté, mais dont il n'hésite pas à biaiser éventuellement le sens pour donner une cohérence à l'ensemble. La cohérence que Galien recrée est tout à fait remarquable. Car la diversité des matériaux n'est plus visible dans la synthèse qu'il opère. Galien reconstitue même à partir de ces matériaux la logique de la pensée d'Hippocrate, pour ne pas dire l'histoire de sa découverte des travaux de la nature. À la base de la découverte

[80] Le traité fait partie de la liste des ouvrages d'Hippocrate chez Érotien en tête de son *Glossaire hippocratique* (= *Gloss.*) (*Vocum Hippocraticarum collectio*, rec. E. NACHMANSON [Göteborg 1918], 9,16). La citation est attribuée aussi à Hippocrate, non seulement par Stéphane, commentateur de Galien (*Commentarii in priorem Galeni librum therapeuticum ad Glauconem*, 220, 5 Dikson = I p.321,35-322,1 Dietz), mais aussi par Jean Philopon, commentateur d'Aristote (*In Aristotelis de generatione et corruptione* 1, 5, CAG XIV 2, p.106,33 sq. Vitelli, et *De aeternitate mundi* 7, 17, p.283,19 sq. Rabe).

se trouve la conception d'une nature prévoyante et technicienne. Puis aussitôt après cela (τοιαύτην δὲ οὖσαν, εὐθὺς ... ὑπέλαβεν), Hippocrate a supposé l'existence de facultés naturelles, attractive et répulsive. Galien recompose, en somme, la genèse de la découverte d'Hippocrate sur la nature, en indiquant un ordre dans la découverte malgré l'immédiateté de la succession.

À la fin du passage qui a servi de base à notre réflexion, Galien oppose cette conception hippocratique de la nature à celle d'Asclépiade, lequel part, non de la continuité, mais de la discontinuité, toute la substance étant, selon lui, naturellement divisée en atomes. Cette opposition entre ces deux médecins prend tout son sens dans une vision plus large sur les deux options possibles que Galien distingue dans la recherche sur la nature. C'est dans un autre passage important d'un autre traité, le *Sur les facultés naturelles*, que Galien développe cette vision d'ensemble. C'est vers lui qu'il faut nous tourner maintenant. La phrase d'introduction montre clairement l'enjeu:

> "Il existe deux sectes en médecine et en philosophie parmi les hommes qui ont fait un exposé sur la nature (τῶν ἀποφηναμένων τι περὶ φύσεως ἀνδρῶν)."[81]

Galien expose ce que sont ces deux sectes et les principes qui les caractérisent. La première pense que la substance formant le substrat des êtres soumis à la génération et à la corruption est une, mais se modifie, et que la nature est antérieure aux corps qu'elle façonne avec art et prévoyance par les facultés dont elle dispose. La seconde divise la matière en atomes immuables et ne croit pas à l'existence d'une nature technicienne et prévoyante disposant de facultés propres. De la seconde secte Galien donne comme exemple Asclépiade, alors qu'Hippocrate inaugure la première voie. À la suite d'Hippocrate, vient Platon, qui se réclame de la méthode d'Hippocrate, puis Aristote que Galien qualifie "d'exégète des raisonnements d'Hippocrate sur la nature" (ἐξηγητὴν

[81] GAL. *Nat.Fac.* 1, 12, *Scripta min.* III p.120,7-9 Helmreich = II 27,1-3 K.

ὄντα τῶν περὶ φύσεως λογισμῶν Ἱπποκράτους Ἀριστοτέλη),[82] ensuite les Stoïciens qui "admettent toutes les opinions d'Hippocrate sur la nature" (ἅπαντα ... τὰ περὶ φύσεως Ἱπποκράτους δόγματα),[83] et bien entendu, *last but not least*, Galien qui se croit encore plus fidèle à Hippocrate qu'Aristote ou les Stoïciens. Seul celui qui étudie la nature selon cette voie mérite le terme de φυσικός.

Galien ne juge même pas digne de nommer ceux qui empruntent l'une des deux voies pour s'en écarter ensuite. Il pense, en particulier, à Érasistrate, lequel prétend suivre l'enseignement des Péripatéticiens sur la nature en la célébrant comme technicienne, mais n'en fait rien dans la réalité. Car affirmer que la nature est technicienne, c'est reconnaître qu'elle ne fait rien au hasard. La formule οὐδὲν ἡ φύσις ἐργάζεται μάτην, revenant dans le *Sur l'utilité des parties* comme une litanie, est trop célèbre pour que l'on y insiste.[84] Or Érasistrate, selon Galien, détruit dans les faits cette proposition, parce qu'il ne perçoit pas la finalité de certains organes.[85] Il ne reconnaît pas non plus l'existence des facultés naturelles mises par la nature dans chacun des organes et ne fait pas la différence entre l'art des hommes et l'art de la nature.[86]

Entre philosophes et médecins, on voit donc que Galien ne fait pas de différence fondamentale dans cette recherche sur la nature, puisque l'initiateur de cette φυσιολογία, définie comme la science qui porte sur les corps soumis à la naissance, à la destruction et en un mot au changement, est un médecin, Hippocrate. "La *physiologia* d'Hippocrate remporte la victoire (ἡ Ἱπποκράτους νικᾷ φυσιολογία) selon Platon, selon les Péripatéticiens

[82] GAL. *MM* 1, 2, X 15,8 sq. K.
[83] GAL. *MM* 1, 2, X 16,8 K.
[84] GAL. *UP* 12, 14, II p.222,14 Helmreich = IV 56,13 K; 13, 2, II p.237,20 Helmreich = IV 78,6 sq. K; 13, 8, II p.263,2 Helmreich = IV 112,6 sq.); 15, 5, II p.359, 8 Helmreich = IV 240,17 K; cf. aussi 15, 4, II p.350,6 Helmreich = IV 228,14 K.
[85] GAL. *Nat.Fac.* 2, 4, *Scripta min.* III p.167,13 Helmreich = II 91,8 sqq. K.
[86] GAL. *Nat.Fac.* 2, 3 et 4, III p.159,5-169,5 Helmreich = II 80,6-93,13 K.

et selon ceux du Portique" est-il dit dans le prologue du *Sur la méthode de soigner.*[87] C'est donc l'œuvre d'un médecin, Hippocrate, qui a été suivie et poursuivie par des philosophes, Platon, Aristote et les Stoïciens, avant d'être reprise par un médecin Galien. Cette manière de présenter l'histoire de la recherche sur la nature en privilégiant le premier, le fondateur, par rapport au second et au troisième me paraît être à l'image de la propre démarche de Galien dans sa recherche sur la nature, où il remonte à ce qui est de premier rang organisé par la nature, pour reprendre ses mots, alors que le reste n'en est qu'une conséquence nécessaire. Cela aboutit à minimiser le rôle des philosophes par rapport à l'initiateur, qui est un médecin, et tout particulièrement la contribution d'Aristote sur la nature par rapport à celle d'Hippocrate.

Exceptionnels, en effet, sont les passages où Hippocrate et Aristote sont sur le même plan, l'un exposant les principes de la médecine et l'autre les principes de la *physiologia.*[88] D'ordinaire, Aristote apparaît en second rang après Hippocrate, quand il n'est pas question de Platon, et il précède éventuellement les Stoïciens, qui viennent en troisième rang.[89] Une formule du traité *Sur les facultés naturelles* est assez significative: "Hippocrate, le premier de tous ceux que nous connaissons, a correctement dit, Aristote, en second, a correctement expliqué".[90] Galien ne reconnaît pas, en s'exprimant de cette manière, tout ce qu'il doit à Aristote dans son vocabulaire et dans sa représentation de la nature démiurge. Car ce n'est pas chez Hippocrate que Galien a trouvé l'expression qui revient si souvent chez lui ἡ φύσις ἐδημιούργησε,[91] mais bien dans les écrits biologiques

[87] GAL. *MM* 1, 2, X 17,2-4 K.

[88] GAL. *Hipp.Elem.* 1, 5, 4, p.92,24-26 De Lacy = I 449,2-4 K.

[89] GAL. *Nat.Fac.* 2, 4, *Scripta min.* III p.168,11 sq. Helmreich = II 92, 14-15 K.

[90] GAL. *Nat.Fac.* 2, 4, III p.166,10-12 Helmreich = II 90,2-3 K.

[91] GAL. *Nat.Fac.* 1, 10, III p.117,18-19 Helmreich = II 23,11 K; 2, 9, p.196,16-17 Helmreich = II 131,11 K; *UP* 1, 18, I p.47,6-7 Helmreich = III 64,14 K; 2, 12, I p.100,22 Helmreich = III 137,9 K; 3, 6, I p.141,24-25 Helmreich = III 193,18 K, etc.

d'Aristote. Si je cite par exemple la formule καὶ ταῦτα πάντα εὐλόγως ἡ φύσις δημιουργεῖ ("la nature organise tout cela avec raison"), on croirait lire du Galien. Et pourtant c'est de l'Aristote![92] Faut-il rappeler aussi que quand Galien dit que "la nature ne fait rien en vain", il ne fait que reprendre l'expression même d'Aristote ἡ φύσις οὐδὲν ποιεῖ μάτην, que l'on rencontre déjà une vingtaine de fois dans l'œuvre du philosophe, notamment dans ses écrits biologiques?[93] Ce n'est pas non plus Hippocrate qui a parlé des œuvres de la nature. C'est chez Aristote que l'on rencontre pour la première fois l'expression τὰ τῆς φύσεως ἔργα.[94] Et par voie de conséquence, ce n'est pas chez Hippocrate, mais chez Aristote que Galien a puisé le thème si récurrent chez lui de la comparaison entre l'art de la nature-démiurge et les arts humains, ainsi que de la supériorité des œuvres de la nature sur celles des humains.[95] Et même cette admiration devant les travaux de la nature, si caractéristique de Galien comme je l'ai souligné précédemment, trouve son origine dans un très beau passage des *Parties des Animaux* d'Aristote dont je retiendrai la formule finale: "Dans tous les travaux de nature il y a quelque chose d'admirablc" (ἐν πᾶσι γὰρ τοῖς φυσικοῖς ἔνεστί τι θαυμαστόν).[96] Je ne veux pas dire, par là, que Galien est un simple exégète d'Aristote. Je ne veux pas dire non plus que Galien n'a pas reconnu les mérites d'Aristote, qu'il connaît bien,[97] car l'œuvre de Galien est si vaste et si complexe qu'il faut toujours

[92] ARIST. *De generatione animalium* 1, 23, 731 a 24.

[93] ARIST. *De incessu animalium* 2, 704 b 15 (avec d'assez nombreuses références données *ad loc.* dans l'éd. P. LOUIS, p.13, n.6, *i.e.* p.155); variante de ἡ φύσις οὐδὲν δημιουργεῖ μάτην en *De incessu animalium* 12, 711 a 18.

[94] ARIST. *De partibus animalium* 1, 1, 639 b 6: ἐν τοῖς τῆς φύσεως ἔργοις, et 1, 5, 645 a 24-25; cf. *De generatione animalium* 5, 778 b 4; *De incessu animalium* 2, 704 b 14; *Meteorologica* 389 b 27-28; voir aussi *Problemata* 10, 45, 895 b 32-33.

[95] Voir chez Aristote, *GA* 2, 6, 743 b 22-25: comparaison de la nature démiurge avec le peintre; *PA* 2, 9, 654 b 29 sqq.: comparaison de la nature démiurge avec les sculpteurs. Pour la supériorité des œuvres de la nature sur celles des arts humains, voir *PA* 1, 1, 639 b 19-21.

[96] ARIST. *PA* 1, 5, 645 a 17 sq.

[97] Pour la connaissance de la philosophie de la nature d'Aristote par Galien, voir P. MORAUX, *Der Aristotelismus bei den Griechen* II (Berlin 1984), 729-791.

introduire des nuances. Galien peut de façon exceptionnelle reconnaître le mérite d'Aristote: "lui qui est pourtant si habile en particulier à exposer l'art de la nature (τέχνην φύσεως)."[98] Mais, ce qui est significatif, c'est que cet éloge intervient en contrepoint pour introduire une critique. Ce que je veux souligner surtout, c'est que Galien, dans la présentation de sa conception téléologique de la nature-démiurge, met Aristote en retrait pour remonter à un Hippocrate, archégète mythique, reconstruit par le médecin de Pergame.[99]

C'est de cette façon que Galien privilégie un médecin dans l'histoire de la recherche sur la nature. Sans doute y a-t-il des différences, dans l'esprit de Galien, entre médecine et philosophie en ce domaine. Certains problèmes débattus par les philosophes sont d'une subtilité trop grande pour des médecins. Par exemple, il y a une légère différence entre Aristote et les Stoïciens sur le problème de savoir si le mélange porte uniquement sur les qualités, comme chez Aristote, ou également sur les corps comme chez les Stoïciens; mais pour Galien, discuter de cette divergence n'est pas utile aux médecins.[100] Inversement, "la recherche de l'utilité des parties... est utile non seulement au médecin, mais beaucoup plus encore qu'au médecin au philosophe qui aspire à acquérir la science de la nature entière (τῆς ὅλης φύσεως ἐπιστήμην); car il doit être initié à ce mystère."[101]

Toutefois il est une question, concernant la nature, qui reste particulière aux médecins et qui leur est essentielle. C'est par là que je terminerai. Alors que la *physiologia* a pour seule fin la contemplation de la nature, la médecine est un art dont la fin est la production du redressement du corps.[102] Quelle est donc

[98] GAL. *UP* 1, 8, I p.11,24-26 Helmreich = III 16,10-12 K.

[99] L'obscurité et la concision d'Hippocrate alléguées par Galien favorisent cette reconstruction.

[100] GAL. *MM* 1, 2, X 16,13-16 K.

[101] GAL. *UP* 17, 1, II p.447,25-448,4 Helmreich = IV 360,15-361,2 K.

[102] Pour cette distinction entre la *physiologia* (ou *physikè*), art contemplatif, et la médecine, art poiétique produisant le redressement du corps, voir les développements sur la diérèse des arts dans *Thras.* 30, *Scripta min.* III pp.71 sqq. Helmreich = V 861 sq. K, et dans *CAM* 1, CMG V 1, 3, p.56,19 sqq. Fortuna = I 227,10 sqq. K.

sa place par rapport à l'œuvre de nature qui produit le corps et aussi le redresse? J'esquisserai simplement l'approche de ce problème, pour ne pas déborder sur la notion d'art, en partant de l'une des affirmations importantes que Galien a relevées chez Hippocrate sur la nature. C'est l'aphorisme d'*Épidémies VI* sur “les natures médecins des maladies”, que j'ai déjà mentionné dans la première partie à propos de la définition de la nature chez les commentateurs alexandrins.[103] Si les natures sont médecins des maladies, l'art de la médecine existe-t-il? Galien se fait l'écho de cette objection que l'on a pu faire à Hippocrate et il y répond dans un long commentaire au passage hippocratique.[104] Selon Galien, il n'y a pas contradiction, mais hiérarchie entre le médecin, l'art et la nature: le médecin est le serviteur de l'art, et c'est là une formule hippocratique;[105] mais Galien ajoute que la médecine est, à son tour, le serviteur de la nature (τὴν ἰατρικὴν αὐτήν, ἥτις πάλιν ὑπηρετεῖ τῇ φύσει),[106] laquelle est le premier et le plus important de tous les arts de la guérison (τὴν φύσιν ἁπασῶν τεχνῶν πρώτην τε καὶ κυριωτάτην ⟨οὖσαν εἰς τὰς⟩ ἰάσεις).[107] On retrouve dans cette définition galénique de la nature médecin, la conception technicienne et démiurgique de la nature, qui n'est jamais explicite chez Hippocrate, mais aussi l'idée que la nature est première et primordiale.

[103] Voir *supra*, p. 234 et n.19.

[104] GAL. *Hipp.Epid.VI*, 5, 1, XVIIB 222-233 K.

[105] HIPP. *Epid.* 1, 5, II p.636,2 Littré (ὁ ἰητρός, ὑπηρέτης τῆς τέχνης).

[106] Pour la médecine serviteur de la nature, voir aussi le développement sur la diérèse des arts dans *Thras.* 30, *Scripta min.* III p.73,6-8 Helmreich = V 862,5-7 K: la nature (ἡ φύσις) fait le corps et le répare quand il est malade, la médecine est au service (ὑπηρετική) de la nature et redresse le corps. Comparer aussi *PHP* 9, 8, 27, p.596,25 sq. De Lacy = V 791,2-3 K, où le médecin est dit “serviteur et imitateur de la nature” dans une affirmation que Galien attribue à Hippocrate. Le glissement est net par une sorte de raccourci: alors que le texte hippocratique dit que le médecin est serviteur de l'art, Galien lui fait dire qu'il est le serviteur de la nature; cf. *Ars Med.* 26, p.358,12 sq. Boudon = I 378,9-10 K: ἡ μὲν φύσις ἐστὶ δημιουργός, ὁ δ' ἰατρὸς ὑπηρέτης.

[107] GAL. *Hipp.Epid.VI*, 5, 1, CMG V 10, 2, 2, p.258,1 sq. et 259,5 sq. Wenkebach = XVIIB 231,12 sq. et 233,6 sq. K.

Par là on rejoint, pour finir, le noyau sémantique de la notion de nature chez Galien que j'ai essayé de dégager, dès la première partie de cet essai, par-delà les diverses acceptions du terme, à savoir ce qui est à la fois premier et primordial.

DISCUSSION

J. Barnes: This rich and stimulating paper encourages numerous questions, only two of which I have time to raise.

1) The first has a very limited scope: when Galen says that κατὰ φύσιν has several meanings, you take this to imply different meanings for the word φύσις, but is it not rather that the preposition κατά may have different forces? In general, something may be κατὰ X if it is directly determined by X, but also if it is an indirect consequence of X.

2) Your paper brings out very clearly the 'creative' nature of much of Galen's interpretation of Hippocrates. Perhaps this phenomenon could be set in a wider context — for in a similar way we find Alexander 'recomposing' Aristotle and Plotinus Plato. Part of the explanation for this is perhaps to be found in the fact that Galen, like Alexander and Plotinus, thought that his author was, very largely, right in what he said. The interpretative question was not "What does he mean?", but rather "Given that what he says is true, what does he mean?".

J. Jouanna: La réponse à votre première question est très délicate, car l'expression prépositionnelle κατὰ φύσιν forme un tout dans lequel il paraît impossible de distinguer ce qui peut venir d'une différenciation du sens de la préposition ou du substantif. Le grec a, du reste, la possibilité d'en faire une expression substantivée τὸ κατὰ φύσιν. Cela pourrait être probablement un peu différent si on avait l'expression avec l'article κατὰ τὴν φύσιν. Quand j'ai rapproché les deux propositions τῆς φύσεως πολλαχῶς λεγομένης et πολλαχῶς δὲ τοῦ κατὰ φύσιν λεγομένου, j'ai pris l'expression κατὰ φύσιν comme un tout ayant plusieurs sens et je ne crois pas avoir dit que la différenciation des sens venait du seul mot φύσιν.

Je vous remercie de souligner que la relecture d'Hippocrate par Galien peut se situer dans un contexte plus large, et que l'on pourrait trouver effectivement des voies de recomposition analogues d'Aristote ou de Platon chez Alexandre d'Aphrodise ou chez Plotin. Vous qualifiez heureusement aussi la méthode d'interprétation qui consiste à expliquer les passages particuliers difficiles en fonction de l'idée générale que les interprètes se font de la doctrine qu'ils considèrent juste dans l'ensemble. J'ajouterai que cette doctrine générale à laquelle l'interprète se réfère est elle-même une recomposition; c'est au moins ce que j'ai voulu montrer pour l'Hippocrate de Galien. Toutefois, par rapport à la relecture d'Aristote par Alexandre ou de Platon par Plotin, il reste une plus grande complexité dans le cas de la lecture d'Hippocrate par Galien, et nécessairement une plus grande recomposition, dans la mesure où les écrits transmis sous le nom d'Hippocrate sont issus de plusieurs auteurs de date différente et que Galien attribue à un même auteur des traités aussi dissemblables, par la date et par les doctrines, que *Nature de l'homme* et *Aliment.*

M. Frede: It seems to me to be extremely helpful to be reminded of the fact that Hippocrates is an authority, perhaps the major authority for Galen, and that Galen when he talks about nature believes he is talking about nature in the sense in which Hippocrates was talking about nature. But I think that the two senses of 'nature' which Prof. Jouanna isolates on the basis of the *Commentary on the Aphorisms* do themselves stand in need of a good deal of explication and explanation to understand how they are related to the way Galen elsewhere uses the term 'nature'. In particular it is difficult to see how either of these two senses can cover the use of 'nature' when it is used interchangeably with 'Demiurge', and so it would be desirable to have some elucidation as to how this third use is related to the first two.

J. Jouanna: Les deux sens de φύσις que j'ai isolés en partant du *Commentaire aux Aphorismes* sont deux sens que Galien a lui-même donnés parmi la pluralité des sens qu'il reconnaît à φύσις. Il n'en a pas donné d'autres dans ce *Commentaire*, parce qu'il n'avait pas besoin de les donner pour l'explication des *Aphorismes*. Et parmi ces sens qu'il n'a pas donnés, il y a évidemment le sens de 'nature démiurgique' auquel vous faites allusion et qui est fondamental chez Galien. J'ai rappelé que les commentateurs alexandrins avaient complété les deux définitions données dans le *Commentaire aux Aphorismes* par deux autres sens parmi lesquels il y a la nature organisatrice. Pour répondre à votre question de la relation entre les deux sens distingués dans le *Commentaire aux Aphorismes* et le troisième sens qui est 'nature démiurgique', si l'on en reste à la perspective que j'ai adoptée, à savoir d'expliquer Galien par Galien, il faudrait posséder la définition de l'ouvrage perdu *Sur les termes médicaux*, où Galien nous dit qu'il avait donné tous les sens de φύσις. Dans l'état actuel de l'œuvre de Galien — car une redécouverte par la tradition arabe reste possible, même si elle est improbable —, Galien est plus préoccupé par la distinction des sens que par le lien qui les unit. En effet, comme j'ai essayé de le montrer, lorsque Galien distingue des sens de φύσις, ce n'est pas pour montrer la genèse de ces sens, mais c'est pour éviter des erreurs d'interprétation dans des passages particuliers par l'application d'un mauvais sens parmi les différents sens possibles. Par ailleurs, l'étude que je propose de la façon dont Galien utilise des matériaux divers et de nature différente écrits par des auteurs différents et de date différente pour reconstruire un seul et même Hippocrate pris comme modèle pour la conception de la nature, creuse l'écart qu'il y a, à l'origine, entre la nature prise comme substance primordiale (premier sens donné dans le *Commentaire aux Aphorismes*) et le sens de nature démiurgique. Cela étant dit, Galien n'a, à aucun moment, l'impression d'une fracture entre ces différents sens. La fracture pour lui est entre deux conceptions de la nature qu'il juge irréconciliables.

D. Manetti: 1) Dalla sua ricca relazione è emersa con grande evidenza una tensione fra due nozioni di natura utilizzate da Galeno e che risultano direttamente ispirate a trattati diversi del

Corpus Hippocraticum, una, che si basa essenzialmente su *De natura hominis* che equivale a *krasis*, l'altra, che si basa invece su trattati come *De alimento*, che è indiscutibilmente legata alla visione platonica di una natura demiurgica. La discussione ha sollevato domande sul modo in cui Galeno poteva conciliare due nozioni simili. Io credo che una possibile via attraverso la quale Galeno poteva, se non assimilare, far convivere queste due nozioni per lui ascrivibili ai due modelli Ippocrate e Platone, è una visione generale dello sviluppo del pensiero, di cui peraltro lei ha già fatto cenno. Intendo dire l'idea che, secondo Galeno, la tradizione filosofico-scientifica procede per esegesi e allargamenti successivi, come è chiaro per esempio dal passo di *Nat.Fac.* 2, 4, II 88,14-89,12 K (Aristotele e Teofrasto hanno spiegato la teoria di Ippocrate su caldo, freddo, secco e umido). Insomma la tradizione è vista come una serie ininterrotta di interpretazioni e reinterpretazioni, senza rotture traumatiche. Forse una tale visione riflette il più generale clima della filosofia del II secolo, basata sostanzialmente sull'esegesi dei grandi maestri come Platone o Aristotele, che vengono fatti in certa misura convergere.

2) Una piccola precisazione a proposito del paragone fra l'uso di φύσις secondo i filosofi e in un passo omerico, da lei citato a p.243: il confronto non è poi cosi paradossale, secondo almeno i criteri interpretativi di Galeno, che nel trattato *Sui nomi medici* (p.26,17 ss. e p.31,15 Meyerhoff-Schacht) indica che per indagare il significato dei nomi bisogna avere tre punti di riferimento: la indicazione interna della parola, cioè l'etimologia, la *synetheia* degli antichi e la *synetheia* dei moderni, la *synetheia* degli antichi in particolare si basa su autori 'non tecnici' come Aristofane. Perciò Galeno considera Omero come parte fondamentale della *synetheia* degli antichi.

J. Jouanna: La première partie de votre intervention, dont je vous remercie, prend très heureusement le relais, après ma réponse à la question de M. Frede. Je terminais en disant qu'il n'y a pas fracture entre les sens de φύσις, mais entre deux voies opposées prises par les philosophes et les médecins sur la notion de nature, à savoir la conception discontinue et atéléologique d'un Démocrite ou d'un Asclépiade et la conception continue et téléologique d'un Hippocrate. Dans cette seconde voie, qui est la bonne pour Galien, il est vrai que l'évolution est vue par Galien comme une succession d'exégèses et d'élargissements, comme vous le soulignez. Moi-même, j'ai mentionné la succession Hippocrate, Platon, Aristote, les Stoïciens dans la seconde voie et j'ai rappelé qu'Aristote, selon Galien, était un exégète de ce que Hippocrate avait correctement écrit. Mais il est un point de votre intervention sur lequel je voudrais revenir et qui me permettra de compléter ce que j'ai dit à propos de l'origine de la nature démiurgique chez Galien. Vous avez parlé de la vision platonicienne de la nature démiurgique ("visione platonica di una natura demiurgica"), et j'imagine que cette manière de s'exprimer doit être partagée par beaucoup, étant donné que Platon dans le *Timée* est le premier philosophe à avoir accordé de l'importance au démiurge. On y trouve et le substantif δημιοῦργος et le verbe dérivé δημιουργέω. Mais, ce qui m'a frappé en partant de l'expression de Galien ἡ φύσις ἐδημιούργησε (cf. aussi dans le *Hipp.Elem.* 11, 6, CMG V 1, 2, p.142,9 De Lacy = I 495,5 sq. K, l'expression ἀγαθός τις οὖσα δημιουργὸς ἡ φύσις), c'est qu'elle n'est pas encore dans le *Timée*. La *physis* n'est pas encore assimilée au démiurge chez Platon. C'est seulement dans les écrits biologiques d'Aristote que l'expression ἡ φύσις ἐδημιούργησε apparaît; c'est la raison pour laquelle j'ai parlé de la vision aristotélicienne de la nature démiurgique. On a là un glissement entre Platon et Aristote qui est l'exemple même d'une évolution non "traumatique", pour reprendre votre mot, mais qui paraît au philologue que je suis, et probablement aussi à l'historien des idées, comme une étape importante dans l'histoire du concept de φύσις en Grèce ancienne.

Votre deuxième remarque sur la justification de la mention d'Homère dans l'histoire de la notion philosophique de φύσις retracée par Galien dans son *Commentaire* de la *Nature de l'homme* est très précieuse, car elle permet de mieux comprendre que la mention d'Homère est moins étonnante qu'il n'y paraît. Il reste que le commentaire de la citation d'Homère amène Galien à employer l'expression αἰσθητὴ φύσις qui, à ma connaissance, ne se retrouve pas dans le reste de son œuvre.

V. Barras: Traiter de la nature chez Galien évoque bien vite dans une perspective d'histoire de la médecine, la question des "six choses non-naturelles". De même que pour la notion de nature, dont vous montrez très clairement la reconstruction par Galien lecteur d'Hippocrate, s'agirait-il aussi de montrer, dans l'élaboration que propose Galien des *six non naturales*, l'importance de la figure d'Hippocrate? Si oui, quel serait le lien que l'on pourrait établir avec la vision de Galien à propos de la nature (je pense en particulier à ce que vous évoquez en conclusion sur le problème spécifiquement médical — par rapport à la *physiologia* — de la production d'"un redressement du corps")?

J. Jouanna Votre question porte sur une classification qui a eu beaucoup de succès dans des articles récents. Et pourtant, je n'en ai pas parlé, car cette classification sous la forme des *six non naturales* ne se trouve pas dans l'œuvre de Galien elle-même, mais appartient au galénisme arabo-latin, même si l'on peut trouver la principale origine de cette classification dans l'*Ars medica* de Galien (voir la note très riche de V. Boudon [éd.], *Galien. Art médical* [Paris 2000], 425-427, sur les discussions modernes concernant l'origine de ces *six non naturales*). Mais dans l'*Art médical* six altérations énumérées ne sont pas encore expressément dites non naturelles. On n'y trouve pas l'expression οὐ κατὰ φύσιν *vel* παρὰ φύσιν pour les qualifier. C'est la raison pour laquelle je n'en ai pas parlé. Pour répondre à votre question, il n'y a aucune chance de retrouver dans cette classification post-galénique une origine hippocratique. De façon plus générale, les classifications que Galien a établies ne sont pas hippocratiques. J'ai eu l'occasion de l'indiquer (*supra*, p.231) à propos de la notion de φύσις au sens de κρᾶσις qui est hippocratique, mais a donné lieu chez Galien à une classification en un nombre défini de huit mélanges mauvais qui ne se trouvent pas chez les médecins du *Corpus hippocratique*.

VII

Véronique Boudon

ART, SCIENCE ET CONJECTURE CHEZ GALIEN

L'attention portée par Galien à la notion de *technè*, à la notion d'art, se dévoile de façon indiscutable à travers les nombreuses pages de ses différents traités. En même temps, cet intérêt authentique pour l'une des catégories conceptuelles majeures de la pensée antique apparaît sans surprise directement lié à une réflexion approfondie sur le statut de la médecine elle-même. Pour le dire en un mot, généralisation et abstraction articulées autour de la notion d'art sont rares chez Galien et n'intéressent le médecin qu'en tant qu'elles lui permettent de penser son art propre, l'art médical. Les titres de quelques-uns de ses traités sont à cet égard révélateurs. Le lecteur de l'*Art médical* comme celui du *À Patrophile, sur la constitution de l'art médical*, du *À Thrasybule, si l'hygiène est une partie de la médecine ou de la gymnastique* ou encore du *Protreptique* (ou *Exhortation à l'étude de la médecine*), n'est pas trompé. À l'intérieur de tous ces traités, comme les titres l'indiquent, et bien que la réflexion sur l'art ne soit jamais absente, c'est en effet d'abord de médecine qu'il est question. Ce même lecteur aura cependant bientôt la surprise de constater que différentes opinions sur l'art en général cohabitent au sein de l'œuvre galénique, où elles sous-tendent à leur tour des conceptions, non pas exactement conflictuelles mais assurément divergentes, sur le statut de l'art médical en particulier. Les différences de point de vue nourries par Galien sur son art propre, la médecine, vont en effet entraîner à leur tour des différences de point de vue notables sur sa conception de l'art en général, les préoccupations du médecin prenant le pas sur les réflexions du théoricien de l'art, et jamais l'inverse. En ce sens, et dans la mesure où c'est indiscutablement la réflexion sur la médecine qui prioritairement guide et détermine la réflexion sur l'art, il y a donc une sorte de légitimité conceptuelle à s'intéresser d'abord à la médecine pensée comme art et à sa place parmi les autres arts, avant d'explorer le statut fondamentalement ambigu d'un art médical écartelé entre *technè*, *épistèmè* et stochastique.

Place de la médecine dans la hiérarchie des arts

Une apparente dichotomie

Il a déjà été noté que la médecine galénique ne jouit pas toujours du même statut dans la hiérarchie des arts.[1] Tantôt, comme dans le *Protreptique* ou le *Que l'excellent médecin est aussi philosophe*, l'art médical occupe l'un des rangs les plus élevés aux côtés de l'astronomie, la géométrie et jusqu'aux arts divins, tantôt, comme dans le *À Patrophile, sur la constitution de l'art médical* ou le *À Thrasybule, si l'hygiène relève de la médecine ou de la gymnastique*, Galien nous décrit la médecine comme ravalée au niveau des arts les plus vulgaires (βάναυσοι), comme celui du ravaudeur.[2] Frappé par ce qu'il considère comme une apparente dichotomie, M. Vegetti a en particulier distingué une médecine

[1] Voir M. Isnardi, "Techne", in *PP* 16 (1961), 257-296, étude qui reste toujours fondamentale sur la notion d'art en général et dont la réflexion s'enracine précisément dans le traité de Galien intitulé *Que l'excellent médecin est aussi philosophe*, qui lui sert de point de départ. Sur la place de la médecine parmi les autres arts, voir les travaux de M. Vegetti, "Modelli di medicina in Galeno", in *Galen. Problems and Prospects*, ed. by V. Nutton (London 1981), 47-63 et "L'immagine del medico e lo statuto epistemologico della medicina in Galeno", in *ANRW* II 37, 2 (Berlin 1994), 1672-1717. Enfin on signalera l'étude de W. Tatarkiewicz, "Classification of Arts in Antiquity", in *Journal of the History of Ideas* 24 (1969), 231-240, qui cependant repose pour Galien sur la seule lecture du *Protreptique* et ne prend donc pas en compte le second modèle de classification représenté par le *À Patrophile, sur la constitution de la médecine* (= *CAM*) et le *À Thrasybule, si l'hygiène relève de la médecine ou de la gymnastique* (= *Thras.*).

[2] Galien a en outre plus ponctuellement abordé ce problème dans l'*Ars medica*. La chronologie des traités ne permet pas de saisir ce qui aurait pu être la trace

dite "de profil haut", anatomo-physiologique, de tradition alexandrine, davantage intellectualisée et théorisée, telle qu'illustrée par un traité comme le *Protreptique*, et une médecine dite "de profil bas", clinico-thérapeutique, de tradition hippocratique, plus empirique et plus tournée vers la pratique, telle que développée dans le *À Patrophile.*[3] J'ai moi-même réfléchi à cette étrange ambivalence de l'art médical galénique dans mon édition du *Protreptique* parue dans la CUF et plus largement je me suis interrogée ailleurs sur la place de la médecine à l'intérieur de la classification des arts.[4] Sans m'attarder davantage, j'indiquerai cependant que l'apparente dichotomie dénoncée par M. Vegetti n'interdit cependant pas une certaine forme de conciliation. Mais avant de s'engager sur cette voie, il convient de rappeler brièvement l'énoncé des deux thèses galéniques en apparence inconciliables et telles qu'exposées à l'intérieur de deux traités pour lesquels nous disposons d'éditions critiques récentes, le *Protreptique* et le *À Patrophile, sur la constitution de l'art médical,* auxquels je limiterai volontairement ici l'emprunt de mes exemples.[5]

d'une évolution dans la pensée de Galien, puisque celui-ci dans le *À Thrasybule*, écrit lors de son second séjour à Rome, c'est-à-dire dans les années 169-180, expose déjà des conceptions fort proches de celles qu'il développera à la fin de sa vie par exemple dans le *À Patrophile.*

[3] Sur ces distinctions, voir M. VEGETTI, *art.cit.*, in *ANRW* II 37, 2 (1994), 1672-1717. Voir aussi J. HANKINSON, "Galen on the foundations of science", in *Galeno: Obra, pensamiento e influencia,* ed. por J.A. LÓPEZ FÉREZ (Madrid 1991), 15-29 et S. FORTUNA, "La definizione della medicina in Galeno", in *PP* 42 (1987), 181-196, qui, bien que sensible à ce qu'elle nomme une embarrassante dichotomie entre τέχνη λογική et τέχνη ποιητική, ne reprend pas totalement à son compte la thèse de M. Vegetti et préfère prôner une réconciliation possible entre les deux courants qui traversent l'œuvre galénique.

[4] Galien. *Exhortation à l'étude de la médecine. Art médical.* Texte établi et traduit par V. BOUDON (Paris 2000); "Les définitions tripartites de la médecine chez Galien", in *ANRW* II 37, 2 (Berlin 1994), 1468-1490; "La place de la médecine à l'intérieur de la classification des arts dans le *Ad Patrophilum, De constitutione artis medicae*", in *Galien. Systématisation de la médecine, à Patrophile,* Actes de la Journée d'Étude organisée par le "Groupe Catégories de la pensée antique" (Université Charles de Gaulle-Lille III, 4 mars 1997) (Paris), 63-86 (à paraître).

[5] Pour le *Protreptique* (= *Protr.*), voir l'édition d'A. BARIGAZZI dans le CMG V 1, 1 (Berlin 1991) et ma propre édition dans la CUF (Paris 2000). Pour le

De fait, ces deux traités, par bien des aspects, apparaissent à la fois curieusement opposés et complémentaires, non seulement par leur contenu mais aussi par l'histoire du texte. Rappelons en effet que du traité *À Patrophile*, à l'origine composé de trois livres et intitulé *Sur la constitution des arts*, ne nous est parvenu que le dernier livre sous le titre *Sur la constitution de la médecine*, les deux premiers livres consacrés aux arts en général étant perdus.[6] Le *Protreptique* quant à lui devait connaître le sort inverse, puisque seule sa partie initiale consacrée à la présentation de tous les arts est aujourd'hui conservée, alors que sa partie finale consacrée à la seule médecine est perdue. Les deux traités diffèrent également quant à leur contenu, le *Protreptique* proposant une hiérarchie des arts au sommet desquels se situent les arts 'logiques' et parmi eux la médecine, alors que le *Sur la constitution de l'art médical* prône l'unité des arts fondée sur l'existence d'une seule et même méthode commune à tous et qui dépend de la notion de fin, classification des arts que l'on qualifiera donc de téléologique et qui, comme on l'a déjà signalé, apparaît également présente dans un autre traité galénique, le *À Thrasybule*.

Selon un schéma bien connu et presque exactement reproduit dans les deux traités, Galien distingue dans le *Sur la constitution de la médecine* (*CAM* 1, p.56,19-26 Fortuna = I 227,10-228,3 K):

À Patrophile, sur la constitution de la médecine (= *CAM*), voir l'édition de S. FORTUNA dans le CMG V 1, 3 (Berlin 1997).

[6] Voir *De libris propriis* 11 (XIX 44,18-45,1 K = *Scripta min.* II p.120,17-18) et CMG V 1, 3, p.45 Fortuna. Une allusion précise au *Sur la constitution des arts* (= *CAM*) se trouve dans le prologue de l'*Ars medica* (I 306,2-7 K = p.275,1-4 Boudon: οὐδεὶς μέντοι ... ἑτέρωθι διήλθομεν). Ouvrage à nouveau cité dans le catalogue final de l'*Ars medica* comme un traité se situant au niveau des principes et non du particulier (*Ars Med.* 37, I 407,8-12 K = p.388,5-8 Boudon). La perte des deux premiers livres dut intervenir assez tôt, avant le VIe siècle, date à laquelle les scholies rassemblées par G. HELMREICH ("Zu Galenos", in *Berliner Philologische Wochenschrift* 16 [1896], col.317-318) et P. MORAUX ("Unbekannte Galen-Scholien", in *ZPE* 27 [1977], 1-63) se réfèrent déjà à notre traité comme à un traité indépendant cité sous le titre *De constitutione artis medicae* (voir CMG V 1, 3, p.46 Fortuna).

1) les arts θεωρητικαί, qui ont leur fin dans la seule contemplation de la nature des choses qu'ils prennent en considération (p.56,19-20 Fortuna: Ἐπειδὴ τῶν τεχνῶν ἔνιαι μὲν ἐν μόνῳ τῷ θεωρῆσαι τὴν φύσιν ὧν ἐπισκοποῦνται πραγμάτων ἔχουσι τὸ τέλος), comme par exemple l'arithmétique, l'astronomie et la *physiologia* (c'est-à-dire la science de la nature);
2) les arts πρακτικαί, qui accomplissent une action comme la danse et l'art du héraut, mais qui ne peuvent présenter aucun résultat de leur action une fois que celle-ci a cessé (p.56,21-23: τινὲς δὲ πράττουσι μέν τινας πράξεις, ὡς ὀρχηστική τε καὶ κηρυκική, δεῖξαι δ' οὐδὲν ἔργον ἑαυτῶν ἔχουσι τοῦ πράττειν παυσάμεναι);
3) les arts ποιητικαί, qui à l'inverse sont capables d'exhiber leur production comme les architectes et les charpentiers (p.56,23-24: τινὲς δ' ἔμπαλιν τούτων ἐπιδείκνυνται δημιουργήματα, καθάπερ οἰκοδομική τε καὶ τεκτονική);
4) et enfin les arts κτητικαί, qui ne produisent rien en eux-mêmes, mais ont pour objet et ambition de pourchasser et acquérir, comme la pêche et la chasse avec un chien, et pour le dire en un mot comme toute sorte de chasse (p.56,24-26: τινὲς δ' οὐδὲν μὲν αὐταὶ δημιουργοῦσιν, ἔργον δ' αὐταῖς ἐστι καὶ σπούδασμα θηρᾶσαί τε καὶ κτήσασθαι, καθάπερ ἥ τε ἁλιευτικὴ καὶ κυνηγετικὴ καὶ συλλήβδην εἰπεῖν ἡ θηρευτικὴ πᾶσα).

Toutes ces distinctions cependant ne valent qu'en vertu d'un principe structurant fort clair qui est la recherche d'une fin, d'un *telos*, en vue de laquelle chaque art est entrepris. Aussi, pour discerner à quelle catégorie appartient un art, suffit-il bien souvent de se demander quel désir nous a poussés à en entreprendre l'apprentissage. Patrophile, interrogé sur ce point par Galien, lui fait cette réponse sans ambiguïté: il s'est tourné vers la médecine dans le but "si possible, de ramener à un état selon la nature les hommes dont le corps était contre nature" (p.56,32-34 = I 228,10-12 K: ἀπεκρίνω δέ μοι βούλεσθαι τοὺς παρὰ φύσιν ἔχοντας ἀνθρώπους τὸ σῶμα μάλιστα μέν, εἰ οἷόν τε, πάντας εἰς τὴν φύσιν ἐπαναγαγεῖν) et si c'était impossible de posséder au moins une certaine connaissance pour distinguer les cas curables de ceux qui ne le sont pas.

Dans la mesure où n'apparaît le résultat de son action qu'une fois que celle-ci a cessé, la médecine fait donc quant à elle partie des arts 'poiétiques' aux côtés de l'art du forgeron, du cordonnier, du constructeur de navire, du charpentier, du sculpteur, du peintre ..., les arts poiétiques étant de loin les plus nombreux que tous les autres. Ils sont en outre de deux sortes, l'art de la médecine appartenant pour sa part aux arts qui corrigent ce qui existe déjà (p.58,16-22 = I 229,17-230,6 K: οὐσῶν δὲ διφυῶν, ὡς ἐδείχθη, τῶν ποιητικῶν ἐκ τῶν ἐπανορθουμένων ἂν εἴη τὸ ἤδη γεγονός, ἣν ζητοῦμεν) comme celui du ravaudeur appliqué aux vieux vêtements ou encore celui du réparateur de vieux souliers (καθάπερ αἵ τε τὰ διερρωγότα τῶν ἱματίων καὶ τὰ διεσπασμένα τῶν ὑποδημάτων συρράπτουσαι), et non aux arts qui produisent ce qui n'existait pas précédemment (οὐκ ἐκ τῶν δημιουργουσῶν, ὃ μήπω πρόσθεν ἦν) comme celui du tisserand ou du cordonnier. D'un point de vue strictement téléologique, si l'on se borne à considérer en vue de quelle fin est exercée la médecine, celle-ci rejoint donc la catégorie des arts dits vulgaires (βάναυσοι), tel celui du ravaudeur.

Exigence scientifique et efficacité rhétorique

La surprise peut donc être grande, à la lecture d'un traité comme le *Protreptique*, de voir se substituer une tout autre hiérarchie des arts où cette fois la médecine occupe la plus haute place. Au schéma arborescent du *À Patrophile* se trouve substituée une représentation concentrique formée des différents cercles (ou chœurs) qui entourent le dieu Hermès, "maître en raison et artisan de tout art" (*Protr.* 3, 1, p.116,24-25 Barigazzi = I 4,15-16 K: λόγου μὲν ὄντα δέσποτην, ἐργατὴν δὲ τέχνης ἁπάσης). Au premier rang des sectateurs de cette divinité figurent en effet en bonne place les géomètres, les mathématiciens, les philosophes, les médecins, les astronomes et les grammairiens. Au deuxième rang, suivent les peintres, les sculpteurs, les maîtres d'école, les charpentiers, les architectes[7] et les lapidaires. Viennent enfin au dernier rang les représentants de tous les autres arts. Cet ordre apparemment si bien établi est cependant bientôt remis en cause par l'existence d'un quatrième groupe dont Galien nous dit, sans plus de précisions, qu'il est placé au plus près du dieu. Ce quatrième cercle rassemble des représentants de tous les arts, distingués pour leur vie vertueuse et bien connus pour exceller dans leur art (5, 2, p.120,4-5 Barigazzi = I 7,15-17 K: τοὺς καλῶς μὲν βιοῦντας, ἐν δὲ ταῖς ἑαυτῶν τέχναις πρωτεύοντας). Cette redistribution de la géographie des arts, si surprenante qu'elle puisse apparaître au premier abord, ne me paraît nullement inconciliable avec la précédente, celle du *À Patrophile*, tant au niveau du contenu que du projet didactique et méthodologique que véhiculent les deux textes. En effet, en ce qui concerne le contenu et à bien lire le *Protreptique*, rien ne s'oppose à ce qu'un médecin côtoie un ravaudeur au sein de ce quatrième cercle réservé aux meilleurs praticiens dans chacun des arts même réputés les plus vils.[8] Ensuite, d'un point de vue purement méthodologique cette fois, les conceptions de Galien exposées dans le *Protreptique* en ce qui concerne la fin visée par tout art apparaissent pleinement conciliables avec celles exposées dans le *À Patrophile*. Galien ne conclut-il pas le *Protreptique* sur la répétition de ce principe à ses yeux absolument intangible, que seul vaut vraiment d'être exercé un art qui ait à la fois "une fin utile à la vie" et puisse durer toute la vie? C'est donc là encore, dans le *À Patrophile* comme dans le *Protreptique*, en fonction de

[7] La comparaison avec l'art de l'architecture tient également une grande place dans le *À Patrophile* (= *CAM*).

[8] À la fin du *Protreptique* (14, 4, p.150,8-10 Barigazzi = I 38,13-15 K), Galien opposera à nouveau les arts rationnels et nobles (λογικαί τε καὶ σεμναί), qui comptent la médecine, la rhétorique, la musique, la géométrie, l'arithmétique, la dialectique, l'astronomie, la grammaire, l'art de légiférer, et éventuellement la peinture et la sculpture, aux arts vulgaires et manuels (βαναύσους τε καὶ χειρωνακτικάς), qui impliquent au cours de leur exercice une peine physique.

la fin assignée à chaque art, fin à partir de laquelle chaque art est constitué,[9] que Galien dans les deux cas détermine son jugement. Certes, l'art médical jouit dans les premières lignes du *Protreptique* du statut d'art noble auquel la comparaison avec l'art du ravaudeur dans le *À Patrophile* peut à juste titre paraître radicalement opposée. Mais au-delà de l'emphase et de l'hyperbole dont les traités du genre 'protreptique' sont de toute façon rarement dépourvus, il convient de souligner l'unité de la réflexion méthodologique de Galien articulée en vue de la notion de fin et indiscutablement commune aux deux traités. Plus profondément, le discours de Galien, dans son argumentation, davantage encore que dans son contenu lui-même, apparaît comme grandement dépendant du public auquel il est destiné. Rien d'étonnant en effet, lorsqu'il s'adresse à l'un de ces jeunes gens encore indécis quant au choix d'une carrière, comme dans le *Protreptique* et non plus à ses amis médecins, Patrophile ou Thrasybule, à ce que Galien s'emploie d'abord à exalter la figure triomphante du médecin fier de son art, au détriment de l'unité de la *technè* guidée par une *methodos* et organisée en vue d'une fin (*telos*). De ce point de vue, l'exigence scientifique cède alors le pas à l'efficacité rhétorique.

En même temps, il convient de rester attentif à la complexité et à l'audace de la réflexion galénique, qui n'hésite pas, dans une juxtaposition volontairement provocatrice, à associer art médical et art du ravaudeur. Selon moi, la dichotomie attribuée à Galien entre une médecine de profil haut et une médecine de profil bas s'explique d'abord par un réel souci d'efficacité rhétorique, lui-même dicté par la nécessité de séduire un vaste public constitué aussi bien de spécialistes déjà initiés à la médecine comme Patrophile que de jeunes gens encore ignorants de quelque art que ce soit comme les destinataires du *Protreptique*. Mais plus fondamentalement, elle apparaît d'abord comme le

[9] Voir la définition donnée dans le *À Patrophile* (= *CAM*): ἐπιδεικνύον, ὅπερ οἱ παλαιοὶ φιλόσοφοι λέγουσι, τὸ πάσῃ τέχνῃ τὴν σύστασιν ἀπὸ τῆς κατὰ τὸ τέλος ἐννοίας γίγνεσθαι (I 227,3-5 K = p.56,13-14 Fortuna).

reflet d'une difficulté épistémologique fondamentale à rendre compte de l'ambiguïté irréductible d'un art comme la médecine. Au-delà des catégories traditionnelles, en grande partie héritées des Stoïciens et ici reprises par Galien, le médecin de Pergame peine visiblement à exprimer la spécificité d'un art qui décidément semble échapper à toute classification. Plus précisément, l'hésitation de Galien à enfermer la médecine dans un cadre précis et univoque fonctionne comme le révélateur d'un malaise plus subtil lié à la difficulté de penser la médecine comme art. En effet, et comme j'essaierai de le montrer à présent, alors même que le statut de la médecine en tant qu'art n'apparaît presque jamais remis en cause, à y regarder de plus près, il est en réalité bien loin d'être clairement admis, la *technè* le disputant sans cesse à l'*épistèmè* et, de façon plus inattendue peut-être, à la *stochastikè*.

Art et savoir

Lien et complémentarité τέχνη / ἐπιστήμη

Là encore, à ne considérer que le titre des traités galéniques, on constate que la médecine est sans ambiguïté désignée comme un art. Tel est le cas en particulier du traité que le médecin de Pergame a spécialement consacré à l'art de la médecine et intitulé *Art médical* (Τέχνη ἰατρική). Après un bref prologue méthodologique, Galien y définit d'emblée la médecine, en des termes directement hérités d'Hérophile, par la formule suivante (*Ars Med.* 1b, 1, p. 276,6-7 Boudon = I 307,5-6 K): Ἰατρική ἐστιν ἐπιστήμη ὑγιεινῶν καὶ νοσωδῶν καὶ οὐδετέρων; "La médecine est la science de ce qui est sain, malsain et neutre", établissant du même coup un lien étroit entre l'art et la science, entre la τέχνη et l'ἐπιστήμη.[10] Or, Galien le

[10] Sur cette définition héritée du médecin alexandrin Hérophile et reprise par Galien, voir mon article "Les définitions tripartites de la médecine chez Galien", in *ANRW* II 37, 2 (Berlin 1994), 1468-1490. Sur Hérophile, voir H. von Staden (Ed.), *Herophilus. The Art of Medicine in Early Alexandria* (Cambridge1989), 90 sqq.

sait bien, ce lien n'a rien d'évident et est loin d'aller de soi. Pour Aristote en particulier, la τέχνη, qui appartient à la sphère de la ποίησις (de la production), est clairement distinguée de l'ἐπιστήμη, qui, elle, relève d'une πρᾶξις, d'une activité démonstrative et déductive qui se déploie du connu à l'inconnu grâce notamment au συλλογισμός et à l'ἐπαγωγή.[11] Aussi, pleinement averti de ces difficultés, Galien éprouve-t-il immédiatement le besoin de préciser à son lecteur en quel sens il convient d'entendre ce mot d'ἐπιστήμη: "Quant au nom de science, il faut l'entendre en un sens général et non particulier" (τοῦ μὲν οὖν τῆς ἐπιστήμης ὀνόματος κοινῶς καὶ οὐκ ἰδίως ἀκούειν χρή).[12] Mais, à ce niveau de l'exposé, Galien ne précisera pas davantage sa pensée et il faudra attendre qu'il dénonce l'existence d'une certaine ambiguïté liée à la définition même de la médecine comme science (*Ars Med.* 1b, 9, p.277, 19 Boudon = I 309,3 sqq. K) pour qu'il revienne sur les différents sens d'ἐπιστήμη. Pour notre propos, et avant de revenir à ce passage fondamental de l'*Art médical*, il conviendra donc de tenter de discerner, chaque fois que nous rencontrerons le terme ἐπιστήμη lié à la notion d'art, ce qui, selon la terminologie galénique de l'*Art médical*, relève du particulier, c'est-à-dire du simple savoir à propos d'un objet donné et clairement défini, de ce qui relève du général, c'est-à-dire cette fois du domaine de la science entendue au sens large. En effet, alors même que l'exercice de l'art médical suppose le recours à l'*épistèmè* en tant que savoir donné sur un sujet particulier, en revanche en tant que science prise en un sens général, l'*épistèmè* entretient avec l'art des relations autrement plus complexes qui, pour ne pas devenir conflictuelles, nécessiteront la médiation d'un troisième terme, désigné par Galien sous le nom de *stochastikè*.

[11] Sur ces distinctions conceptuelles ici seulement esquissées, voir M. ISNARDI, *art.cit.*, 269 sqq. Voir en particulier Aristote, *Éthique à Nicomaque* 6, 3, 1139 b; 6, 10, 1143 a et *Politique* 4, 1, 1288 b. Il convient en outre de noter que si chez Aristote la distinction conceptuelle entre *technè* et *épistèmè* apparaît claire, leur attribution aux différents domaines de la pensée est beaucoup plus fluctuante. La médecine en particulier est également qualifiée d'ἐπιστήμη κατὰ μέρος dans l'*Éthique à Nicomaque* (6, 10, 1143 a 3) et de τέχνη dans la *Politique* (6, 1, 1288 b 19-21) à côté de l'art de la navigation et du tailleur.

[12] *Ars Med.* 1b, 1 (I 307,7-8 K = p.276,8-9 Boudon).

L'ἐπιστήμη comme fondement de la τέχνη

Comme le proclame triomphalement Galien, l'art suppose un savoir qui se transmet par un enseignement. Là réside d'ailleurs pour une grande part la grandeur de l'humanité à propos de laquelle Galien n'hésite pas à proclamer dans le *Protreptique*: "L'homme seul étant capable de science, apprend l'art qu'il désire" (καὶ ὅτι μόνος ἄνθρωπος, ἐπιστήμης ἐπιδεκτικός, ἣν ἂν ἐθελήσῃ τέχνην μανθάνει).[13]

Aussi celui qui s'y connaît dans l'art de la médecine est-il d'abord désigné comme le détenteur d'un savoir qui fonde sa supériorité. Et des expressions comme τὸν τῆς ὑγιεινῆς τέχνης ἐπιστήμονα (*San.Tu.* 1, 7, VI 32,10-11 K); τὸν ἐπιστήμονα καὶ ὑγιεινῆς ἁπάσης τέχνης (*San.Tu.* 1, 15, VI 77,14 K); σεμνῆς οὕτω τέχνης ἐπιστήμονι (*San.Tu.* 3, 13, VI 228,16 K); ὥστε χρὴ ... ἁπάσης ἐπιστήμονα τῆς περὶ τὸ σῶμα τέχνης γενέσθαι (*San.Tu.* 5, 2, VI 318,11-14 K) revêtent une valeur laudative manifeste sous la plume de Galien.[14]

Le médecin de Pergame nous donne ailleurs des renseignements précis sur le contenu de ce savoir indissociable de l'art médical. Certaines parties de l'art sont ainsi désignées comme faisant prioritairement l'objet d'un savoir. Tel est le cas de l'hygiène, dont l'art de la gymnastique (entendu comme art des exercices) ne constitue pas la moindre part: τῆς ὑγιεινῆς ἐπιστήμης οὐ φαυλότατόν ἐστι μόριον ἡ περὶ τὰ γυμνάσια τέχνη.[15] Ou encore de la pharmacologie qui suppose là encore un savoir précis à propos des médicaments.[16] Un passage du *Sur*

[13] *Protr.* 1 (I 2,3-5 K = p.84,10-12 Boudon).

[14] Voir aussi le jugement de Galien à propos des sectateurs d'Athénée d'Attale qui s'y connaissent en fièvres, à l'exception de celles dites "éphémères" sur lesquelles Galien a une opinion divergente: κινδυνεύει γὰρ οὖν δοξάζειν ὧδε καὶ ὁ τῶν ἀπ' Ἀθηναίου χορός, ἄνδρες οὐχὶ φαυλότατοι τά τ' ἄλλα τῆς τέχνης καὶ οὐχ ἥκιστα πυρετῶν ἐπιστήμης, περὶ ὧν κἀγὼ τό γε πλεῖστον αὐτοῖς σύμφημι, πλὴν ἕν τι παρίημι, τοὺς ἐφημέρους ὀνομαζομένους πυρετούς (*Diff.Feb.* 1, 7, VII 295,11-15 K).

[15] *San.Tu.* 4, 1, VI 234,17-18 K.

[16] *De simplicium medicamentorum temperamentis ac facultatibus* 6, prol. (XI 795,8 sqq. K): "La plus grande partie de l'usage des médicaments se trouve traitée dans les ouvrages de thérapeutique eux-mêmes qu'ont rédigés les anciens, ainsi

la constitution de la médecine 13 insiste tout particulièrement sur l'importance de ce savoir au service de l'art thérapeutique: "Celui qui possède la connaissance de toute la matière particulière des remèdes (ὁ … τῆς κατὰ μέρος ὕλης ἁπάσης ἐπιστήμην ἔχων *sc.* βοηθημάτων), non seulement de leur faculté, mais aussi de leur usage, celui-là aura parachevé toutes les causes salutaires, sans rien négliger de ce qui constitue l'art de la thérapeutique (τὴν τῆς θεραπευτικῆς τέχνης σύστασιν), qui consiste en ces deux points principaux, la connaissance (τὴν γνῶσιν) des corps auxquels sont appliqués les remèdes et la nature même des remèdes (καὶ αὐτὴν τὴν τῶν βοηθημάτων φύσιν)".[17] De ce point de vue, un savoir plus vaste peut englober des savoirs plus restreints. Tel est le cas du savoir relatif au régime dont Galien écrit dans le *Sur la méthode thérapeutique* qu'il ne constitue pas la moindre partie de l'art de la médecine, qui est grand, puisqu'il repose sur la connaissance des remèdes (on retrouve ici la pharmacologie), mais aussi des aliments et des boissons, des lotions, des cataplasmes et des clystères: ἀλλ' ὅλης οὔσης μεγάλης τῆς τέχνης ἕν τι τῶν μερῶν αὐτῆς οὐ τὸ φαυλότατόν ἐστιν ἐπιστήμη διαίτης, ἥτις ἐκ τούτων μάλιστα συμπληροῦται τῶν βοηθημάτων, τροφῶν καὶ πομάτων ἐπιβροχῶν τε καὶ καταπλασμάτων καὶ κλυστήρων.[18]

Plus encore, le fait de posséder un savoir dans un art autre que la médecine peut aider à la compréhension des préceptes du médecin. Tel est le sens de l'intervention de Galien quand dans le petit traité intitulé *Conseil pour un enfant épileptique* il fait part de ses réticences au père de l'enfant. Celui-ci, n'étant pas lui-même médecin, saura-t-il bien interpréter les conseils qui lui seront donnés? N'y a-t-il pas quelque danger à s'adresser à quel-

qu'en outre presque tous les modernes. Et de fait bien des choses ont été dites par Hippocrate, et aussi par Euryphon, Dieuchès, Dioclès, Pleistonax, Praxagoras et Hérophile, et il n'est aucun ancien qui n'ait plus ou moins contribué à l'art pour ce qui est de la science des médicaments" (795,14-15: καὶ οὐκ ἔστιν οὐδεὶς ἀνὴρ παλαιὸς ὃς οὐ συνεβάλλετό τι τῇ τέχνῃ μεῖζον ἢ μεῖον εἰς ἐπιστήμην φαρμάκων).

[17] *CAM* 13, 7, I 271,7-14 K = CMG V 1, 3, p.96,14-20 Fortuna.

[18] *MM* 11, 15, X 780,12-16 K.

qu'un qui n'est pas un homme de l'art et qui donc pourra ne pas comprendre ou mal comprendre les recommandations du médecin, notamment en ce qui concerne la mesure et l'occasion (le μέτρον et le καῖρος) dans l'administration des remèdes? Galien consentira cependant à poursuivre la rédaction de sa missive eu égard aux connaissances de son correspondant dans le domaine de la logique, cette formation représentant finalement à ses yeux un gage suffisant: "Ce n'est assurément pas pour les premiers venus des médecins que j'ai écrit mon ouvrage sur la méthode thérapeutique, mais toi et tous les autres qui êtes savants dans les arts logiques, tout en étant profanes en médecine, je pense que vous pourriez peut-être également retirer quelque utilité de cet écrit" (*Puer.Epil.* 1, XI 359,15-360,2 K: ἐκείνοις [*sc.* οὐδὲ τοὺς ἐπιτυχόντας τῶν ἰατρῶν] μὲν οὖν ἡ τῆς θεραπευτικῆς μεθόδου πραγματεία γέγραπται, σοὶ δὲ καὶ τοῖς ἄλλοις ὅσοι τεχνῶν μὲν τινῶν ἐστὲ λογικῶν ἐπιστήμονες, ἰδιῶται δὲ τῆς ἰατρικῆς, γένοιτ' ἂν ἴσως, οἶμαι, καὶ παρὰ τοῦδε τοῦ γράμματος ὠφέλεια).

Ce qui autorise ainsi Galien à s'adresser au père du jeune épileptique, c'est la certitude qu'il saura user d'une méthode logique sûre et infaillible. Car, aux yeux du médecin de Pergame, ce qui fonde le lien art/savoir c'est précisément l'existence d'une méthode. Dans ce même traité *Sur la méthode thérapeutique* 9, 6 (X 628), auquel Galien vient justement de faire référence dans le *Conseil pour un enfant épileptique*, Galien, après avoir traité des différents types de fièvres et de leurs causes, rappelle qu'il n'est pas possible d'acquérir la connaissance d'un art quel qu'il soit sans recourir d'une part à la méthode qui procède de ce qu'on appelle des théorèmes relatifs au général, et d'autre part à l'exercice qui s'appuie sur des exemples particuliers. Méthode et exercice étant inséparables et symbolisant les deux jambes sur lesquelles le médecin doit nécessairement s'appuyer pour atteindre la fin assignée à l'art quel qu'il soit, sinon il s'expose tel un boîteux (σκάζων), poursuit Galien, à beaucoup errer et se tromper en chemin.[19]

[19] *MM* 9, 6, X 628,10-17 K: εὖ εἰδότες ὡς οὐχ οἷόν τ' ἐστὶ τέχνης οὐδεμιᾶς ἐπιστήμην κτήσασθαι χωρὶς τοῦ μέθοδον μέν τινα διὰ τῶν καθόλου λεγομένων

On notera qu'en définissant l'art comme dépendant à la fois d'une méthode et d'un exercice, Galien introduit du même coup la thématique particulièrement féconde du général et du particulier.

À cette étape de la réflexion, on pourra donc conclure que l'*épistèmè* au sens de savoir particulier dans un domaine donné, loin de s'opposer à la *technè*, constitue au contraire le fondement de l'art, son θεμέλιον. Tel est en effet le terme même utilisé par Galien dans le prologue de son *Commentaire à la Nature de l'Homme,* quand, après avoir fustigé ceux qui refusent d'y voir un authentique traité d'Hippocrate,[20] il conclut: "De même que ces gens-là ne cessent de mal agir, de même nous ne cessons de leur rappeler de se souvenir de ce qui est exposé dans chacun de ses ouvrages, et qu'ils n'aillent pas, lorsque nous montrons qu'Hippocrate dans tous ses ouvrages a établi le fondement (θεμέλιον) de son art dans la connaissance des éléments qu'il avait découverts (*i.e.* le chaud, froid, sec et humide), délaissant cela, se mettre en quête de leur vérité".[21]

On ne s'étonnera donc pas qu'après avoir posé l'*épistèmè* comme fondement de la *technè*, Galien aille dans certains de ses écrits jusqu'à poser l'équation *technè/épistèmè*, les deux termes apparaissant presque comme interchangeables. Ainsi dans un passage du *Sur la constitution de l'art médical*, après s'être interrogé sur le statut exact de l'hygiène (ὑγιεινόν) à l'intérieur de l'art médical, se demandant si elle appartient au genre conservateur des états présents (φυλακτικόν) ou si plutôt elle ne diffère

θεωρημάτων, ἄσκησιν δὲ διὰ τῶν ἐν μέρει λαμβάνειν παραδειγμάτων· οὔτε γὰρ οἷόν τε χωρὶς τοῦ γυμνάσασθαι πολυειδῶς ἐν τοῖς κατὰ μέρος ἐπὶ τῶν καμνόντων ἃ χρὴ πράττειν· οὔτ' αὐτὴν τὴν γυμνασίαν ἐγχωρεῖ γίγνεσθαι προσηκόντως ἄνευ τῆς τοῦ καθόλου γνώσεως· ἐν ἐκείνοις μὲν γὰρ ἡ μέθοδος, ἡ δ' ἄσκησις ἐν τοῖς κατὰ μέρος.

[20] La *Nature de l'homme* est en réalité l'œuvre de Polybe, mais Galien attribue sa première partie sur les humeurs à Hippocrate.

[21] *HNH* 1, prol., XV 15,17-16,5 K: ὥσπερ οὖν ἐκεῖνοι κακουργοῦντες οὐ παύονται, οὕτω καὶ ἡμεῖς μεμνῆσθαι τῶν προκειμένων ἐν ἑκάστῳ τῶν ὑπομνημάτων ἀναμιμνήσκειν αὐτοὺς καὶ μήθ' ὅταν ἀποδεικνύωμεν Ἱπποκράτην κατὰ πάντα τὰ συγγράμματα θεμέλιον τῆς ἑαυτοῦ τέχνης τιθέμενον ἐν τῇ περὶ τῶν εὑρημένων στοιχείων ἐπιστήμῃ, καταλιπόντες τοῦτο, περὶ τῆς ἀληθείας αὐτῶν ζητῶσι … .

pas de la thérapeutique (θεραπευτικόν) par cela seulement qu'elle introduit de maigres corrections là où la thérapeutique, elle, en introduit de plus grandes, Galien conclut sur la nécessité pour tout homme de pouvoir disposer d'un art qui l'assiste: "Un corps qui conserverait son état précédent ne saurait avoir besoin d'un art (τέχνης) pour l'assister; mais la raison même pour laquelle il a besoin d'un savoir (ἐπιστήμης) qui puisse prendre soin de lui tient au fait qu'il est soumis à la corruption et ne demeure pas tel qu'il était précédemment".[22] Cet art et ce savoir ici confondus dans l'esprit de Galien, c'est bien sûr l'art médical dont aucun homme ne saurait longtemps faire l'économie.

Pour autant, si l'art médical peut parfois être confondu avec les différents savoirs particuliers qui en constituent le fondement, la médecine, précisément parce qu'elle a affaire au particulier, ne saurait sans difficulté épistémologique majeure être assimilée à l'*épistèmè* pris cette fois au sens général et aristotélicien de science.

Art et science

La médecine: art ou science?

La question du statut de la médecine, art ou science, appartient à un débat traditionnel, déjà alimenté par les prédécesseurs mêmes de Galien et tel qu'un traité apocryphe comme l'*Introduction ou le médecin* (XIV 674-797 K) s'est fait l'écho. Aussi, et avant même d'examiner la conception galénique telle qu'elle apparaît analysée et exposée dans l'*Art médical*, convient-il de faire un détour par l'*Introduction*, vraisemblablement antérieure d'un siècle à la rédaction du corpus galénique.[23]

[22] *CAM* 19, I 301,13-302,1 K = p.126,14-17 Fortuna: οὐ γὰρ δὴ διαφυλλάτοντί γε τῷ σώματι τὴν ἔμπροσθεν ἕξιν ἐπιστατούσης ἐδέησε τέχνης· ἀλλ' αὐτὸ τοῦτ' ἔστιν αἴτιον τοῦ δεῖσθαι τῆς προνοησομένης ἐπιστήμης, ὅτι διαφθείρεταί τε καὶ οὐ διαμένει τοιοῦτον, οἷον ἔμπροσθεν ἦν.

[23] Voir J. KOLLESCH, *Untersuchungen zu den Pseudogalenischen Definitiones Medicae* (Berlin 1973), 30-35.

Le chapitre 5 de ce traité, intitulé "La médecine, science ou art?" (684, 11 Εἰ ἐπιστήμη ἡ ἰατρική, ἢ τέχνη), est en effet entièrement consacré à la question qui nous intéresse ici. L'auteur de l'*Introduction* choisit d'abord de rapporter l'opinion de ceux qui considèrent la médecine comme une *épistèmè* (employé ici au sens général de science et non plus de savoir particulier). Mais aussitôt après, soulignant l'absence d'accord entre les médecins sur ce statut de science dévolu à la médecine, il introduit le terme de stochastique, avant même celui de *technè*, signe, s'il en était besoin, que le débat *technè/épistèmè* s'est désormais déplacé au profit d'un débat *épistèmè/stochastikè*.

"Certains des <médecins> logiques, écrit en effet l'auteur de l'*Introduction*, parmi lesquels Érasistrate, ont supposé que la médecine tenait en partie de la science (ὑπέλαβον τὸ μέν τι ἐπιστημονικὸν ἔχειν τὴν ἰατρικήν), par exemple les domaines de l'étiologie et de la physiologie, et en partie de la conjecture (τὸ δὲ στοχαστικόν), par exemple les domaines de la thérapeutique et de la sémiologie. Mais les méthodiques prétendent qu'elle est une science à part entière (οἱ δὲ μεθοδικοὶ καὶ δι' ὅλου ἐπιστήμην αὐτὴν ἀποκαλοῦσιν); tous deux se sont écartés du vrai, surtout les méthodiques."

On remarquera ici que la réflexion sur le statut de l'art apparaît liée d'emblée à la différenciation de différents domaines à l'intérieur de la médecine (étiologie, physiologie ou connaissance de la nature, thérapeutique et sémiologie). Qui plus est, en posant le problème du statut de la médecine en relation à la science d'une part, et à la conjecture d'autre part, la véritable question est de savoir non pas si la médecine est une science ou un art, mais si d'abord elle tient davantage de la science ou de la conjecture, les différentes écoles médicales ayant apporté sur ce point, selon le degré d'infaillibilité qu'elles accordent à la médecine, des réponses également divergentes. Encore faut-il, pour progresser à l'intérieur d'un tel débat, s'entendre sur une définition exacte de l'*épistèmè* ainsi revendiquée. Aussi l'auteur de l'*Introduction* va-t-il immédiatement s'employer à nous en donner une, définition largement influencée par les conceptions stoïciennes et à laquelle bien évidemment ne saurait répondre la médecine: “Une science en effet est une connaissance bien enracinée, solide, inébranlable par la raison (ἐπιστήμη γάρ ἐστι γνῶσις ἀραρυῖα καὶ βεβαία καὶ ἀμετάπτωτος ὑπὸ λόγου)”. On aura reconnu là la définition de l’*épistèmè* popularisée par Chrysippe en des termes presque exactement équivalents.[24] Or, commente l’auteur de l’*Introduction*, “cette conception de l’*épistèmè* ne peut exister chez les philosophes, encore moins dans le domaine de la connaissance de la nature (μάλιστα ἐν τῷ φυσιολογεῖν); à plus forte raison, ne saurait-elle se trouver dans la médecine, et même elle ne descend pas du tout au niveau des hommes”. Si cependant la médecine n’est certainement pas une science, elle ne peut non plus être que conjecture. Face à cette aporie, l’auteur de l’*Introduction* va donc proposer sa solution, en des termes là encore directement hérités de la philosophie stoïcienne: ni *épistèmè*, ni *stochastikè*, la médecine est d’abord une *technè*, ce dernier mot étant employé ici en un sens extrêmement précis: “C’est pourquoi ‘art’, conclut en effet l’auteur de l’*Introduction*, serait un nom juste pour la médecine (685,2-3: διὸ τέχνη εἰκότως ἂν λέγοιτο ἡ ἰατρική); un art en effet est un système résultant de conceptions et de notions, éprouvées relativement à la qualité et la quantité, et tendant vers une fin utile à la vie (τέχνη γάρ ἐστι σύστημα ἐγκαταλήψεων καὶ διανοιῶν, ποιόν τε καὶ ποσὸν συγγεγυμνασμένων, πρός τι τέλος νευουσῶν χρήσιμον τῷ βίῳ)”.[25] Telle est ici la définition proposée pour l’art, si du moins le texte grec de l’édition Kühn est correct.[26] Elle apparaît en tout cas directement influencée là encore

[24] *SVF* I 68, *ap*. Stob. *Ecl.* II p.73,19 W.: εἶναι τὴν ἐπιστήμην κατάληψιν ἀσφαλῆ καὶ ἀμετάπτωτον ὑπὸ λόγου.

[25] Je cite ici non pas exactement le texte de Kühn, mais celui établi par C. Petit qui prépare une édition de ce traité de Galien et qui, après collation des manuscrits, propose de lire συγγεγυμνασμένων donné par le manuscrit V plus ancien, au lieu de συγγεγυμνασμένον.

[26] Rapprochant ce passage du Ps.Galien de la définition canonique stoïcienne, M. Isnardi, *art.cit.*, 263, corrige en effet le texte de la façon suivante: τέχνη γάρ ἐστι σύστημα ἐκ καταλήψεων καὶ διανοιῶν, κατὰ ποιόν τε καὶ ποσὸν γεγυμνασμένων, πρός τε τέλος νευουσῶν χρήσιμον [lege χρήσιμον pro χρήσιμου donné par erreur] τῷ βίῳ.

par la définition de la *technè* donnée conjointement par Zénon et Chrysippe.[27] Or cette définition ne saurait mieux correspondre à la médecine qui précisément repose sur un ensemble de principes cohérents au sujet de l'homme et qui, pour l'auteur de *l'Introduction* comme pour Galien lui-même, a vu le jour "pour sauver et maintenir les hommes en bonne santé" (ἐπὶ γὰρ τὸ σώζειν καὶ ὑγιάζειν τοὺς ἀνθρώπους παρῆλθεν εἰς τὸν βίον). Ce bel accord sur la finalité de l'art masque mal cependant une difficulté essentielle liée au problème de l'infaillibilité de l'art et qui n'est toujours pas résolu. Car il faut bien reconnaître, et l'auteur de l'*Introduction* en convient immédiatement après, que certains arts atteignent toujours la fin qu'ils visent (menuiserie, construction navale, architecture), alors que d'autres "manquent leur fin, comme on manque un but, et ne la trouvent pas toujours, mais seulement la plupart du temps". Ces derniers sont alors qualifiés de conjecturaux (στοχαστικαί), comme précisément la médecine, la rhétorique, l'art du pilotage et le tir à l'arc. Enfin, et avant de conclure, notre auteur se fait l'écho d'une seconde distinction entre les arts, venant comme se superposer à la précédente (686,1-2: ἔστι δὲ καὶ ἑτέρα διαφορὰ τῶν τεχνῶν, διττὴ καὶ αὐτή) entre arts conjecturaux et non conjecturaux, distinction directement liée à la réalisation de la fin visée par l'art en question et qui peut être soit présente (art de la danse, cithare, lutte et tous les arts musicaux, la danse cessant quand le danseur s'arrête), soit future (statuaire, peinture, architecture et médecine, dont les effets se font ressentir après l'intervention du médecin). D'après ce témoignage, la pensée médicale antérieure à Galien, sans remettre directement en question le statut de la médecine en tant qu'art, semble ainsi avoir distingué deux niveaux de réflexion, entre arts conjecturaux et non conjecturaux d'abord, entre fin présente ou fin future ensuite. Ce sont ces deux niveaux d'analyse, peut-être issus de deux traditions distinctes, et en tout cas antérieures à Galien, qui seront repris et

[27] *SVF* I 73; II 95: τέχνη ἐστὶ σύστημα ἐκ καταλήψεων συγγεγυμνασμένων, πρός τι τέλος εὔχρηστον τῶν ἐν τῷ βίῳ.

enrichis dans son œuvre avec des variantes, des aménagements originaux, mais aussi de nouveaux prolongements.

La médecine est la science des choses telles et telles (τὸ ὁποίων)

La question du statut de la médecine, art ou science, apparaît directement liée pour l'auteur de l'*Introduction* au problème de sa fiabilité. Ignorant volontairement ce problème épistémologique majeur et s'en tenant au seul niveau de la théorie, Galien nous livre dans l'*Art médical* une définition de l'*épistèmè* aussi prudente que conciliante.

L'*Art médical*, nous l'avons dit, s'ouvre sur une définition de la médecine comme "science de ce qui est sain, malsain et neutre" (Ἰατρική ἐστιν ἐπιστήμη ὑγιεινῶν καὶ νοσωδῶν καὶ οὐδετέρων), *épistèmè* devant être entendu ici, selon les recommandations mêmes de Galien, "en un sens général et non particulier" (κοινῶς καὶ οὐκ ἰδίως), c'est-à-dire, nous l'avons vu, au sens de science, et non de simple savoir. Ces affirmations liminaires, Galien le perçoit lui-même, ne sauraient cependant se passer de quelque éclaircissement. Car, le médecin de Pergame en est bien conscient, la définition ainsi proposée de la médecine n'est pas exempte d'une certaine ambiguïté (Ib, 9, I 309,3-8 K): "Mais en ce qui concerne l'ensemble de la définition, il existe une certaine ambiguïté dans les termes (ἀμφιβολία τις) qu'il nous faut elle aussi éclaircir. En disant en effet que la médecine est la science (ἐπιστήμην) de ce qui est sain, malsain et neutre, on l'entend par là comme la science de toutes les particularités (σημαίνεται μὲν καὶ τὸ πάντων τῶν κατὰ μέρος), comme celle de certaines (τό τινων) ou comme celle de telles ou telles (τὸ ὁποίων)." Or à chacun de ces différents sens s'attachent des enjeux épistémologiques également différents. Si l'on assigne à la médecine la mission de rendre compte de toutes les particularités (τὸ πάντων), son domaine devient du même coup illimité et impossible à concevoir (ἀπεριόριστόν τε καὶ ἀδύνατον); si au contraire elle se limite à certains cas seulement (τὸ δέ τινων), son domaine est incomplet et n'obéit pas aux règles de l'art (ἐλλιπές τε καὶ οὐ τεχνικόν); si enfin elle se limite à tels ou tels cas pour lesquels seuls elle a compétence (τὸ δὲ ὁποίων), alors son domaine est cette fois "conforme aux règles de l'art et en même temps suffisant pour comprendre absolument toutes les parties qui composent l'art (τεχνικόν τε ἅμα καὶ διαρκὲς εἰς ἅπαντα τῆς τέχνης τὰ κατὰ μέρος)".

À lire ici Galien, il n'existe pas de difficulté majeure à qualifier la médecine d'*épistèmè*, il suffit seulement d'en définir strictement le domaine d'application à la connaissance des seuls faits qui relèvent de la compétence de la médecine. *Technè* et *épistèmè* se trouvent donc du même coup indissolublement liés, la seule définition de l'*épistèmè* réellement recevable étant celle qui se révèle précisément conciliable avec les exigences de l'art, c'est-à-dire la définition τὸ ὁποίων. Échappant à la critique aristotélicienne pour laquelle il ne saurait y avoir de science que du général, Galien, sans pour autant limiter le domaine de la médecine au traitement des seuls cas particuliers, lui assigne ce moyen terme qu'est la connaissance des seuls cas relevant de sa compétence. Ce faisant, il choisit fort habilement d'ignorer la difficulté majeure soulevée par l'auteur de l'*Introduction*, à savoir la question du caractère faillible de l'art médical. Or, un art qui parfois ne remplit pas sa fin peut-il encore être qualifié d'art ou de science? C'est à cette question, dictée par toute pratique médicale quotidienne, que Galien se devra d'apporter une réponse théorique originale et nuancée en accord cette fois non pas tant avec les critiques aristotéliciennes qu'avec les exigences stoïciennes.

Art et conjecture

La conjecture dite technique

C'est en effet confronté aux difficultés de la pratique médicale que Galien se verra contraint d'infléchir ses positions théoriques les plus marquées pour recourir dans le *Sur les lieux affectés* 3, 4 à ce que l'on nomme une "conjecture technique" (VIII

145,12-13 K: τῷ καλουμένῳ τεχνικῷ στοχασμῷ), c'est-à-dire "une conjecture fondée sur l'art", réalisant ainsi une curieuse alliance de mots entre *technè* et *stochastikè*.[28]

Pour mieux comprendre ce que Galien entend par là, il convient en effet de se référer à son traité *Sur les lieux affectés*, qui traite des lésions cachées plus que tout autres susceptibles de mettre en échec l'art et le savoir du médecin.[29] Dans ces cas difficiles, la stochastique apparaît moins comme une remise en cause directe de la *technè* et de l'*épistèmè* que comme un troisième terme susceptible de leur servir de relais. Prenons l'exemple des différents cas d'ischurie, c'est-à-dire de rétention d'urine, que peut avoir à connaître un médecin et dont la cause n'est pas toujours aisée à déterminer. Galien rapporte ainsi dans le *Sur les lieux affectés* 1, 1 qu'un homme ayant été frappé violemment à la partie appelée périnée, il s'ensuivit une inflammation qui entraîna une ischurie. Dans de tels cas, précédés d'un traumatisme connu et identifié, "nous diagnostiquons nettement la cause, commente Galien, mais dans certains autres peu nettement ... Nous mettons alors à profit la conjecture technique, selon l'expression habituelle, conjecture tenant le milieu entre une connaissance exacte et une ignorance complète."[30] La conjecture ici définie comme un moyen terme entre connaissance exacte et ignorance complète ne saurait donc se

[28] Signalons également cette autre curieuse alliance de mots dans le *Praes.Puls.* 1, 1, IX 216,16-18 K, où il est dit qu'en ces matières et en ces circonstances la vérité doit être explorée et conjecturée de tout côté: ἐν μὲν δὴ τοῖς τοιούτοις καιροῖς ἀναγκαῖόν ἐστι πανταχόθεν ἐπιτεχνᾶσθαί τε καὶ στοχάζεσθαι τἀληθοῦς.

[29] Après l'achèvement de ce papier, j'ai pu prendre connaissance de l'article consacré par S. FORTUNA aux différents modes de diagnostic chez Galien: "Il metodo della diagnosi in Galeno (*De locis affectis*, VIII, 1-452 K.)", in *Elenchos* 22 (2001), 281-304. La dernière partie de cette étude qui s'interroge sur les modalités d'un diagnostic "stochastique" rejoint pour l'essentiel mes propres conclusions.

[30] *Loc.Aff.* 1, 1, VIII 14,7-12 K: ἐπὶ μὲν δὴ τῶν τοιούτων ἐναργῶς ἡμῖν ἡ τῆς ἰσχουρίας αἰτία διαγινώσκεται· κατ' ἔνια δὲ τῶν ἄλλων οὐκ ἐναργῶς, ἀλλ' ὁ συνήθως ὀνομαζόμενος ὑπὸ πάντων ἤδη χρήσιμος ἡμῖν τεχνικὸς στοχασμός, ὃς ἐν τῷ μεταξύ πώς ἐστιν ἀκριβοῦς τε γνώσεως καὶ παντελοῦς ἀγνοίας.

passer du raisonnement. Bien au contraire, elle suppose le médecin capable d'exercer ce raisonnement (γεγυμνάσθαι χρὴ τὸν λόγον) pour "nettement distinguer non seulement quelle est l'affection, mais encore quel est le lieu affecté". En même temps, le recours à la conjecture exige de poser des limites précises à ce raisonnement en l'orientant vers un objet également précis et clairement défini: "Mais pour l'exercer convenablement, on n'ira pas rechercher s'il faut dire que c'est le col de la vessie qui est affecté par l'obstruction que cause la pierre ou le caillot, ou que c'est la fonction qui est lésée, tandis que le col est exempt d'affection. Telles sont les questions que se pose Archimède, questions bien inutiles pour l'art (περιττὰ πρὸς τὴν τέχνην). D'autres diront que ce n'est pas la fonction même qui est lésée, substituant au mot lésion le mot empêchement (ἐμποδίζεσθαι). Comme si ce faisant, ils rendaient service à l'art médical!..." De semblables errements sont sévèrement fustigés par Galien. Ce sont là des recherches purement spéculatives (1, 1, VIII 15,17-18 K: αἱ μὲν δὴ τοιαῦται ζητήσεις, ὡς ἔφην, λογικαί τινές εἰσιν καὶ γυμνάζουσι τὸν λογισμόν), qui exercent le raisonnement sans aider ni au diagnostic des affections ni à la découverte des lieux affectés. Or la conjecture technique, en se mettant au seul service de l'art, se gardera également de l'élucubration et de la spéculation. S'appuyant sur de solides connaissances anatomiques, elle s'efforcera ainsi d'échapper à ce qui, au-delà de ses mérites propres, constitue il est vrai son principal inconvénient, sa propension à générer de longues discussions (19,1: καὶ διὰ ταῦτά γε μακρὸς ὁ λόγος γίγνεται).

*Domaines respectifs de la conjecture et de l'*épistèmè *à l'intérieur de la* technè

Le recours à la conjecture, loin de ruiner les prétentions de l'art à l'exactitude, apparaît en effet comme un relais possible de l'ἐπιστήμη confrontée à des réalités médicales particulièrement imprévisibles. En ce sens, à l'intérieur de la médecine définie comme τέχνη, certains domaines relèveront naturellement soit du στοχάζεσθαι, soit de l'ἐπιστήμη.[31]

L'établissement du pronostic en particulier constitue l'un des domaines privilégiés de l'exercice de la conjecture. Confronté à la difficulté de connaître et prévoir les paroxysmes et les constitutions des maladies (τοὺς δὲ παροξυσμοὺς καὶ τὰς καταστάσιας) Galien déclare, dans le *Commentaire aux Aphorismes* 1, 12, XVIIB 380 sqq., qu'il est en général possible de diagnostiquer la force ou la vigueur du malade (τῆς δυνάμεως τοῦ κάμνοντος) par exemple en prenant le pouls et en recourant à tout ce qui est recommandé dans le *Pronostic*. Mais en revanche il n'est pas toujours possible d'identifier l'intensité de cette vigueur ou résistance du malade de façon parfaitement exacte. Il faut alors tenter de s'en approcher au plus près en recourant à "une conjecture technique" (τῷ τεχνικῷ γοῦν στοχασμῷ πλησίον ἀφικνεῖσθαι), Galien faisant ici d'Hippocrate le champion avant la lettre de toute conjecture technique.[32] Confronté à de nombreuses maladies, ce dernier, selon Galien, s'est en effet très souvent révélé capable d'en acquérir une connaissance exacte, et pour ainsi dire scientifique (πολλάκις μὲν ἀκριβῶς καὶ ὡς ἂν εἴπῃ τις ἐπιστημονικῶς), mais assez souvent également il en a acquis une connaissance conjecturale, et pour autant non contraire à l'art, ni éloignée de la vérité, mais qui au contraire puisse nous permettre de nous en approcher de fort près.[33]

[31] Selon une partition entre les différents domaines de l'art médical déjà évoquée par l'auteur de l'*Introductio sive medicus.*

[32] *Hipp.Aph.* 1, 12, XVIIB 382,7-18 K: ὅθεν οὐδὲ ἀδύνατον ἔφησέ τις εἶναι διαγνῶναι μέγεθος δυνάμεως· ἀλλ' εἰ καὶ μὴ δυνατὸν ἀκριβῶς αὐτῆς ἐξευρεῖν τὸ ποσόν, τῷ τεχνικῷ γοῦν στοχασμῷ πλησίον ἀφικνεῖσθαι συγχωροῦσιν ἅπαντες· τὴν δὲ τοῦ νοσήματος κατάστασιν ὁποία τις ἔσται καὶ τοὺς κατὰ μέρος παροξυσμοὺς πολλοῖς τῶν ἰατρῶν ἀδύνατον ἔδοξε διαγνῶναι, οὐ μὴν Ἱπποκράτει γε· ἀλλὰ κἀνταῦθα καθάπερ ἐπὶ τῶν ἄλλων, πολλάκις μὲν ἀκριβῶς καὶ ὡς ἂν εἴπῃ τις ἐπιστημονικῶς, πολλάκις δὲ στοχαστικῶς μέν, ἀλλ' οὐκ ἀτέχνως, οὐδὲ πόρρω τῆς ἀληθείας, ἀλλ' ἐγγὺς καὶ πλησίον ἀφιξόμεθα, τήν τε μέλλουσαν ἀκμὴν προγινώσκοντες καὶ τὰς ἀνταποδόσεις τῶν παροξυσμῶν.

[33] Il convient cependant de noter que, dans le *Corpus hippocratique*, le verbe στοχάζεσθαι ne désigne pas encore la conjecture au sens galénique du terme, mais

Car bien loin de déprécier l'art, le recours à la conjecture en fait partie intégrante et celui qui s'avèrerait incapable d'y recourir, ne serait ni plus ni moins qu'un mauvais médecin. Ainsi dans le *Contre ceux qui ont écrit sur le cours des maladies* est réaffirmée l'absolue nécessité pour le médecin, s'il veut être utile au malade, d'être capable de pronostiquer les paroxysmes des maladies, et ce particulièrement à propos des fièvres récurrentes, tierces ou quartes. Or nul autre moyen n'est plus approprié pour parvenir à ce résultat que le recours à la conjecture.[34] L'art de la conjecture cependant n'est pas toujours aisé. Le médecin qui ne parviendrait pas dès le début à manier correctement la conjecture se voit donc encouragé par Galien à y parvenir avec l'aide du temps (480,3: προϊόντος δὲ τοῦ χρόνου). Mais celui qui, faute de savoir recourir à la conjecture, continuerait d'être tenu en échec dans son pronostic des crises, alors celui-là est sévèrement désigné par Galien comme un de ces médecins qui ignorent une partie importante de leur art (480,16: πολὺ μέρος οὗτος τῆς τέχνης ἀγνοεῖ). Cette connaissance, ainsi que le recours à la conjecture technique qui en est la condition même, fait donc non seulement partie de l'art mais, aux yeux de Galien, en constitue une part revendiquée comme importante.[35]

le simple effort du médecin pour 'viser juste' et atteindre son but. L'idée de conjecture, elle, est exprimée par un autre verbe, τεκμαίρεσθαι. Voir sur ce point ma communication au XIe Colloque International Hippocratique de Newcastle (28-30 août 2002) intitulée "Art, science et conjecture d'Hippocrate à Platon et Aristote".

34 *Adv.Typ.Scr.* 2, VII 479,16-480,2 K: 'Επεὶ τοίνυν οὐδὲν οὕτω χρήσιμόν ἐστι, καὶ μάλιστα ἐν τοῖς πυρετοῖς, ὡς τὸ προγινώσκειν τὰς ἀρχὰς τῶν ἐσομένων παροξυσμῶν, ἐὰν μέν τις ἀπ' ἀρχῆς οἷός τε ᾖ στοχασμῷ τεχνικῷ τοῦτ' ἐξεργάζεσθαι, μέγιστα τὸν κάμνοντα δι' ὅλου τοῦ νοσήματος ὠφελήσει.

35 Le *De locis affectis* 3, 4, VIII 145 K, fait ainsi allusion à deux types de diagnostic possibles: un diagnostic scientifique (145,11: ἐπιστημονικὴν διάγνωσιν) et un diagnostic qui relève de la conjecture dite technique (145,12-13: τῷ καλουμένῳ τεχνικῷ στοχασμῷ) et dont les conclusions se vérifient généralement, tant est grande la puissance de la conjecture technique. La même idée est à nouveau abordée et développée dans le *De plenitudine* 11, 37, VII 581 K (= p.76,26 éd. C. Otte) où il est dit que pour établir son diagnostic, le médecin se base: 1) sur des signes scientifiques (582,14-15 K = p.78,16 Otte: ἔνια μὲν γὰρ τῶν γνωρισμάτων ἐστὶν ἐπιστημονικά) tels que la tension, le poids, le gonflement des veines, la couleur, le mouvement du pouls; 2) sur des signes qui le sont moins

Complexité de la conjecture technique

Aussi convient-il à présent d'examiner précisément en quoi consiste cette complexité de la conjecture technique et pourquoi le pronostic, dont la thérapeutique elle-même dépend dans une large mesure, relève nécessairement de la stochastique. Galien n'est certes pas le premier médecin à développer une telle théorie de la conjecture et de ce point de vue la comparaison avec les conceptions d'un Alexandre d'Aphrodise sur la médecine considérée comme art stochastique pourront s'avérer fructueuses.[36] Mais la richesse des analyses galéniques sur ce thème apparaît de façon originale dans l'effort manifesté par le médecin de Pergame pour dépasser le simple niveau théorique d'une réflexion générale sur la stochastique au profit d'un exposé clair et précis consacré aux diverses modalités pratiques de l'application de la *stochastikè technè* aux différents cas particuliers rencontrés. Aussi, dans le *Sur la constitution de l'art médical*, *CAM* 17 (I 289,1 sqq. K = p.112,13 sqq. Fortuna), saisit-il l'occasion de revenir sur la difficulté liée à l'établissement de tout pronostic. Celui qui veut rassembler (constituer) l'art pronostic (τῷ μὲν οὖν πρῶτον βουλομένῳ συστήσασθαι τέχνην προγνωστικὴν) doit en effet d'abord être conscient, rappelle Galien, qu'une maladie dont la guérison intervient naturellement au bout de deux mois ne peut se résoudre en quatre jours. Mais comme de plus en plus de médecins établissent des pronostics, les profanes

(582,18-583,3 K: ἔνια δὲ ἀπολείπεται τούτων) tels que rétention des excrétions, vie inactive, aliments trop nombreux et trop nourrissants et bains après le repas qui, s'ils se trouvent réunis aux premiers, atteignent à un statut proche de celui des signes dits scientifiques (p.78,20-21: συνιόντα μέντοι τὰ σύμπαντα τοῖς ἐπιστημονικοῖς ἐγγὺς ἥκει); 3) sur des signes liés au caractère habituel de l'affection (le fait que le patient soit fréquemment la proie des maladies pléthoriques) et tout ce qui relève des lieux et des saisons. Les catégories 2 et 3 relèvent du stochastique avec une plus grande proximité avec le scientifique pour la catégorie 2. On a ainsi trois degrés d'exactitude scientifique, de 1 à 3, de l'*épistèmè* au stochastique.

[36] Voir en particulier l'article de K. IERODIAKONOU, "Alexander of Aphrodisias on medicine as a stochastic art", in *Ancient Medicine in its Socio-Cultural Context*, ed. by Ph.J. VAN DER EIJK, H.F.J. HORSTMANSHOFF, P.H. SCHRIJVERS (Amsterdam-Atlanta 1995), II 473-485.

ne s'interrogent même plus pour savoir si un pronostic est possible ou non, mais tiennent tous la chose pour possible et s'enquièrent auprès des médecins pour savoir quel jour la maladie se résoudra. Or il n'en va pas du tout ainsi et un pronostic n'est possible qu'à certaines conditions que Galien va s'employer à définir, n'hésitant pas au passage à briguer le titre de premier médecin à avoir véritablement constitué l'art du pronostic (οὐδὲν ἂν εἴη χεῖρον ὑποθέσθαι νῦν πρῶτον ἡμᾶς συνίστασθαι τέχνην προγνωστικήν). "Il faut en particulier nécessairement, pour qu'un pronostic puisse être réalisé, que certains faits adviennent de façon assurée dans le futur (Ἓν μὲν δὴ καὶ πρῶτον ἀναγκαῖον, εἴπερ εἴη τις πρόγνωσις, εἶναί τινα βεβαίως ἐσόμενα κατὰ τὸν μέλλοντα χρόνον). Et il faut s'efforcer de découvrir quels sont les faits de cette nature et en quel nombre (τίνα τε καὶ πόσα τὰ τοιαῦτά ἐστιν)". Le problème vient cependant du fait que tout ce qui est susceptible de concerner le malade n'a pas pour autant une existence nécessaire (οὐ γὰρ δὴ πάντα γε τὰ γενησόμενα περὶ τὸν κάμνοντα τὴν γένεσιν ἀναγκαίαν ἔχει). Et Galien de donner des exemples de ces événements non nécessaires qui sont cependant susceptibles d'influer sur le cours de la maladie: le bruit des voisins la nuit, les aboiements des chiens peuvent rendre le malade insomniaque, mais non nécessairement, ce qui rend également le pronostic non assuré (290,7-8 K = p.114,2-3 Fortuna: ὧν οὐδὲν οὔτ' ἀναγκαίαν ἔχει τὴν γένεσιν οὔτε βεβαίαν τὴν πρόγνωσιν). Autre exemple, une humeur superflue peut s'écouler à l'intérieur du corps envahissant une partie nécessaire à la vie, comme elle peut aussi bien se déplacer d'une partie importante à une partie non importante. De l'humeur passée dans la partie importante résultera nécessairement un danger extrême, tandis que de celle déplacée vers une partie non importante résultera la guérison instantanée et imprévisible du malade (290,15-17 K = p.114,9-10 Fortuna: τῷ μεταστάντι δ' ἐξαιφνίδιός τε καὶ ἀπροσδόκητος ἡ τοῦ κάμνοντος σωτηρία). "Aussi, dans de telles constitutions, ne peut-on établir de pronostic que de ce qui est mal assuré et incertain, sans qu'il soit possible de découvrir avec exactitude quelle fin en résultera" (290,17-291,3 K = p.114,11-13

Fortuna: Τῶν μὲν δὴ τοιούτων καταστάσεων αὐτὸ τοῦτο μόνον ἔστι προγνῶναι, τὸ ἀβέβαιόν τε καὶ σφαλερόν, οὐ μὴν ἐς ὅ τι τελευτήσει δυνατὸν ἀκριβῶς ἐξευρεῖν). Mais si le médecin peut disposer d'un seul point fixe et assuré, à la manière d'un Archimède pour poser son levier, comme par exemple l'assurance que les humeurs superflues ne s'écoulent plus mais demeurent dans le lieu qu'elles occupent, alors il lui devient possible d'établir un pronostic (ἐγχωρεῖ προγνῶναι τὸ μέλλον). En effet, dans la mesure où nous connaissons la nature de chacune des humeurs et où la coction de chacune d'elles, en dehors des cas de pléthore, se fait en un temps fixé d'avance (291,9-10 K = p.114,18 Fortuna: καὶ ταῦτα προθεσμίαν ἕξει πέψεως ἰδίαν ἕκαστον), dans ces conditions, il sera possible de faire quelque conjecture technique sur leur coction, si évidemment tout ce qui regarde le soin du malade est fait correctement (p.114,19: οὕτω γὰρ ἐγχωρήσει τι καὶ περὶ τῆς πέψεως αὐτῶν στοχάσασθαι τεχνικῶς ἁπάντων γε δηλονότι τῶν περὶ τὸν κάμνοντα πραττομένων ὀρθῶς). Car toute faute commise (sous-entendu au cours du traitement) constitue une cause susceptible de retarder la résolution de la maladie ou d'anticiper la mort (et donc de mettre le pronostic en défaut). En conclusion, seuls se réaliseront les pronostics de l'excellent médecin quand il soigne lui-même un malade qui, pour sa part, ne commet aucune erreur relativement aux prescriptions du médecin (291,16-292,1 K = p.114,24-25 Fortuna: μόνου γὰρ αἱ προγνώσεις ἀποβήσονται τοῦ ἀρίστου ἰατροῦ, θεραπεύοντος αὐτοῦ τὸν κάμνοντα μηδὲν ἁμαρτάνοντα).

L'utilité de la conjecture technique, au sein de l'art médical, se manifeste ainsi de façon privilégiée dans les cas les plus susceptibles de mettre en échec les ressources de l'*épistèmè*, en tant que connaissance ferme et assurée (γνῶσις βεβαῖα). Loin de nier le caractère faillible de la médecine, le médecin pleinement conscient de son art saura en effet puiser dans les ressources de la conjecture dite technique, c'est-à-dire réalisée selon les règles de l'art, un nouveau titre de gloire. Mais surtout et en même temps, en abordant le cas de chaque patient de façon individuelle, il se sera donné les moyens d'apprécier ce qui, dans le cadre d'un savoir général, ressort de la connaissance de données particulières.

La médecine art du particulier et de l'individualité

Confronté à la nécessité de conjuguer les exigences d'un savoir général sur la médecine avec les réalités individuelles rencontrées lors de sa pratique médicale, Galien a bien compris que la résolution de la dichotomie art/science ne pourrait se réaliser qu'à l'intérieur du champ plus vaste de la méthode. Aussi la réflexion de Galien sur ce thème apparaît-elle comme fortement dépendante du débat qui agite alors les tenants des différentes écoles médicales de son temps, empirique et surtout méthodique. Ainsi, dans le *Sur la méthode thérapeutique* 3, 7, la critique des méthodiques qui succède à celle des empiriques (3, 6) sert d'introduction aux propres conceptions galéniques sur la véritable méthode (*MM* 3, 6, X 204,6 K: τὴν ὄντως δηλονότι μέθοδον). Les méthodiques que Galien se plaît à désigner comme paradoxalement "dépourvus de méthode" (ἀμέθοδοι), usent d'une méthode qui n'est en réalité qu'un vain mot, vidé de tout contenu (3, 7, X 204,7 Τὴν γὰρ τῶν ἀμεθόδων Θεσσαλείων μέθοδον ὄνομα μόνον οἶσθα δήπου κενόν, ἔρημον ἔργου παντός). "Ils s'imaginent en effet, parce qu'ils disent que les plaies creuses (*i.e.* les ulcères) ont besoin d'être comblées, que ce qui est comblé a besoin de cicatrisation, qu'un excès de chair a besoin d'être réduit, que d'autre part ce qui est souillé a besoin d'être nettoyé, ce qui est nettoyé a besoin de cicatrisation et ce qui est sanglant a besoin d'être rapproché, avoir exposé une méthode pour la guérison des plaies. Tant ils sont éloignés de savoir qu'aux natures plus humides sont utiles les médicaments moins desséchants, et aux natures plus sèches les plus desséchants". Galien annonce alors qu'il a pris l'exemple de la cicatrisation des plaies, mais que ces remarques vaudront pour l'art de guérir dans son ensemble (3, 7, X 205,8-9 K: περὶ πάσης ὁμοῦ τῆς ἰάσεως ἐν τῷ καθόλου). Car la remarque de Galien sur la nécessité de considérer si les natures sont sèches ou humides ne se comprend en réalité qu'en référence à cette observation fondamentale qui non seulement repose sur un fondement logique, mais aussi sur l'expérience, à savoir que "toute nature ne demande pas les mêmes médicaments" (205,11: οὐ τῶν αὐτῶν ἅπασα φύσις δεομένη φαρμάκων). Le corollaire immédiat de cette observation, assénée comme une vérité fondamentale, sera qu'il faut considérer la nature de chaque malade pour adapter chaque traitement à chaque nature individuelle (205,17-206,1: ὅτι τε τὴν φύσιν ἐπισκεπτέον ἐστὶ τοῦ κάμνοντος, ὅτι τε καθ' ἕκαστον ἄνθρωπον ἰδίᾳ τίς ἐστι θεραπεία). Enfin, conséquence immédiate de cet état de fait, étant donné que le caractère individuel de chaque nature est indicible et insaisissable dans la perspective d'une science exacte, le meilleur médecin de toutes les maladies particulières est celui qui sera en possession d'une méthode qui lui permette à la fois de diagnostiquer les natures (*i.e.* les natures individuelles) et conjecturer les remèdes propres à chacune (3, 7, 206,1-6 K: καὶ τρίτον ἐπὶ τούτοις ὡς ἐπειδὴ τὸ τῆς ἑκάστου φύσεως ἴδιον ἄρρητόν ἐστι καὶ πρὸς τὴν ἀκριβεστάτην ἐπιστήμην ἄληπτον, οὗτος ἂν ἄριστος ἰατρὸς εἴη τῶν κατὰ μέρος ἁπάντων νοσημάτων, ὁ μέθοδόν τινα πορισάμενος ἐξ ἧς διαγνωστικὸς μὲν τῶν φύσεων ἔσοιτο, στοχαστικὸς δὲ τῶν ἑκάστης ἰδίων ἰαμάτων).

Car penser qu'il puisse y avoir un traitement commun pour tous les hommes, comme le pensent les méthodiques, est en réalité de la dernière bêtise (ἐσχάτως ἠλιθιόν). De fait, assène Galien à son lecteur qui n'aurait encore pas compris, "ce n'est pas le genre humain en général qu'on soigne, mais chacun d'entre nous, l'un ayant bien évidemment un tempérament et une nature, et l'autre un autre" (206,14-17: θεραπεύεται μὲν γὰρ οὐχ ὁ κοινὸς καὶ γενικὸς ἄνθρωπος, ἀλλ' ἡμῶν ἕκαστος, ἄλλος ἄλλην ἔχων δηλονότι κρᾶσίν τε καὶ φύσιν). Et Galien de poursuivre: "Car si je savais exactement trouver la nature propre de chacun, je serais tel, je suppose, que fut Asclépios; mais puisque c'est impossible, en revanche pour ce qui est de s'en approcher le plus près qu'il est possible à un homme, j'ai moi-même appris à m'y exercer et j'engage les autres à le faire" (207,1-5: ἐγὼ δ' εἰ καὶ τὴν ἑκάστου φύσιν ἀκριβῶς ἠπιστάμην ἐξευρίσκειν, οἷον ἐπινοῶ τὸν Ἀσκληπιόν, αὐτὸς ἂν ἦν τοιοῦτος· ἐπεὶ δ' ἀδύνατον τοῦτο, τὸ γοῦν ἐγγυτάτω προσιέναι καθόσον ἀνθρώπῳ δυνατὸν αὐτός τε ἀσκεῖν ἔγνωκα καὶ τοῖς ἄλλοις παρακελεύομαι).

Pour le dire autrement, en matière de médecine, l'exactitude scientifique est de l'ordre du divin, seule la conjecture appartient à l'humain. De ce point de vue, le recours à la stochastique, en rendant compte de l'irréductible singularité du vivant, offre un fondement épistémologique indiscutable à la supériorité en quelque sorte ontologique de la médecine, seule de tous les autres arts à avoir affaire à l'humain.

DISCUSSION

J. Barnes: Your polished and lucid paper is very persuasive in its general lines. But in one or two specific places I am inclined to read the texts in a slightly different way, for example: (1) The two senses of ἐπιστήμη, κοινῶς and ἰδίως are surely an example of a common phenomenon: a word has a 'generic' and a 'specific' sense (many names for animals in English — cf. 'duck', 'goose' — are like that). The word ἐπιστήμη in the generic sense is any organized body of knowledge; ἐπιστήμη in the specific sense is any organized body of theoretical knowledge. (2) The threefold ἀμφιβολία at *Ars Med.* 1(I 309,4 K) perhaps alludes to, and answers a stark sceptical objection to definitions of this type 'X is a science of Ys': of every individual Y? — No, there are infinitely many individuals. Then of some individuals Ys? — No, for thus it would not be a science. The sceptic concludes that the definition is bad. Galen replies by insisting that X is not knowledge of individual Ys but of sorts of Y. And in this he is thoroughly Aristotelician.

V. Boudon: En ce qui concerne votre première remarque sur le sens 'générique' ou 'spécifique' que peut revêtir un même mot selon les contextes, il me semble utile de la rapprocher du commentaire du médecin égyptien Ali ibn Ridwan (in *Articella,* Venise 1523), nourri de philosophie aristotélicienne, qui recommande en effet d'entendre ici κοινῶς en tant que genre commun qui regroupe tous les arts relatifs aux sciences naturelles (*genus est commune non proprium istis artibus*). Cette interprétation ne me semble pas inconciliable avec les deux traductions d'ἐπιστήμη que j'ai proposées, à savoir 'la science' entendue en un sens général, à distinguer du 'savoir' entendu en un sens particulier. En ce qui concerne le second point, Galien reste assez vague sur ce qu'il faut entendre par τὸ πάντων τῶν κατὰ μέρος, τό τινων et τὸ ὁποίων. Ali ibn Ridwan, là encore, comprend qu'il s'agit d'une part de la science que l'on peut tirer des différents cas eux-mêmes dépendant des différentes parties de la médecine (*scientiam ex partibus medicine*), et d'autre part de celle relative aux cas individuels, qui sont en nombre infini (*individua infinita*), le recours à un ensemble de règles et de canons (*canones et regulae*) permettant seul d'aborder les cas particuliers en les classant à l'intérieur de différentes catégories déjà connues (τὸ ὁποίων). Il faut d'ailleurs signaler que ce passage a très tôt donné lieu à des interprétations divergentes.

M. Frede: I think it might help to see Galen's conception of the art of medicine as a stochastic art against the background of discussions since the end of the 5th century B.C. concerning the question whether medicine is a τέχνη at all, given, for instance the fact that doctors often fail to cure the patient. The response is that it lies in the nature of the art of medicine that one can fail to cure a patient without this reflecting badly on the competence of the doctor or of the state of the art of medicine. To say that the art of medicine is conjectural is to say that even if medical science were perfected and the doctor had completely mastered the art of medicine, the exercize of the art in the individual case would involve a conjectural element, given which success is not guaranteed. One tries to capture this by distinguishing between the τέλος and the σκόπος of the art. Curing the patient is the τέλος, doing the humanly possible to cure the patient is the σκόπος. One can do the humanly possible without managing to cure the patient. There are different possible views as to why this is so. One set of views relies on the limits of human knowledge and turns even on the limits of knowledge of the perfect doctor; the other set of views relies on the assumption that some of the empirical facts relevant to the cure by their very nature cannot be known, rather than in virtue of some limitation of human knowledge.

V. Boudon: Il est certain que la question du statut de l'art a très tôt été posée en relation étroite avec son caractère faillible ou infaillible. L'auteur du traité hippocratique *De l'art* 4, 1, p.227,8-10 Jouanna, déplore déjà que "du fait que tous ne guérissent pas, pour cette raison l'art est désormais blâmé". Mais c'est aussitôt pour ajouter (6, 4, p.230,18-20 Jouanna) que "la médecine, elle, dans la mesure où elle est de l'ordre du pourquoi et de la prévision, a et aura manifestement toujours une réalité". À l'intérieur de ce débat, la distinction τέλος / σκόπος sur laquelle s'ouvre le *De sectis ingredientibus* de Galien (1, I 64,1-2: "L'art médical a pour but la santé, pour fin, son acquisition"), apparaît d'autant plus fondamentale qu'elle entre dans la définition même de l'art, chaque art étant constitué en vue d'une fin (voir sur ce thème le *De constitutione artis medicae*). Et je vous remercie, précisément à propos de l'impossible infaillibilité de l'art médical, d'avoir mis cette difficulté en relation avec le débat consacré aux limites de la connaissance humaine.

R.J. Hankinson: Merci bien pour votre communication à la fois très intéressante, très claire et très riche. I have a few small observations to make. In particular it seems to me that there is a text you did not cite which is particularly relevant from *De optima secta*, a text which I am sure is not by Galen, but since you discussed in some detail the *Introductio* which is also not authentic, it seems permissible to do so. Towards the beginning of that text (*Opt.Sect.* 4, I 112-15 K), the author is discussing the status of medical theorems, and asks whether, medicine being a *technê stochastikê*, its stochastic nature is to be discovered in the theorems themselves, or in the application of them. And indeed the first possibility might itself be distinguished as follows, following the sorts of distinctions made by Michael Frede: are the theorems stochastic because the world itself is metaphysically indeterminate in some way, or is it simply for epistemic reasons (this mirrors the question in the Peripatetic tradition as to whether Aristotle's "for the most part" propositions are merely provisional and could in principle be replaced by exceptionless generalizations, or whether they actually represent the real nature of things)? But the author clearly comes down on the side of taking the theorems themselves to be universal generalizations, and the stochastic nature of the art to enter at the level of their application, which fits well what Galen himself says elsewhere, for instance in the pharmacology, that it is difficult accurately to determine precise temperatures, and the precise *dunameis* of various drugs, and also in the book on the *kairoi* of diseases that it is hard to estimate exactly the appropriate times. Again the problem seems to arise at the level of practice and this seems to me to follow in a very long tradition, stretching all the way back at least to the Hippocratic.

V. Boudon: Merci beaucoup pour cette référence et pour vos remarques sur la difficulté pour le médecin à penser le passage de la théorie à la pratique, le recours à la stochastique figurant sans nul doute un des outils de prédilection du praticien en pareil cas.

T. Tieleman: You refer to the Stoic definition of τέχνη as used by the author of the pseudo-Galenic *Introductio sive medicus* (XIV 685 K). Its emphasis on a useful goal, you suggest, also suits Galen's concept of medicine. You further argue that the Stoic definition involves a difficulty — for Galen, as I take it — because medicine is obviously not an infaillible art. I have one remark and one question. 1) Insofar as the Stoic definition is concerned, it should be noted that it does not imply infaillibility on the level of practical application. On the contrary, the Stoic insisted that rational choice does not guarantee that its intended effect is achieved. This does not detract from the correctness of the decision, nor from the knowledge and/or art which underlies the decision. In other words, one may be a perfectly wise person while not achieving one's aims in the practical sphere. Seen in this light, the Stoic definition is even better suited to medical theorists such as Galen. 2) Could you expatiate a little on Galen's response to the Stoic definition? You do imply that he responded to it. As it is, you now refer to a pseudo-Galenic treatise only.

V. Boudon: Merci pour votre remarque à laquelle je souscris pleinement. Je pense en particulier à ce passage attribué à Chrysippe (*SVF* III 6 d'après Alexandre d'Aphrodise, *Quaest.* 2, 16, p.61,1 Bruns) sur la στοχαστικὴ τέχνη à l'intérieur duquel il examine pourquoi les arts stochastiques réalisent leur fin d'une tout autre manière que les arts non stochastiques. L'une des réponses proposées, en particulier, est que pour les arts conjecturaux, la fin ne consiste pas à atteindre tel ou tel objet, mais d'abord à agir en tout selon les règles de l'art (κατὰ τὴν τέχνην), et ce, même si le succès ne suit pas toujours. En effet, il convient d'être averti que la réussite dans certains cas dépend de conditions qui ne relèvent pas toutes de l'art (ἃ μὴ ἔστιν ἐπὶ μόνῃ τῇ τέχνῃ). En ce qui concerne votre question, je répondrai que l'apport de Galien (je préfère parler d'apport plutôt que de réponse, dans la mesure où je ne discerne pas de véritable antagonisme entre les positions galénique et stoïcienne) consiste dans un effort de définition du champ d'application de la conjecture technique et de ses outils conceptuels, effort particulièrement sensible dans un traité comme le *De locis affectis*.

D. Manetti: Ho l'impressione che nel passo di *Introductio* 5 (XIV 684,11 ss. K) siano rispecchiate due nozioni un po' diverse del termine *stochastikon*. Nella prima definizione di medicina (attribuita a Erasistrato) i due termini *to epistemonikon* e *to stochastikon* sono opposti l'uno all'altro, come se lo *stochastikon* fosse alternativo a *techne*. Poco dopo invece l'autore riporta una diversa classificazione, dove le arti sono distinte in *stochastikai* e non *stochastikai*. Se questo è vero, lo statuto del termine *stochastikon*, nella discussione precedente a Galeno, aveva una certa ambiguità potendo collocarsi sia come qualificazione di un certo tipo di *technai*, sia come un livello di sapere alla pari e distinto da *techne*. Le chiedo se questa interpretazione del passo di *Int.* le pare accettabile, e, se sì, se Galeno abbia tenuto conto di questa discussione a lui precedente e nell'usare l'espressione *stochasmos technikos* (*Loc.Aff.* 3, 4, VIII 145,12-13 K) abbia fatto il tentativo di non lasciare spazio alle ambiguità.

V. Boudon: Je ne pense pas que dans la première définition attribuée à Érasistrate le *stochastikon* représente une véritable alternative à la *technè*. Je comprends plutôt qu'à l'intérieur de la *technè* prise comme un tout, certains domaines relèvent de l'*épistèmonikon*, tandis que d'autres relèvent du *stochastikon*. Il est assez probable cependant que dans la réflexion médicale antérieure à Galien une certaine ambiguïté ait été attachée au terme *stochastikon*, employé à la fois pour désigner un niveau de savoir à l'intérieur de la *technè* et pour qualifier un certain type de *technè* dite stochastique dans la mesure où elle n'atteint pas toujours nécessairement son but. Dans cette perspective, il n'est sans doute pas interdit de voir dans la curieuse expression *stochasmos technikos* un effort de Galien pour bannir toute ambiguïté et clairement signifier au lecteur que, dans le *Corpus* galénique, le terme *stochasmos* est désormais employé en un sens technique (*technikos*) pour désigner une procédure d'enquête précise et nettement définie à l'intérieur même de la *technè*. En ce sens, le *stochasmos technikos* n'est donc pas très éloigné de la première définition érasistratéenne, même si l'effort de Galien pour en codifier nettement les différentes étapes lui a sans doute beaucoup fait gagner en technicité.

V. Barras: Votre démonstration de l'ambiguïté à laquelle est confronté Galien lorsqu'il ordonne, ou tente d'ordonner, la médecine dans la hiérarchie des arts me paraît très convaincante. Elle esquisse par ailleurs une (ré)conciliation possible entre une médecine 'haute' et une médecine 'basse', tempérant ainsi la dichotomie que met en exergue M. Vegetti. Si, comme vous le montrez, la prise en compte de la stochastique permet d'offrir un fondement épistémologique à la supériorité ontologique de la médecine, pensez-vous qu'il s'agit là d'un apport singulier de Galien (en rapport peut-être avec sa 'théologie')? Quelles seraient, sinon, les influences que l'on pourrait suspecter dans la tradition médicale antérieure?

V. Boudon: La question de l'originalité de la position de Galien par rapport à ses prédécesseurs est une question aussi vaste que difficile et qui se pose dans de très nombreux domaines de sa pensée médicale et philosophique. Dans le cas particulier du rôle dévolu à la conjecture, j'ai tenté d'apporter un embryon de réponse en évoquant, aussi prudemment que possible, les données de la philosophie stoïcienne qui indéniablement sert de toile de fond à la réflexion galénique. De ce point de vue, l'étude de M. Isnardi sur la notion de *technè*, que j'ai citée en note, reste toujours fondamentale. La véritable originalité de Galien, dans ce domaine comme dans d'autres, me semble cependant avoir consisté dans ce mouvement commun, et qui lui est si propre, à la fois de rationalisation des données antérieures sur la conjecture, et d'uniformisation à l'intérieur du système médical galénique fondé sur l'unité de la *technè*.

VIII

Gotthard Strohmaier

DIE ETHIK GALENS UND IHRE REZEPTION IN DER WELT DES ISLAMS

Anders als sein berühmter Landsmann Ailios Aristeides war Galen nicht davon überzeugt, daß sich die Römer dadurch auszeichneten, daß sie im Gegensatz zu den früheren Weltreichen "Herrscher über Freie" seien.[1] In seinem Kommentar zu der Hippokratesschrift *De aere aquis locis*, der nur in einer arabischen Fassung erhalten ist, erwähnt er beiläufig die Bewohner der Berge Pisidiens und Mysiens, die nach seinen Worten in den Tagen des Hippokrates frei waren, nun aber seien sie "die Sklaven von anderen", d.h. der Römer.[2] An einer anderen Stelle des Kommentars beschreibt er eine Diskussion, die er mit einer Gruppe von Römern über Fragen des Kalenders und der Astronomie führte. Er fand sie ein wenig begriffsstutzig, denn sie hätten ihn angestaunt, als ob er von "weißen Raben" erzählen wollte. Überhaupt fand er das, was die Römer, d.h. deren staatstragende Schicht, von der Mathematik zu lernen pflegten, als

[1] Μόνοι γὰρ τῶν πώποτε ἐλευθέρων ἄρχετε (*Or.* 26, 36 Keil), vgl. dazu J. Bleicken, *Der Preis des Aelius Aristides auf das römische Weltreich (or. 26 K)*, Nachrichten der Akademie der Wissenschaften in Göttingen, Philol.-hist. Kl., 1966, 7 (Göttingen 1966), 234-263.

[2] Handschrift Kairo, Ṭalʿat, ṭibb 550 (s. F. Sezgin, *Geschichte des arabischen Schrifttums* III [Leiden 1970], 37 u. 123f.), fol. 83ᵛ5-7; Faksimileedition v. F. Sezgin, *Galen's Commentary on the Hippocratic Treatise On Airs, Waters, Places* (Περὶ ἀέρων, ὑδάτων, τόπων) *in Arabic Translation*, Publications of the Institute for the History of Arabic-Islamic Science, Series C: Facsimile Editions 65 (Frankfurt a.M. 2001), 112.

ungenügend. Sie beschränkten sich auf Euklid, aber gingen von da nicht zur Astronomie weiter, hingegen seien sie sehr von der Astrologie eingenommen.[3]

Galen huldigte einem strengen Hellenozentrismus. Eine kleine Nuance in einer bekannten Philosophenanekdote, die er in seinem *Protreptikos* nacherzählt, ist bezeichnend. Aristipp von Kyrene, es kann auch ein anderer Weiser gewesen sein, fand sich nach einem Schiffbruch am Strand einer unbekannten Insel wieder. Da sah er in den Sand gezeichnete geometrische Figuren und fühlte sich erleichtert, denn es waren "Spuren von Menschen (*hominum vestigia*)", so jedenfalls in der Version der Geschichte bei Cicero und Vitruv.[4] Bei Galen hingegen zieht der Philosoph den Schluß, daß er zu Griechen gekommen sei und nicht zu Barbaren.[5] Angesichts dieser reservierten Haltung gegenüber den Beherrschern der Ökumene könnte man sich fragen, warum er ausgerechnet in Rom Karriere gemacht hat. Er lobt Hippokrates, indem er auf die Legende verweist, wie dieser die Einladung des Perserkönigs ausschlug, dessen Volk wegen einer ausgebrochenen Pest zu behandeln, vielmehr habe er es vorgezogen, seinen Landsleuten zu dienen.[6] Damit wurde schon damals ein schwieriges Problem medizinischer Deontologie angesprochen. Denn was soll man beispielsweise heutzutage tun, wenn nach einem Attentat der Angreifer schwerer verwundet daliegt als seine unschuldigen Opfer und die Möglichkeiten der ersten Hilfe begrenzt sind? Galen sieht das Problem allein unter einem pekuniären Blickwinkel. Nach seiner Meinung wollte

[3] Ebenda, fol. 73^{r}20-74^{r}11 (in der Faksimileedition S.91-93); der Passus wurde bereits herausgegeben und übersetzt von G.J. TOOMER, "Galen on the astronomers and astrologers", in *Archive for the History of Exact Sciences* 32 (1985), 193-206.

[4] VITR. 6, *prooem.* 1; CIC. *Rep.* 1, 29.

[5] *Protr.* 5, 3, I 8,12-13 K = CMG V 1, 1, S.120f.

[6] *Opt.Med.* 3, I 58,4-10 K = *Scripta min.* II p.5,6-13; F. ROSENTHAL, "An Ancient Commentary on the Hippocratic Oath", in *Bulletin of the History of Medicine* 30 (1956), 77-79 (Nachdruck in DERS., *Science and Medicine in Islam: a collection of essays* [Aldershot 1990], Nr. III); vgl. J. RUBIN PINAULT, *Hippocratic Lives and Legends* (Leiden 1992), 79-93.

Hippokrates lieber den Armen in Kranon und Thasos helfen, er entschied sich gegen die Liebe zum Geld.[7]

Als Erbe eines beachtlichen Vermögens war Galen unabhängig, und der pekuniäre Aspekt war für ihn nicht entscheidend. Er war wirklich in erster Linie ein Mann der Wissenschaft, und die Hauptstadt gab ihm die Möglichkeit, zu beobachten und mit den Vertretern der verschiedenen philosophischen und medizinischen Schulen zusammenzutreffen. In einem zehnten Buch zu *De placitis Hippocratis et Platonis*, von dem wir nur dürftige Spuren in der arabischen Tradition vorfinden,[8] bezeichnet er die Hauptstadt als einen "Mikrokosmos".[9]

Die Abneigung muß aber gegenseitig gewesen sein. Galen hat in der lateinischen Literatur so gut wie keine Spuren hinterlassen. Macrobius zitiert in seinen *Saturnalia* verschiedene medizinische Autoritäten der Griechen, aber Galen ist nicht unter ihnen. Man braucht auch nur einen Blick in die Indizes der Editionen des Censorinus oder des Marcellus Empiricus zu werfen, um das gleiche festzustellen.[10] Galen hat in Rom keine Schule begründet. Hingegen bildeten in der Folgezeit die Ärzte des Ostens, in Byzanz wie in der islamischen Welt, eine einzige galenische Sekte. Dies ist sogar an der nichtmedizinischen Literatur abzulesen. Hieronymus bezeichnet in seiner Streitschrift

[7] Vgl. J. JOUANNA, "La lecture de l'éthique hippocratique chez Galien", in *Médecine et morale dans l'Antiquité*, Entretiens sur l'Antiquité classique 43 (Vandœuvres 1997), 233f.

[8] Siehe mein Kapitel über die arabische Tradition in *PHP*, CMG V 4, 1, 2, I S.44f.

[9] Zitiert bei al-Fārābī, *Kitāb al-ḫiṭāba*, hrsg. v. J. LANGHADE, in *Mélanges de l'Université Saint-Joseph* (Beirut) 43 (1967), 129,1f. (Übers. s. Anm.8, S.44); für vergleichbare Bezeichnungen in der zeitgenössischen Literatur vgl. F. UNRUH, *Das Bild des Imperium Romanum im Spiegel der Literatur an der Wende vom 2. zum 3. Jh. n.Chr.*, (Bonn 1991), 106.

[10] Macrobius, *Saturnalia*, hrsg. v. J. WILLIS (Leipzig 1973); Censorinus, *De die natali liber*, hrsg. v. K. SALLMANN (Leipzig 1983); Marcellus Empiricus, *De medicamentis liber*, hrsg. v. M. NIEDERMANN u. E. LIECHTENHAN (Berlin 1965), 2 Bde. (Corpus Medicorum Latinorum V).

Adversus Iovinianum Galen als einen *vir doctissimus, Hippocratis interpres.* Das schrieb er zwar in Latein, aber im Osten in der Stadt Bethlehem.[11] Gesios, um das Jahr 500 ein hochverehrter Professor in Alexandrien, erscheint in einer Hagiographie des Bischofs Sophronios als ein Anhänger von Hippokrates, Galen und Demokrit.[12] Auch in der schönen Literatur des arabischen Mittelalters ist *Ǧālīnūs* eine wohlbekannte Persönlichkeit, sie erscheint sogar in den Märchen aus *Tausendundeiner Nacht.*[13] Und als sein Name schließlich im Abendland in der *Commedia* Dantes auftaucht, ist er von zwei muslimischen Denkern eingerahmt:

> Ipocràte, Avicenna e Galieno,
> Averoìs, che 'l gran comento feo. (*Inf.* IV 143-144)

Galen war tatsächlich zur Zeit des großen Florentiners ein Teil der griechischen Tradition, die von der arabischen Kultur herüberkam.

Die Ursache für seine Rezeption im Orient ist in den besonderen Verhältnissen der Schule von Alexandrien zu suchen. Hier empfahl sich Galen wegen seiner philosophischen Ambitionen und seiner grundsätzlichen Nähe zur aristotelischen Naturphilosophie. Johannes Philoponus rühmt ihn in seiner Schrift *De aeternitate mundi contra Proclum* als einen Mediziner, der zur gleichen Zeit ein wahrer Philosoph war.[14] Die Intelligenz der syrischen Region war seit der Zeit des Hellenismus zweisprachig und unter dem starken Einfluß der alexandrinischen Schule. Sergios von Rēšʿainā (gestorben 536), der erste uns

[11] 2, 11, in *Patrologia Latina* 23, Sp.300 B.

[12] *Narratio miraculorum ss. Cyri et Joannis* 30, in *Patrologia Graeca* 87,3, Sp.3513-3520; vgl. W. Wolska-Conus, "Stéphanos d'Athènes et Stéphanos d'Alexandrie", in *REByz* 47 (1989), 47-59.

[13] 58. Nacht (Ausg. Kairo, I 272,19).

[14] 17, 5, S.599,24-26 Rabe (Leipzig 1899; Nachdr. Hildesheim 1963): ἀνὴρ φυσικώτατός τε καὶ οὐδὲν ἧττον τῆς ἰδίας ἐπιστήμης τὰ κατὰ φιλοσοφίαν ἠκριβωκὼς θεωρήματα.

bekannte Übersetzer der Werke Galens ins Syrische, hatte in Alexandrien studiert.[15]

Nach dem Sieg der Abbasiden kam es in der neugegründeten Hauptstadt Bagdad im neunten Jahrhundert zunächst zu einem erneuten Aufblühen der syrischen Studien, und die christlichen Hofärzte bestellten für sich neue Galenübersetzungen in ihrer Sprache. Auf Grund des nachfolgenden Niedergangs der syrischen Kultur unter dem Islam sind diese Übersetzungen fast völlig untergegangen. Jedoch hatten hochgebildete und an allen Wissenschaften interessierte muslimische Hofbeamte fast zeitgleich für sich arabische Übersetzungen in Auftrag gegeben. So ist die allgemeine Überlieferungssituation die, daß ein gewisser Teil der Werke Galens sowohl in der griechischen Originalfassung wie in arabischer Übersetzung erhalten ist, ein anderer Teil nur auf griechisch und ein anderer nur auf arabisch.[16] Dabei ist hervorzuheben, daß sich das Interesse der Übersetzer und ihrer Klienten nicht auf die medizinischen Schriften beschränkte, sondern daß seine philosophischen Schriften den gleichen Widerhall fanden. Sie wurden diskutiert, manchmal in durchaus kontroverser Weise, und aus diesem Grunde finden sich Zitate und Resümees unerwartet an manchmal sehr entlegenen Stellen in der ungeheuren arabischen Literatur des arabischen Mittelalters.

Galen taucht hier sogar in den volkstümlichen Sammlungen ethischer Weisheitssprüche und Anekdoten, den sogenannten *Gnomologien*, auf,[17] was sich für den griechischen Raum noch

[15] H. HUGONNARD-ROCHE, "Note sur Sergius de Rešʿainā, traducteur du grec en syriaque et commentateur d'Aristote", in *The Ancient Tradition in Christian and Islamic Hellenism. Studies on the Transmission of Greek Philosophy and Sciences dedicated to H. J. Drossaart Lulofs on his ninetieth birthday*, ed. by G. ENDRESS and R. KRUK (Leiden 1997), 121-143.

[16] G. STROHMAIER, "Der syrische und der arabische Galen", in *ANRW* II 37, 2 (Berlin 1994), 1987-2017.

[17] Vgl. z.B. Ḥunain ibn Isḥāq, *Ādāb al-falāsifa*, hrsg. v. ʿA. BADAWI (Kuwait 1985), 122f.; Al-Mubaššir ibn Fātik, *Muḫtār al-ḥikam wa-maḥāsin al-kalim*, hrsg. v. ʿA. BADAWI (Madrid 1958), 293-296.

nicht feststellen läßt. Aber in dieser Literatur herrscht ein derartiges Chaos, daß man bei der Auswertung sehr vorsichtig sein muß.[18] Nur sehr selten läßt sich eine Anekdote oder eine Sentenz in den originalen Schriften der Autorität aufspüren, der sie zugeschrieben wird. In einem Fall jedoch ist das möglich. In dem *Gnomologium* von al-Mubaššir liest man unter dem Namen Galens die folgende Geschichte: "Er sah einen Mann, den die Könige wegen der Stärke seines Körpers ehrten, und da fragte er, was er Außerordentliches getan hätte. Sie antworteten: 'Er hat einen geschlachteten Ochsen aus der Mitte des Palastes bis nach draußen getragen'. Da sagte er ihnen: 'Und derselbe Ochse hat ihn getragen, ohne daß dem Tier daraus ein Verdienst zukam'."[19] Das stammt mit einer beträchtlichen Umformung und Zuspitzung aus dem *Protreptikos*, wo von dem Athleten Milon von Kroton die Rede ist, der einen Ochsen quer durch ein Stadion trug und später wegen seiner leichtsinnigen Dummheit ums Leben kam.[20] Die ethische Tendenz ist aber hier wie dort dieselbe, nämlich daß der rohen Körperkraft im Rahmen der menschlichen Existenz keine Bedeutung zukommen sollte.

Das starke Interesse an den ethischen Verlautbarungen Galens ist auch damit zu erklären, daß er der Gegenstand einer regelrechten Hagiographie geworden ist. Ibn abī Uṣaibiʿa (gest. 1270), der Verfasser der ungewöhnlich reichhaltigen *Quellen der Nachrichten über die Klassen der Ärzte*, beginnt die Biographie Galens mit der Feststellung, daß er von der Elite wie von der breiten Masse als "das Siegel (*ḫātim*) der großen lehrenden Ärzte" angesehen werde.[21] Diese Rede ist in ihrem islamischen

[18] G. STROHMAIER, "Das Gnomologium als Forschungsaufgabe", in *Dissertatiunculae criticae: Festschrift für Günther Christian Hansen*, hrsg. v. Chr.-Fr. COLLATZ, J. DUMMER, J. KOLLESCH u. M.-L. WERLITZ (Würzburg 1998), 461-471 (Nachdr. in DERS., *Hellas im Islam. Beiträge zu Ikonographie, Wissenschaft und Religionsgeschichte* [Wiesbaden; im Druck]).

[19] Al-Mubaššir… (s.o. Anm.17), 296,6-8.

[20] *Protr.* 13, 3, I 34,3-11 K = CMG V 1, 1, S.144-147.

[21] *ʿUyūn al-anbāʾ fī ṭabaqāti l-aṭibbāʾ*, hrsg. v. August MÜLLER (Kairo 1882), I 71,10f.

Kontext zu verstehen, und zwar in dem gleichen Sinne, wie Mohammed "das Siegel der Propheten" war, der die Reihe der Gottgesandten abschloß und nach dem kein weiterer Prophet mehr kommen konnte. Das schloß natürlich jede Idee eines weiteren Fortschritts aus, der übrigens den Ärzten der abbasidischen Blütezeit keineswegs fremd war. Aber bereits ʿAlī ibn Riḍwān (gest. 1068), ein Leibarzt der ägyptischen Fatimidendynastie, erklärt in seinem kleinen Traktat *Über den Weg zur Glückseligkeit durch den ärztlichen Beruf*, daß Gott den Asklepios gesandt habe, damit er die Mitglieder seiner Familie die Medizin lehre. Nachdem sie sich aber über diesen Rahmen hinaus verbreitete, habe sich ihr Zustand verschlechtert, bis Galen kam und sie zu ihrer ursprünglichen Größe wiederherstellte.[22] Galen selber hatte solchen Gedanken Vorschub geleistet, wenn er in *De anatomicis administrationibus*, das auch ins Arabische übersetzt war, erklärt: "Indem die Kunst aus dem Asklepiadengeschlecht herausfiel und danach unter den vielen Nachfolgern sich immer mehr verschlechterte, bedurfte sie schriftlicher Aufzeichnungen, welche die Lehre bewahren sollten".[23]

Eine Eigentümlichkeit der muslimischen Traditionswissenschaft, welche die Erinnerung an die Aussprüche und Handlungen des Propheten bewahrte, war die, daß man großen Wert auf die moralische Integrität der einzelnen Überlieferer legte. Man sammelte ihre Biographien und ordnete sie in 'Klassen' nach chronologischen und geographischen Gesichtspunkten. Das ließ sich auf die Medizin und ihre Geschichte übertragen. Der Terminus der 'Klassen' taucht nicht umsonst auch in den Kompilationen zur Geschichte der Wissenschaften auf. Das Interesse an dem ethischen Standard der Überlieferungsträger paßte gut zu dem, was Galen von sich selber zu erzählen wußte. Ibn abī Uṣaibiʿa als großer Kenner seiner Schriften zitiert daraus

[22] Hrsg. v. A. DIETRICH, Abhandlungen der Akademie der Wissenschaften in Göttingen, Philol.-hist. Kl., 3. Folge, Nr.129 (Göttingen 1982), 26f.

[23] *AA* 2, 1, II 281,14-17 K = ed. I. GAROFALO (Napoli 1986), S.71,17-20.

einschlägige Stellen, darunter solche, die sonst verloren sind. Max Meyerhof hat sie in seinem 1929 erschienenen Aufsatz "Autobiographische Bruchstücke Galens aus arabischen Quellen" zusammengestellt.[24] Andere Zitate können an den erhaltenen echten Schriften überprüft werden, und sie geben Zeugnis von der exakten Arbeitsweise. Von dem Traktat *De optimo medico cognoscendo* fanden sich später zwei arabische Handschriften, und die umfänglichen Exzerpte Ibn abī Uṣaibiʿas erwiesen sich als so zuverlässig, daß sie Albert Z. Iskandar, unser Herausgeber im *Corpus Medicorum Graecorum*, als Textzeugen zusammen mit den Handschriften verwenden konnte.[25]

Aus einem anderweitig verlorenen Traktat *Daß die Besten der Menschen von ihren Feinden Nutzen haben* zitiert er eine Behauptung Galens, daß er weder von seinen Schülern noch von den Patienten Geld nehme, er schenke ihnen im Gegenteil wenn nötig die Arzneien und beschaffe ihnen das Pflegepersonal, wenn sie keine Bedienung haben, und lasse ihnen sogar die erforderlich Nahrung zubereiten.[26] Über den weiteren Inhalt kann man nur Vermutungen anstellen; Meyerhof verweist auf den ähnlichen Titel Πῶς ἄν τις ἀπ' ἐχθρῶν ὠφελοῖτο im Korpus der Schriften des Plutarch.[27] In einer anderen Schrift unter dem Titel *Über die schwer heilbaren Krankheiten* konnte man lesen, wie Galen in der Öffentlichkeit einem Scharlatan das Handwerk legte. Der Mann zog Leuten, die an Zahnweh litten, Würmer aus dem Mund, wo er sie vorher geschickt hineinpraktiziert hatte. Galen wurde aber wahrscheinlich zu dem Vorgehen provoziert, weil der

[24] In *Archiv für Geschichte der Medizin* 22 (1929), 72-86 (Nachdr. in *Galen in the Arabic Tradition. Texts and Studies* III, ed. by F. SEZGIN, Publications of the Institute for the History of Arabic-Islamic Science: Islamic Medicine 20 [Frankfurt a.M. 1996], 208-222).

[25] CMG Suppl. Or. IV, vgl. die Einleitung, S.15f.

[26] Ibn abī Uṣaibiʿa... (s.o. Anm.21), S.86,32-87,8.

[27] S.o. Anm.24, S.84.

Mann behauptete, einer seiner Schüler zu sein.[28] Eine Distanz zu dem persönlichen Verhalten Galens findet sich höchstens bei den Philosophen. Er war den Prügelknabe der arabischen Peripatetiker, die seine gelegentliche Kritik an Aristoteles nicht schätzten. Al-Fārābī (gest. 950) rügt die unsachliche Polemik gegen Thessalos, dem Galen seine niedrige Herkunft vorwarf.[29]

Im folgenden soll eine kurze und notgedrungen unvollständige Übersicht über das gegeben werden, was die arabische Überlieferung an Neuem gegenüber dem auf griechisch Zugänglichen bietet. Dies sei in vier Themenkreisen gruppiert, erstens dem der ärztlichen Deontologie, zweitens dem einer philosophischen Ethik, die sich um das seelische Gleichgewicht bemüht, wobei die Harmonie des Körpers als Vergleich dient, drittens den Fragen, die mit dem Einfluß des Körpers auf die Seele zusammenhängen, und viertens der von Platon übernommenen Dreiteilung der Seele und ihrer hierarchischen Struktur. Von Fall zu Fall sollen die Reaktionen arabischer Autoren angefügt werden, wobei natürlich auch die Äußerungen Galens einzubeziehen sind, die uns aus der griechischen Tradition bekannt sind.

Ibn abī Uṣaibiʿa und andere Autoren haben uns Fragmente eines Kommentars zum hippokratischen Eid erhalten,[30] unter denen leider die Bemerkungen zu dem Hauptteil der ethischen Vorschriften fehlen. Ich hatte zugunsten der Echtheit argumentiert,[31] was die Mehrheit der Forscher jetzt mit leichten

[28] Zu den verschiedenen Versionen s. G. STROHMAIER, "Der Arzt in der römischen Gesellschaft. Neues aus der arabischen Galenüberlieferung", in *Acta Conventus XI Eirene* (Warszawa 1971), 70f. (Nachdruck in *Von Demokrit bis Dante. Die Bewahrung antiken Erbes in der arabischen Kultur*, Olms Studien 43 [Hildesheim 1996], 84f.).

[29] S.o. Anm.9, S.127 (Übers. s.o. Anm.8, S.44); vgl. *MM* 1,2, X 10,4-16 K.

[30] Gesammelt von F. ROSENTHAL (s.o. Anm.6), 52-87.

[31] "Asklepios und das Ei. Zur Ikonographie in einem arabisch erhaltenen Kommentar zum hippokratischen Eid", in *Beiträge zur Alten Geschichte und deren Nachleben. Festschrift für Franz Altheim*, hrsg. v. R. STIEHL u. H.E. STIER, II (Berlin 1970), 143-153, 448-454 (Nachdr. in *Hellas im Islam* [s.o. Anm.18]).

Bedenken akzeptiert hat, die auch ich durchaus zu teilen geneigt bin. Auf jeden Fall aber hat Ḥunain den Kommentar unter den authentischen Schriften aufgeführt,[32] und es ist vielleicht der Autorität Galens zuzuschreiben, daß der Eid eine offizielle Funktion erlangte, die er in der Antike unseres Wissens nie gehabt hat. Handbücher für den *muḥtasib*, den Marktaufseher, enthalten Vorschriften wie diese: "Es obliegt dem Aufseher, alle Ärzte den Eid des Hippokrates ablegen zu lassen, wobei sie schwören sollen, niemandem ein schädliches Medikament zu verabreichen, kein Gift herzustellen, niemandem im Volk die Rezeptur eines Giftes mitzuteilen, niemandem die Herstellung eines Amuletts zu beschreiben, den Frauen keine Rezeptur zu nennen, die einen Abort herbeiführt, und den Männern keine, die eine Unfruchtbarkeit verursacht. Sie sollen ihre Blicke von den Zimmern der Frauen abwenden, wenn sie in das Haus des Kranken eintreten, keine Geheimnisse ausplaudern und keinen Schleier aufheben."[33]

Die Schrift *De optimo medico cognoscendo*, von der sogar der griechische Titel unbekannt ist, trug bei den arabischen Autoren verschiedene Titel, der am meisten verbreitete, aber sicher nicht ursprüngliche, lautete *Über die Prüfung des Arztes* (*Fī miḥnati ṭ-ṭabīb*). Dies war kein Handbuch für irgendeine amtliche Autorität, sondern nur eine Anleitung für den Laien, wie er einen guten Arzt von einem schlechten unterscheiden könne. Galen geißelt hier das Verhalten stadtrömischer Kollegen, die es vorzogen, bei den Reichen ihre Aufwartung zu machen, anstatt ihre Zeit dem Studium zu widmen. Er beschreibt auch die besonderen Bedingungen für die ärztliche Praxis in der großen Stadt.

[32] Ḥunain ibn Isḥāq, *Über die syrischen und arabischen Galen-Übersetzungen*, hrsg. v. G. BERGSTRÄSSER, Abhandlungen für die Kunde des Morgenlandes 17,2 (Leipzig 1925), Nr.87.

[33] ʿAbd ar-Raḥmān ibn Naṣr aš-Šaizarī, *Nihāyat ar-rutba fī ṭalab al-ḥisba* (*The book of the Islamic market inspector*), übers. v. R P. BUCKLEY, *Journal of Semitic Studies*, Supplement 9 (Oxford 1999), 115; vgl. dazu M. MEYERHOF, "La surveillance des professions médicales et para-médicales chez les Arabes", in DERS., *Studies in Medieval Arabic Medicine. Theory and Practice*, hrsg. v. P. JOHNSTONE (London 1984), XI 129.

Die Menschen leben hier isoliert voneinander, und wenn ein Patient stirbt, erfahren die Nachbarn nichts von der Ursache seines Ablebens und auch nicht, welcher Arzt ihn zuletzt behandelt hat. Galen sieht die Ursache dafür in der Gier der Bewohner nach Geld und Würden.[34] Ibn Ǧumaiʿ, ein jüdischer Leibarzt des Sultans Saladin, der von 1169 bis 1193 regierte, schrieb einen kleinen Traktat *Über die Wiederbelebung der ärztlichen Kunst*, den er seinem Souverän widmete. Hier beklagt er sich auch über das Verhalten der Ärzte, aber er tut das mit einer so engen Anlehnung an den Galenischen Wortlaut in *De optimo medico cognoscendo*, daß man zweifeln muß, ob er wirklich die Verhältnisse in seiner Umgebung beschreibt.[35]

Obwohl Galen jede Art der Anbiederung und ein Eingehen auf unvernünftige Wünsche des Patienten scharf verurteilte, hat er doch generell nach dem Vorbild des Hippokrates ein liebenswürdiges Auftreten empfohlen.[36] Der große Kliniker Rhazes (854-925 oder 935) hat an diese Prinzipien angeknüpft, indem er bestimmte Konzessionen gestattet, um den Kranken bei guter Laune zu halten, indem ihm beispielsweise eine Diät zugeteilt wird, an die er gewohnt war, obwohl sie eigentlich als schwerer verdaulich und nicht als das Optimum einer Krankendiät anzusehen wäre. Diese Gedanken hat er in einer kleinen Schrift dargelegt, der Karl Deichgräber den lateinischen Titel *De indulgentia medici* gegeben hat.[37]

[34] G. STROHMAIER, "Galen über die Vereinsamung des Menschen in der Großstadt", in *Forschungen und Berichte der Staatlichen Museen (Berlin)* 18 (1977), 197f. (Nachdr. in DERS., *Hellas im Islam* [s.o. Anm.18]).

[35] Ibn Jumayʿ, *Treatise to Ṣalāḥ ad-Dīn on the Revival of the Art of Medicine*, hrsg. v. H. FÄHNDRICH, Abhandlungen für die Kunde des Morgenlandes 46,3 (Wiesbaden 1983), §87f., 100-103, 106; vgl. dazu die Einleitung zu *Opt.Med.Cogn.*, CMG Suppl. Or. IV, S.22.

[36] K. DEICHGRÄBER, *Medicus gratiosus. Untersuchungen zu einem griechischen Arztbild*, Akademie der Wissenschaften und der Literatur Mainz, Abhandlungen der geistes- u. sozialwissenschaftlichen Klasse 1970, 3 (Mainz 1970).

[37] *Ibid.*, 108-113 (Übersetzung von Ch. BÜRGEL).

In seiner Eigenschaft als Philosoph hat Galen mehrere ethische Traktate verfaßt, wo er empfiehlt, ein seelisches Gleichgewicht zu bewahren und die Extreme der Freude, des Ärgers und des Zornes zu meiden, dies verbunden mit dem Ratschlag, eine zornige Reaktion eine Weile aufzuschieben, um sie nicht zu heftig ausfallen zu lassen und man hinterher darüber Reue empfinden muß. Der Arzt Sinān ibn Ṯābit (gest. 942) hat so den Emir Abu l-Ḥusain Baḥkam von seinen Tobsuchtsanfällen geheilt, und man hat vermutet, daß Galen mit seiner Schrift *De animi cuiuslibet affectuum dignotione et curatione* dazu die Anleitung gegeben hat.[38] Diese Erörterungen, die in stoischer und platonischer Tradition die Seele als eine selbständige Größe vorführen, stehen, wie Luis García Ballester richtig gesehen hat, unverbunden neben der naturalistischen Betrachtung psychischer Vorgänge in den medizinischen Schriften.[39]

In einem Traktat mit dem Titel *Über die Vertreibung des Kummers* (*Fī nafyi l-ġamm*), den Galen im Verzeichnis seiner Schriften als Περὶ ἀλυπίας angibt,[40] erzählt er, wie er durch den Brand des Friedenstempels im Jahr 192 viele seiner wertvollen Bücher verlor.[41] Weiteres Material aus dieser Schrift, das aber dem Charakter des Gnomologiums angepaßt erscheint und darum nicht ganz wörtlich zu nehmen ist, findet sich in der *Medizin der Seelen* (*Ṭibb an-nufūs*) des Maimonidesschülers Ibn ʿAqnīn (gest. 1226).[42]

[38] Fady HAJAL, "Galen's Ethical Psychotherapy: Its Influence on a Medieval Near Eastern Physician", in *Journal of the History of Medicine and Allied Sciences* 38 (1983), 320-333; vgl. Ibn abī Uṣaibiʿa… (s.o. Anm.21), S.222,23-224,8.

[39] "Lo médico y lo filosófico-moral en las relaciones entre alma y enfermedad: el pensamiento de Galeno", in *Asclepio* 20 (1968), 99-134; "Diseases of the Soul (νοσήματα τῆς ψυχῆς) in Galen. The Impossibility of a Galenic Psychotherapy", in *Clio Medica* 9 (1974), 35-43.

[40] *Lib.Prop.* 12, XIX 45,13 K = *Scripta min.* II S.121,11; vgl. Ḥunain… (s.o. Anm.32), Nr.120.

[41] Ibn abī Uṣaibiʿa… (s.o. Anm.21), S.84,31-85,5; MEYERHOF (s.o. Anm.24), 85f.

[42] A.S. HALKIN, "Classical and Arabic material in Ibn ʿAḳnīn's 'Hygiene of the soul'", in *Proceedings of the American Academy for Jewish Research* 14 (1944), 60-65 u. Nr.181-186; zu möglichen Ergänzungen, die aus der hebräischen

Die Abhandlung *Quod animi mores corporis temperamenta sequantur* ist unter anderem dem Thema gewidmet, wie das Gleichgewicht der Seele von dem Gleichgewicht des Körpers abhängig ist, und dieses wiederum von dem ausgeglichenen Charakter der geographischen Umwelt.[43] Manche Denker des islamischen Mittelalters waren damit nicht ganz einverstanden, indem sie auch die Selbständigkeit der Seele betonten, die ihrerseits die körperliche Verfassung beeinflußt.[44] Galen führt in der genannten Schrift aus, daß der Erdboden Skythiens nur einen einzigen Philosophen hervorgebracht habe, die Stadt Athen hingegen viele. Er brauchte seiner kundigen Leserschaft den Namen des Anacharsis nicht eigens zu nennen; Ḥunain fügt ihn in seiner arabischen Übersetzung hinzu.[45] Für andere griechische Autoren war jener ein Beweis, daß auch die Barbaren fähig seien, Philosophen zu werden. Galen sieht in ihm eine Ausnahme von der Regel und in seiner Vereinzelung den Beweis für die Inferiorität der ganzen Region. Nach einer Mitteilung des Polyhistors al-Masʿūdī (gest. 956), der jedoch leider die Schrift nicht nennt, aus der er sie genommen haben will, hatte Galen neben der Kennzeichnung der körperlichen Merkmale der Schwarzen auch die Behauptung aufgestellt, daß sie wegen eines Schadens an ihrem Gehirn sorglos und schwachsinnig seien.[46] Der Historiker Ibn Ḫaldūn (1332-1382) ist dieser Behauptung entgegengetreten, indem er auf die Wärme der Luft verweist, die z.B.

Popularphilosophie des Mittelalters gewonnen werden können, s. M. ZONTA, *Un interprete ebreo della filosofia di Galeno. Gli scritti filosofici di Galeno nell'opera di Shem Tob ibn Falaquera* (Torino 1995), 113-123.

43 *QAM* 8 f., IV 798-808 K = *Scripta min.* II S.57-67.

44 H.H. BIESTERFELDT, *Ǧālīnūs Quwā n-nafs*. Zitiert, adaptiert, korrigiert, in *Der Islam* 63 (1986), 119-136.

45 *QAM* 11, IV 822,3-6 K = *Scripta min.* II S.79,21-23; vgl. Galens Traktat *Daß die Kräfte der Seele den Mischungen des Körpers folgen* in arabischer Übersetzung, hrsg. v. H.H. BIESTERFELDT, Abhandlungen für die Kunde des Morgenlandes 40,4 (Wiesbaden 1973), 43,18f. (Übers. S.78).

46 *wa-innamā ġalaba ʿala l-aswad aṭ-ṭarab li-fasādi dimāġihi fa-ḍaʿufa li-ḏālika ʿaqluhu*: s. *Kitāb murūǧ aḏ-ḏahab wa-maʿādin al-ǧauhar*, Kap. 62, hrsg. v. C. BARBIER DE MEYNARD u. A.J.B. PAVET DE COURTEILLE, revidiert v. CH. PELLAT, Kap. 7: I (Beirut 1966), §170; Übers.: I (Paris 1962), §170.

auch bei den Ägyptern einen gewissen Leichtsinn verursacht.[47] Zuzutrauen ist sie Galen auf jeden Fall, wenn man sich erinnert, wie er unsere germanischen Vorfahren mit Löwen, Bären und Wildschweinen auf eine Stufe gestellt hat.[48]

Möglicherweise hat Galen hierin einen Einfluß auf den türkischstämmigen Philosophen al-Fārābī ausgeübt, der in seinem *Buch der Staatsleitung* (*Kitāb as-siyāsati l-madanīya*) über die Bewohner der Regionen im äußersten Norden und äußersten Süden folgendermaßen urteilt: "Man muß mit ihnen verfahren wie mit Tieren. Diejenigen, die Haustieren ähneln und zu irgendeinem Zweck in den Städten zu verwenden sind, sollte man am Leben lassen, sie zu Sklaven machen und sie wie Tiere verwenden. Mit denjenigen, die zu nichts nütze oder die schädlich sind, ist so zu verfahren wie mit schädlichen Tieren."[49] Moses Maimonides, ein Anhänger al-Fārābīs, teilt in seinem *Führer der Verirrten* dessen Meinung über die Türken im hohen Norden und die Schwarzen im tiefen Süden: "Jene sind als unvernünftige Tiere anzusehen; ich setze sie nicht mit Menschen gleich, denn sie nehmen unter den Lebewesen einen niedrigeren Platz ein als der Mensch und einen höheren als der Affe, denn sie haben die Gestalt und die Gesichtszüge des Menschen und ein Urteilsvermögen oberhalb des Affen."[50]

Galens Interesse an der Platonischen Philosophie und an der in ihr vertretenen Dreiteilung der menschlichen Seele zeigt sich daran, daß er Kompendien oder Kurzkommentare zu den Dialogen verfaßt hat, von denen sich in der griechischen Überlieferung nichts erhalten hat, während im Arabischen wenigstens der

[47] *Muqaddima*, 4. Aufl., o.J. o.O., S.87; The Muqaddimah, übers. v. F. ROSENTHAL (New York 1958), I 174-176.

[48] *San.Tu.* 1, 10, 17, VI 51,7ff. K = CMG V 4, 2, S.24,22-24; vgl. G. STROHMAIER, "Araber, Römer und Germanen im Urteil eines griechischen Mediziners", in *Das Altertum* 38 (1992), 105-108 (Nachdruck in DERS., *Hellas im Islam* [s.o. Anm.18]).

[49] Hrsg. v. F.M. Naǧǧār (Beirut 1964), 87.

[50] *Guide des égarés* III 51, übers. v. S. MUNK (Paris 1963), III 434.

Timaioskommentar und von den übrigen einige Fragmente erhalten sind.[51] Verschiedentlich wird in der arabischen Literatur nach einem dieser Kompendien, die Galen gelegentlich durch eigene Bemerkungen bereichert hat, eine Beurteilung der Christen zitiert, die nach seiner Meinung an Fabeln und Mythen glauben, aber dennoch in ihrer Askese und ihrer Todesverachtung das Leben von Philosophen führen.[52] Christliche Autoren wollen diese Stellungnahme dem Kompendium des *Phaidon* entnommen haben, muslimische hingegen dem der *Politeia.* Stephen Gero hat in einem längeren Aufsatz nachzuweisen versucht, daß nur das erstere richtig sein kann.[53] Nach meiner Meinung schließt das eine das andere nicht aus; warum soll Galen nicht zweimal auf ein aktuelles Thema eingegangen sein? Auf jeden Fall ist die Bemerkung im Lichte der Platonischen Psychologie und Staatslehre zu verstehen. Auch die Wächterkaste, die zwischen den führenden Weisen und dem erwerbstätigen Volk steht, soll an Fabeln und Mythen glauben, aber dennoch ein philosophisches Leben führen.

Dort, wo Galen sich mehr nach Platon richtet, hat er auch eine andere ethische Konzeption vertreten als nur die der goldenen Mitte zwischen den Extremen. Die Aufgabe besteht nunmehr nur darin, daß der oberste vernünftige Seelenteil, das *logistikon*, die beiden unteren beherrscht oder vielmehr den untersten begierigen, das *epithymetikon*, mit Hilfe des mittleren 'mutartigen', des *thymoeides.* Die primitiven Völker wie die Skythen oder die Kelten definiert er in diesem Rahmen als solche, in denen der mutartige Seelenteil über den vernünftigen die

[51] Ḥunain... (s.o. Anm.32), Nr.124; *Galeni Compendium Timaei Platonis aliorumque dialogorum synopsis quae extant fragmenta*, edd. P. KRAUS et R. WALZER, Corpus Platonicum Medii Aevi, Plato Arabus, I (London 1951); vgl. jetzt auch D. GUTAS, "Galen's synopsis of Plato's Laws and Fārābī's *Talḫīṣ*", in *The Ancient Tradition ...*, ed. by G. ENDRESS and R. KRUK (s.o. Anm.15), 101-119.

[52] R. WALZER, *Galen on Jews and Christians* (Oxford 1949), 15f.; vgl. dazu R. KÖBERT, "Das nur in arabischer Überlieferung erhaltene Urteil Galens über die Christen", in *Orientalia* N.S. 25 (1956), 404-409.

[53] "Galen on the Christians. A Reappraisal of the Arabic Evidence", in *Orientalia Christiana Periodica* 56 (1990), 371-411.

Oberhand hat.[54] Die Annäherung an Platon zeigt sich besonders deutlich in *De placitis Hippocratis et Platonis*, daneben in *De moribus* (Περὶ ἠθῶν), das in einer arabischen Abkürzung erhalten ist. Nach der Edition von Paul Kraus[55] sind immer wieder neue Stücke gefunden worden, zuletzt auch in der hebräischen Popularphilosophie des Mittelalters, die ihrerseits von der arabischen Literatur abhängig ist.[56] Sie stammen zum Teil nicht aus der Abkürzung, sondern aus dem vollständigen Text.[57] Es ist noch zu früh, eine zusammenfassende Edition in Angriff zu nehmen, da man damit rechnen muß, daß weiteres Material hinzukommt.

Die platonisch inspirierte Ethik erscheint hier in einem besonderen Maße akzentuiert, indem als Ziel die Isolierung des vernünftigen Seelenteils von den beiden niederen und seine Annäherung an die Götter vorgegeben wird. Ob er damit seine Unsterblichkeit befördern kann, wird von Galen zwar mit seiner auch sonst oft geäußerten Skepsis offengelassen, dennoch

[54] *PHP* 3, 3, 6, V 303,13-16 K = CMG V 4, 1, 2, I S.186,1f.

[55] *Kitāb al-aḫlāq li-Ǧālīnūs*, in *Maǧalla kullīyati l-ādāb bi-l-ǧāmiʿati l-miṣrīya* 5 (1937), 1 51 (die Edition von ʿA. BADAWI, *Ǧālīnūs, Muḫtaṣar kitāb al-aḫlāq* [Beirut 1981] war mir nicht zugänglich); eine Übersetzung von J.N. MATTOCK, "A Translation of the Arabic Epitome of Galen's Book Περὶ ἠθῶν", in *Islamic Philosophy and the Classical Tradition.* Essays presented to... Richard Walzer, ed. by S M. STERN, A. HOURANI and V. BROWN (Oxford 1972), 235-260; vgl. die Interpretationen von R. WALZER, "New Light on Galen's Moral Philosophy", in *CQ* 43 (1949), 82-96 (Nachdr. in DERS., *Greek into Arabic* [Oxford 1962], 142-163), und "A Diatribe of Galen", in *HThR* 47 (1954), 243-254 (Nachdr. *ibid.*, 164-174); F. RUNDGREN, "Das Muxtaṣar min Kitāb al'Axlāq des Galenos", in *Orientalia Suecana* 23-24 (1974-75), 84-105; M. MARÓTH, "Galen als Seelenheiler", in *Galen und das hellenistische Erbe.* Verhandlungen des IV. Internationalen Galen-Symposiums... Berlin 18.-20. September 1989, hrsg. von J. KOLLESCH u. D. NICKEL, Sudhoffs Archiv, Beihefte, 32 (Stuttgart 1993), 145-155.

[56] M. ZONTA, *op.cit.* (s.o. Anm.42), 29-80.

[57] Vgl. G. LEVI DELLA VIDA, "Two fragments of Galen in Arabic Translation", in *Journal of the Amer.Orient.Soc.* 70 (1950), 182-187 (vgl. dazu F. ALTHEIM u. R. STIEHL, "Eutychios' Annalen", in *Geschichte der Hunnen* V [Berlin 1962], 127-129); S.M. STERN, "Some fragments of Galen's On Dispositions (Περὶ ἠθῶν) in Arabic", in *CQ* N.S. 6 (1956), 91-101 (Nachdr. in S.M. STERN, *Medieval Arabic and Hebrew Thought*, ed. by F.W. ZIMMERMANN [London 1983], III).

solle man so leben, als ob dies möglich wäre. Denn ein Mensch bliebe ein Mensch, auch wenn er alle seine Körperteile und auch die zu ihrem Funktionieren notwendigen unteren Seelenteile verlieren würde.[58] Paul Moraux hat auf Grund dieser Stelle Zweifel an der Echtheit der Schrift geäußert oder zumindest eine verfälschende Bearbeitung durch den Epitomator in Erwägung gezogen,[59] was jedoch von Mauro Zonta unter Heranziehung einer hebräischen Parallelversion, die auf dem vollständigen arabischen Text beruht, zurückgewiesen wird.[60]

Galens unsichere Haltung in weltanschaulichen Fragen, die eben auch eine Offenheit gegenüber der Volksreligion einschloß, kommt besonders in seinem Spätwerk *De propriis placitis* zum Ausdruck. Ein arabisches Testimonium hilft dabei, eine Stelle zu verstehen, die in der erhaltenen hebräischen und lateinischen Version bislang unklar geblieben ist. Verschiedene Indizien haben Galen bewogen, doch an das Walten der Götter oder des einen Demiurgen zu glauben, darunter auch eine Erscheinung, die er bei einer Schiffsreise selbst erlebt hat. Es handelte sich um das sogenannte Elmsfeuer, das bei gewittriger Wetterlage an den Mastspitzen von Schiffen auftritt und das der Volksglaube als Zeichen eines helfenden Eingreifens der Dioskuren bei Seenot ansah. Die büschelförmigen elektrischen Entladungen machen in der Tat einen numinosen Eindruck.[61] Das Testimonium stammt von al-Bīrūnī (973-1048), der das Phänomen ausführlicher beschreibt und sich dabei auch auf Galen beruft, den er in der arabischen Fassung gelesen hat.[62]

[58] *Kitāb al-aḫlāq*... (s.o. Anm.55), 39,20-40,10 (Übers. v. J.N. MATTOCK, 248).
[59] *Der Aristotelismus bei den Griechen* II (Berlin 1984), 775, Anm.364.
[60] *Op.cit.* (s.o. Anm.42), 59.
[61] *Plac.Prop.* 2, CMG V 3, 2, S.58f., vgl. den Kommentar.
[62] A.B. CHALIDOV, "Dopolnenija k tekstu"Chronologii"al-Bīrūnī po leningradskoj i stambul'skoj rukopisjam", in *Palestinskij Sbornik* 1959, Heft 4 (67), 160,13-21; Übers. in: Al-Bīrūnī. *In den Gärten der Wissenschaft. Ausgewählte Texte aus den Werken des muslimischen Universalgelehrten*, übers. u. erläutert v. G. STROHMAIER, 3. neubearbeitete Aufl., Reclam-Bibliothek 20045 (Leipzig 2002), Nr.30.

Der Einfluß der Platonischen Psychologie und die Rolle, die dabei Galen als Vermittler gespielt hat, macht sich besonders bei dem obenerwähnten Rhazes bemerkbar, dem größten Ketzer im mittelalterlichen Islam, der alle Propheten der offenbarten Religionen als Betrüger abtat und statt dessen Sokrates als seinen *imām* erwählte, während er zur gleichen Zeit eine gewisse Neigung zum Manichäismus bekundete.[63] Sein unabhängiger Geist verrät sich auch in einer Schrift, der man den lateinischen Titel *Dubitationes in Galenum* gegeben hat.[64] Hier distanziert er sich in einer vornehmen Art von Galens Behauptung, daß alle nichtgriechischen Sprachen den Lauten von Schweinen, Fröschen, Dohlen und Raben glichen.[65] Meir M. Bar-Asher hat in einer ausführlichen Studie gezeigt,[66] wie sich der Einfluß Galens in zwei anderen Schriften bemerkbar macht, nämlich in der *Medizin des Geistes* (*Aṭ-ṭibb ar-rūḥānī*)[67] und einer Abhandlung mit dem Titel *Der philosophische Lebenswandel* (*Kitāb as-sīrati l-falsafīya*),[68] und zwar in einer verschiedenen Weise. In der *Medizin des Geistes* teilt er Galens Skepsis hinsichtlich der Unsterblichkeit der menschlichen Seele und empfiehlt eine mehr

[63] G. STROHMAIER, "Al-Bīrūnī (973-1048) über Mani und die Manichäer", in *Studia Manichaica*. IV. Internationaler Kongress zum Manichäismus, Berlin, 14.-18. Juli 1997, hrsg. v. R.E. EMMERICK, W. SUNDERMANN u. P. ZIEME, Berlin-Brandenburgische Akademie der Wissenschaften, Berichte und Abhandlungen, Sonderband 4 (Berlin 2000), 591-600 (Nachdr. in *Hellas im Islam* [s.o. Anm.18]).

[64] G. STROHMAIER, "Bekannte und unbekannte Zitate in den *Zweifeln an Galen* des Rhazes", in *Text and Tradition. Studies in Ancient Medicine and its Transmission presented to Jutta Kollesch*, ed. by K.-D. FISCHER, D. NICKEL, P. POTTER, Studies in Ancient Medicine 18 (Leiden 1998), 263-287.

[65] Muḥammad ibn Zakarīyā ar-Rāzī, *Aš-šukūk ʿalā Ǧālīnūs*, hrsg. v. M. MOHAGHEGH (Teheran 1413 A.H.; 1992/1993 n.Chr.), 87,3-10; eine entschiedenere Zurückweisung bei dem Theologen Ibn Ḥazm, *Al-iḥkām fī uṣūli l-aḥkām* (Kairo 1984), I 36,3-6; vgl. *Diff.Puls.* 2, 5, VIII 585,19-586,6 K.

[66] "Quelques aspects de l'éthique d'Abu Bakr al-Razi et ses origines dans l'œuvre de Galien", in *Studia Islamica* 69 (1989), 5-38 u. 119-147.

[67] Ar-Rāzī, *Rasāʾil falsafīya*, hrsg. v. Paul KRAUS (Kairo 1939), 15-96.

[68] *Ibid.*, 97-111, übers. v. Paul KRAUS, "La Conduite du Philosophe. Traité d'éthique d'Abū Muḥammad b. Zakariyyā al-Rāzī", in *Orientalia* N.S. 4 (1935), 300-334 (Nachdr. in P. KRAUS, *Alchemie, Ketzerei, Apokryphen im frühen Islam*, hrsg. v. R. BRAGUE [Hildesheim 1994], 221-255).

utilitaristische Ethik, die eine goldene Mitte zwischen den Extremen einzuhalten sucht. Originell ist bei ihm dabei eine Theorie, die jegliche Lustempfindung nur als Rückkehr von einem unangenehmen Zustand zur Normalität auffaßt. In der Schrift *Der philosophische Lebenswandel* vertritt er hingegen, auch hier wieder Galen folgend, die Hierarchie der Seelenteile und die Aufgabe des *logistikon*, sich Gott anzunähern, und dies hier mit einer Perspektive über das irdische Leben hinaus.

Da Rhazes manche Schriften noch in ihrer vollständigen Fassung lesen konnte, ist manchmal schwer oder auch gar nicht zu entscheiden, ob irgendetwas, was er unter Berufung auf Galen mitteilt, ein neues Faktum darstellt oder ob er es nur ungenau nach dem Gedächtnis vorträgt. An einer unwichtigen Einzelheit sei das verdeutlicht. Als Beispiel für ein jähzorniges Verhalten nennt er Galens Mutter, die nicht nur ihre Sklaven, sondern auch einmal in einen Türriegel gebissen hat, der sich nicht öffnen lassen wollte.[69] Hat er das wirklich in einem uns unzugänglichen Passus gelesen oder hat er es nur aus *De animi cuiuslibet affectuum dignotione et curatione* herausgesponnen, wo allgemein von Leuten die Rede ist, die mit dem Fuß gegen die Tür treten und in den Riegel beißen?[70]

Avicenna (980 oder eher — 1037) hat in seiner allegorischen Erzählung *Ḥayy ibn Yaqẓān* (*Der Lebendige, der Sohn des Wachenden*)[71] in dichterisch verschlüsselter Form die Lehre der Seelenteile aufgenommen, die als unsympathische Freunde den Ich-Erzähler begleiten, der das *logistikon* verkörpert. Wie bei Platon und Galen werden sie mit Tieren verglichen, so das *thymoeides* mit einer Löwin und das *epithymetikon* mit einem Schwein.[72]

[69] *Rasā'il falsafiya* ... (s.o. Anm.67), 55,13f.; s. Meir M. BAR-ASHER, *art.cit.* (s.o. Anm.66), 140.

[70] *Aff.Dig.* 4,5 u. 5,2f., V 16,3-10 u. 22,8-17 = CMG V 4, 1, 1, S.12,11-17 u. 16,7-16.

[71] H. CORBIN, *Avicenna and the Visionary Recital* (Princeton N.J. 1960), 137-150.

[72] *Ibid.*, 139; vgl. PL. *Rep.* 9, 588 d u. e, 589 b; GAL. *PHP* 6, 2, 3f., V 515,3-7 K = CMG V 4, 1, 2, II S.368,13-16; *Kitāb al-aḫlāq* ... (s.o. Anm.55), 37,1 (Übers. v. J.N. MATTOCK, 246).

Aber im Unterschied zu den beiden Griechen ist nicht mehr von einer strengen Hierarchie der Teile die Rede, denn der Titelheld, der den aktiven Intellekt der Aristotelischen Seelenlehre verkörpert, gibt den Rat, die beiden unteren Seelenteile gegeneinander auszuspielen, zwar mit Hilfe des 'mutvollen' den 'begierigen' zu unterdrücken, aber auch jenen mit Hilfe des untersten zu verführen und so seinen Zorn zu besänftigen.[73] Avicenna hat damit die Gedanken Platons und Galens auf eine originelle Weise weitergeführt, wie sie übrigens auch seinem eigenen Lebensstil entsprach.[74]

[73] H. CORBIN, *op.cit.* (s.o. Anm.71),140.
[74] G. STROHMAIER, *Avicenna* (München 1999), 39 u. 82-86.

DISCUSSION

V. Boudon: Vous avez fait allusion dans votre exposé à trois figures d'intellectuels et de sportifs, Aristippe de Cyrène, le Scythe Anacharsis et l'athlète Milon de Crotone. Ma question porte sur la source des trois anecdotes relatives à ces trois personnages utilisée par les auteurs arabes. Vous savez bien sûr que ces trois figures se trouvent déjà réunies, avec d'autres, dans le *Protreptique* de Galien. Pensez-vous qu'il ait pu y avoir une transmission directe de Galien aux Arabes concernant le récit de ces trois anecdotes ou bien s'agit-il d'emprunts à d'autres sources (Diogène Laërce, etc.), si du moins une telle question peut être tranchée?

G. Strohmaier: Galen hat gnomologisches Material benutzt, das auch von den Arabern unabhängig von ihm in vielfältiger Weise übersetzt und rezipiert wurde, z.B. die Anekdote vom Schiffbruch des Aristipp. Diogenes Laertios wurde übrigens nicht übersetzt. In *Quod animi mores...* erwähnt er nur beiläufig und ohne Namensnennung die Person des Anacharsis, aber der Übersetzer kannte ihn entweder aus den *Gnomologien* oder aus dem *Protreptikos* und konnte darum den Namen einsetzen. Im Falle des Athleten Milon von Kroton ist das Verhältnis anders. Die Geschichte, die Galen im *Protreptikos* nacherzählt, ist keine Chreia, aber im arabischen *Gnomologium* ist daraus eine solche mit einer richtigen Pointe gestaltet worden.

V. Barras: Votre exposé, très intéressant, mentionne, comme l'un des exemples de la réception de Galien dans le monde arabe, celui d'al-Fārābī, suggérant la possibilité d'une 'extermination' ou d'une instrumentalisation pour le moins poussée des 'sauvages' provenant des régions situées au nord ou au sud des régions tempérées, en raison de leur nature 'subhumaine', comme on le ferait des bêtes nocives. Cet exemple évoque, par association, celui de Galien dans son traité *Quod animi mores* (*QAM* 11, IV 815,14 sqq. K = *Scripta min.* II p.74,8 sqq.), où il est suggéré qu'une frange d'humains incurables et nocifs (parce que leur nature est ainsi), ne devrait pas être tenue pour responsable de ses actes, mais traitée comme le sont les animaux nocifs, c'est-à-dire éliminée. La solution 'éthique' préconisée est similaire! Avez-vous quelques indices d'une réception de ce passage de Galien dans le monde arabe? Le passage d'al-Fārābī que vous évoquez est-il, à votre avis, inspiré en partie du *QAM* de Galien?

G. Strohmaier: Es ist denkbar, daß al-Fārābī, der sonst von Galen nicht viel hielt, durch den genannten Passus in *QAM* mit angeregt wurde; der Text war ja übersetzt und ist sogar erhalten und von H.H. Biesterfeldt herausgegeben worden. Was in *QAM* jedoch noch fehlt, ist die Verknüpfung mit der Zonentheorie, wodurch der extreme Norden und der extreme Süden wegen des dort herrschenden Klimas keine richtigen Menschen hervorbringen können. Galen erwähnt in dem *Kommentar* zu *De aere aquis locis* die Einteilung der nördlichen Hemisphäre in die Zonen, aber auch hier ohne die anthropologische Verknüpfung.

J. Jouanna: Dans votre exposé, qui apporte beaucoup de témoignages sur la réception de Galien dans le monde islamique, j'ai été particulièrement intéressé par ce que vous avez dit de Jean Philopon, qui vante Galien comme un authentique médecin et un vrai philosophe. En préparant ma propre communication, j'ai remarqué que l'expression technique κατὰ πρῶτον λόγον (opposée à κατὰ συμβεβηκός), caractéristique de Galien, se retrouve après lui non seulement chez les commentateurs alexandrins d'Hippocrate et de Galien, mais aussi chez Jean Philopon (et pas ailleurs). On aurait là un témoignage d'une connaissance approfondie de Galien chez Jean Philopon. Y a-t-il d'autres indices d'un intérêt pour la médecine galénique chez cet auteur?

G. Strohmaier: Johannes Philoponus war tatsächlich an der galenischen Medizin interessiert; das wird besonders deutlich an einem unikalen Text, der sich in Gotha befindet und der einen Kurzkommentar zum elften Buch von *De usu partium* enthält; ein Aufsatz über die vermutliche Echtheit erscheint in der obengenannten Sammlung *Hellas im Islam*.

J. Barnes: Thank you for a paper from which, as from all your work, I have learned a very great deal. I have one, familiar, question about the alleged fragment of Galen's commentary on the *Republic*. The first sentence, which criticizes the Christians, has good Galenic parallels. It is the second part, where Galen praises the Christians — and, if your interpretation is correct, praises them extravagantly —, which has no close parallel in Galen or in any other pagan text. Is it not reasonable to suggest that this second part is connected with those Arabic texts which make Galen a Christian and a contemporary of Jesus Christ?

G. Strohmaier: Die arabischen Autoren, welche die Bemerkung über die Christen zitieren, tun dies gerade aus dem Grunde, weil sie die Legende widerlegen wollen, daß Galen ein Zeitgenosse Jesu war, indem sie darauf hinweisen, daß die (mönchische) Askese eine spätere Erscheinung in der Geschichte der Kirche war. Sie haben also die halb negative, halb positive Bemerkung über die Christen so vorgefunden. Und wer sollte den ihnen vorliegenden Text manipuliert haben? Die christlichen Übersetzer der Ḥunainschule sicher nicht, denn sonst hätten sie die negative Beurteilung eher unterdrückt, was sie aber bei den analogen Äußerungen Galens auch nicht getan haben. Eine tendenziöse Interpolation, welche die Askese hervorhob, konnte im arabischen Text nur von Muslimen vorgenommen worden sein und dann noch möglichst in allen umlaufenden Kopien, was schlicht undenkbar ist. Galen hat auch sonst in seinem *Politeia*kompendium Bemerkungen zu Einzelheiten angefügt, wie aus den polemischen Bemerkungen des Averroes in seinem *Politeiakommentar* zu sehen ist.

INDEX

A. GALIEN

B. AUTEURS ET TEXTES ANCIENS

C. AUTEURS ARABES ET SYRIAQUES

D. AUTEURS MODERNES

De la mi-février à la fin d'octobre, la Fondation Hardt pour l'étude de l'Antiquité classique accueille pour des séjours d'étude de deux à quatre semaines commes hôtes des spécialistes des sciences de l'Antiquité. Pour une somme journalière modique, ils sont logés et nourris, et ont accès à une riche bibliothèque spécialisée. Les intéressés trouveront des informations et les conditions d'admission sur le site internet de la Fondation:

http://fondationhardt.isuisse.com

ACHEVÉ D'IMPRIMER
SUR LES PRESSES
DE N.V. PEETERS S.A.
SEPTEMBRE 2003